Oxford Guide to Brief and Low Intensity Interventions for Children and Young People

OXFORD GUIDES TO
COGNITIVE BEHAVIOURAL THERAPY

Oxford Guide to the Treatment of Mental Contamination
Rachman, Coughtrey, Shafran, and Radomsky

Oxford Guide to Low Intensity CBT Interventions
Bennett-Levy, Richards, Farrand, Christensen, Griffiths, Kavanagh, Klein, Lau, Proudfoot, Ritterband, White, and Williams

Oxford Guide to Surviving as a CBT Therapist
Mueller, Kennerley, McManus, and Westbrook

Oxford Guide to Metaphors in CBT
Stott, Mansell, Salkovskis, Lavender, and Cartwright-Hatton

Oxford Guide to Brief and Low Intensity Interventions for Children and Young People

Edited by

SOPHIE D. BENNETT

PAMELA MYLES-HOOTON

JESSICA L. SCHLEIDER

ROZ SHAFRAN

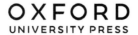

OXFORD
UNIVERSITY PRESS

Great Clarendon Street, Oxford, OX2 6DP,
United Kingdom

Oxford University Press is a department of the University of Oxford.
It furthers the University's objective of excellence in research, scholarship,
and education by publishing worldwide. Oxford is a registered trade mark of
Oxford University Press in the UK and in certain other countries

First Edition published in 2022

Impression: 1

Published in the United States of America by Oxford University Press
198 Madison Avenue, New York, NY 10016, United States of America

British Library Cataloguing in Publication Data

Data available

Library of Congress Control Number: 2022937637

ISBN 978–0–19–886779–1

DOI: 10.1093/med-psych/9780198867791.001.0001

Printed and bound by
CPI Group (UK) Ltd, Croydon, CR0 4YY

We would like to dedicate this book to our patients, family, friends and colleagues who have supported and inspired us throughout our careers.

Preface

Millions of children across the world will experience mental health difficulties. If it were your child, what would you want for them? Access to early treatment with therapies that have been shown to work? Treatment delivered in a way that suited your child and that minimized disruption to your child's life at school and at home, the lives of your other children, and your own commitments at work or home? You almost certainly would not want to be told your child can't access support for several months or years, or that their difficulties are 'too mild' and to wait until a more serious problem develops.

Yet many families across the world are in precisely this situation—unable to access evidence-based support and frequently facing extensive waiting lists for children and young people's mental health services, which are increasingly overstretched. Brief and low intensity (LI) interventions are one way to increase access to essential evidence-based therapies and are now recommended by several national guidelines as first-line interventions for many mental health difficulties. The purpose of this book is to provide a comprehensive resource for therapists, services, and clinical training providers regarding the use, delivery, and implementation of brief and LI evidence-based psychological interventions for children and young people. We define children and young people broadly as under 18s, but we did not want to constrain chapter authors as many agencies consider young people to be up to 25 years old. Chapter authors may refer to children, adolescents, young people, and youth, and define their own terms within their chapters. Similarly, brief and LI evidence-based interventions are not easy to define and Chapter 1 discusses this issue in more depth.

In the UK, there are new workforces trained specifically in such interventions—'children's well-being practitioners' and 'education mental health practitioners'. We have provided a practical focus throughout the book as a resource for these practitioners. However, many countries do not have practitioners trained specifically in LI approaches (e.g. the US) and this book provides an overview of how they may be implemented alongside traditional higher intensity therapies. The chapters are intended as concise overviews of topic areas to demonstrate the wide variety of difficulties and settings that LI approaches may cover. Each chapter includes recommended reading so that readers can investigate topics of interest in more depth.

The book is divided into four sections.

Section 1 provides an overview of brief and LI interventions: what it is (Chapter 1), why it is helpful (Chapter 2), the current evidence base (Chapter 3), its use in prevention/early interventions (Chapter 4), the health economic argument (i.e. cost-effectiveness) (Chapter 5), and recognizing and understanding the side effects (or 'negative effects') (Chapter 6). This short section is a useful overview for anyone wanting to know more about brief and LI interventions.

Section 2 is practically focused for practitioners, including case examples and relevant record and homework sheets. Section 2A details the common elements in LI interventions: assessment (Chapter 7), using routine outcome monitoring (Chapter 8), and implementing interventions with fidelity while maintaining flexibility to respond to clients' needs (Chapter 9). Section 2B then considers problem-specific interventions, beginning with longer chapters for some of the most common mental health difficulties in children and young people, which are the focus of training for the new workforces in the UK: anxiety (Chapter 10), depression (Chapter 11), behavioural problems (Chapter 12), and sleep difficulties (Chapter 13). The chapters that follow also provide a practical overview of brief and LI interventions for obsessive–compulsive disorder (Chapter 14), autism (Chapter 15), Tourette syndrome and tic disorders (Chapter 16), chronic physical illness (Chapter 17), and psychosis (Chapter 18).

Section 3 considers what is needed from a service perspective, from supervision requirements and the practicalities of delivering supervision for brief and LI interventions (Chapter 19), to considerations about implementation in services (Chapter 20), and understanding current models of delivery (stepped care—Chapter 21, and an overview of the model in England—Chapter 22).

Finally, *Section 4* looks to the future with chapters about exciting developments in the area: providing single sessions of interventions (Chapter 23), using computer games (Chapter 24), providing sessions 'one at a time' (Chapter 25), using peer support (Chapter 26), and using apps (Chapter 27) to deliver interventions. Finally, Chapter 28 considers how brief and LI interventions may be used to target transdiagnostic mechanisms.

There are not enough pages in one book to cover all of the advances in brief and LI interventions for children and young people but we hope that the book provides a snapshot of why and how LI interventions can play a role within children and young people's mental health.

We want to make sure that all children and young people who have mental health difficulties are able to access treatment that works, when they need it, and in the way they want it. We want them to go on to live happy and fulfilled lives. We hope that this book inspires you to think about how brief and LI interventions may be one tool that can help achieve this.

Contents

SECTION 4. BRIEF AND LOW INTENSITY INTERVENTIONS
FOR THE TWENTY-FIRST CENTURY

Abbreviations

ADHD	attention deficit hyperactivity disorder
BA	behavioural activation
BFS	Behavior and Feelings Survey
BIP	*Barninternetprojektet*
CAMHS	child and adolescent mental health services
CBIT	comprehensive behavioural intervention for tics
CBT	cognitive behavioural therapy
CBT-I	cognitive behavioural therapy for insomnia
CCAL	Camp-Cope-A-Lot
cCBT	computerized cognitive behavioural therapy
CD	conduct disorder
COVID-19	coronavirus 2019
CWP	children's well-being practitioner
CYP	children and young people
EBI	evidence-based intervention
EBP	evidence-based practice
EQ-5D	EuroQol Five Dimensions
EMA	ecological momentary assessment
EMHP	education mental health practitioner
ERP	exposure and response prevention
FEP	first-episode psychosis
GBO	Goals-Based Outcome
HASQ	Helpful Aspects of Supervision Questionnaire
HRT	habit reversal training
IAPT	Improving Access to Psychological Therapies
ICBT	internet cognitive behavioural therapy
IS	implementation science
IY	Incredible Years
LI	low intensity
MATCH	Modular Approach to Therapy for Children with Anxiety, Depression, Trauma, or Conduct Problems
mHealth	mobile health
MHST	mental health support team
NHS	National Health Service
NICE	National Institute for Health and Care Excellence
OAATT	one-at-a-time therapy
OCD	obsessive–compulsive disorder
ODD	oppositional defiant disorder
QALY	quality-adjusted life year
RCADS	Revised Child and Adolescent Anxiety and Depression Scales
RCT	randomized controlled trial
REM	rapid eye movement
ROM	routine outcome measure

SDQ	Strengths and Difficulties Questionnaire
SF-6D	Short-Form Six Dimensions
SPARX	Smart, Positive, Active, Realistic, X-factor thoughts
STIC	Show That I Can
TDI	technologically delivered intervention
TPA	Top Problems Assessment
YGTSS	Yale Global Tic Severity Scale
ZPD	zone of proximal development

Contributors

Isaac Ahuvia
Stony Brook University
New York, USA

Morgan S. Anvari
University of Maryland
College Park, MD, USA

Abby Bailin
Harvard University
Cambridge, MA, USA

Rinad Beidas
University of Pennsylvania
Philadelphia, PA, USA

Sophie D. Bennett
UCL Great Ormond Street Institute of
Child Health
London, UK

Matteo Catanzano
UCL Great Ormond Street Hospital for Children
London, UK

Chloe Chessell
University of Reading
Reading, UK

Anna Coughtrey
UCL Great Ormond Street Institute of
Child Health
London, UK

Margaret E. Crane
Temple University
Philadelphia, PA, USA

Cathy Creswell
University of Oxford
Oxford, UK

Lauren Croucher
UCL Great Ormond Street Institute of
Child Health
London, UK

Vicki Curry
Anna Freud Centre
London, UK

Windy Dryden
Goldsmiths, University of London
London, UK

Colin A. Espie
University of Oxford
Oxford, UK

Peter Felsman
Stony Brook University
New York, USA

Julia W. Felton
Michigan State University
East Lansing, MI, USA

Olivia Fitzpatrick
Harvard University
Cambridge, MA, USA

Theresa M. Fleming
Victoria University of Wellington
Wellington, New Zealand

Lesley French
Anna Freud Centre
London, UK

Catherine Gallop
University of Exeter
Exeter, UK

Dimitri Gavriloff
University of Oxford
Oxford, UK

Joseph Giacomantonio
Stony Brook University
New York, USA

Ann Hagell
Association of Young People's Health
London, UK

Charlotte L. Hall
University of Nottingham
Nottingham, UK

Claire Hill
University of Oxford
Oxford, UK

Philip C. Kendall
Temple University
Philadelphia, PA, USA

Martin Knapp
London School of Economics and Political
Science
London, UK

Georgina Krebs
Institute of Psychiatry, Psychology &
Neuroscience
King's College London
London, UK

Duncan Law
Anna Freud Centre
London, UK

Carl W. Lejuez
University of Connecticut
Storrs, CT, USA

Matthew D. Lerner
Stony Brook University
New York, USA

Angela Lewis
Institute of Psychiatry, Psychology &
Neuroscience
King's College London
OCD, BDD, and Related Disorders Clinic for
Young People
South London and Maudsley NHS
Foundation Trust
London, UK

Erin J. Libsack
Stony Brook University
New York, USA

Dan I. Lubman
Monash University
Melbourne, Australia

Mathijs F. G. Lucassen
The Open University
London, UK

Jessica F. Magidson
University of Maryland
College Park, MD, USA

Colleen A. Maxwell
Temple University
Philadelphia, PA, USA

Terence V. McCann
Monash University
Melbourne, Australia

Lauren F. McLellan
Macquarie University
Sydney, Australia

Morgan L. McNair
Stony Brook University
New York, USA

Sally N. Merry
The University of Auckland
Auckland, New Zealand

Elif Mertan
UCL Great Ormond Street Institute of
Child Health
London, UK

Wendy Minhinnett
Rollercoaster Family Support
County Durham, UK
Charlie Waller Trust
Berkshire, UK

Tara Murphy
Great Ormond Street Hospital for Children
London, UK

Lindsay B. Myerberg
Temple University
Philadelphia, PA, USA

Pamela Myles-Hooton
Bespoke Mental Health
Reading, UK

Lauran O'Neill
Great Ormond Street Hospital for Children
London, UK

Jonathan Parker
University of Exeter
Exeter, UK

Jonathan C. Rabner
Temple University
Philadelphia, PA, USA

Alexander Rozental
Uppsala University
Uppsala, Sweden

Charlotte Sanderson
Great Ormond Street Hospital for Children
London, UK

Jessica L. Schleider
Stony Brook University
New York, USA

Carolyn Schniering
Macquarie University
Sydney, Australia

Simone Schriger
University of Pennsylvania
Philadelphia, PA, USA

Roz Shafran
UCL Great Ormond Street Institute of
Child Health
London, UK

Matthew J. Shepherd
Massey University of New Zealand
Palmerston North, New Zealand

Paul Stallard
University of Bath
Bath, UK

Karolina Stasiak
The University of Auckland
Auckland, New Zealand

Jenna Sung
Stony Brook University
New York, USA

Katherine Venturo-Conerly
Harvard University
Cambridge, MA, USA

Hannah Vickery (née Whitney)
The Charlie Waller Institute
University of Reading
Reading, UK

Felicity Waite
University of Oxford
Oxford, UK

Polly Waite
University of Oxford
Oxford, UK

Melissa Wei
Harvard University
Cambridge, MA, USA

John Weisz
Harvard University
Cambridge, MA, USA

Zuzanna K. Wojcieszak
Temple University
Philadelphia, PA, USA

Gloria Wong
The University of Hong Kong
Hong Kong

Viviana Wuthrich
Macquarie University
Sydney, Australia

SECTION 1
AN OVERVIEW

1

Brief and low intensity cognitive behavioural therapy for children and young people

Definitions and applications

Pamela Myles-Hooton

Learning objectives

- To describe the prevalence of mental health problems in children and young people.
- To understand the historical context and current need for low intensity cognitive behavioural therapy.
- To appreciate the complexities of diversity applications of interventions under the umbrella term 'brief cognitive behavioural therapy.
- To understand the importance of reaching a consensus of low intensity cognitive behavioural therapy for research and clinical purposes.

Introduction

Low intensity cognitive behavioural therapy (LICBT) is a relatively new approach to delivering evidence-based psychological interventions for adults presenting with common mental health problems, and an even newer approach for working with children and young people. Over recent years, empirically validated LI psychological treatments for children and young people have started to emerge.

In this book, readers will learn about a myriad of applications of LICBT for children and young people, including LICBT approaches using diverse delivery methods (online, face-to-face, bibliotherapy, and telehealth) and targeting widely varying clinical problems (from depression and anxiety to behavioural problems and autism spectrum disorder). In many respects, the potential utility of LICBT for children and young people appears endless, but to date, information about these LI supports has not been collated into a single source.

A key reason for producing this *Oxford Guide to Brief and Low Intensity Interventions for Children and Young People* is to do just that: to create a go-to guide for providing efficient, brief, and effective treatment to children and young people with mental health needs. The interventions described in the upcoming chapters are diverse in form and function, yet all are evidence-based treatments intentionally designed to help broaden the accessibility of appropriate supports to young people and their carers. By consolidating information on the delivery of LICBT, this book may support more therapists in providing such services thus broadening the availability of LI support to far more children and young people than traditional, longer-term CBT could accommodate.

There has been an increase in research into the effectiveness of these more cost-effective approaches over the past 40 years. Rather than practitioners needing to have completed many years of training to deliver evidence-based approaches, there has been a shift towards briefer, more targeted training in specific interventions across a wide range of mental health professionals from varied backgrounds. Over the decades, there has been significant development of self-help books and online materials based on the principles of CBT. There has been a gradual move towards using remote communication technologies for therapeutic contact which exploded with the arrival of COVID-19 which rendered face-to-face interaction inaccessible for a significant period of time. There has also been a societal shift towards 'democratizing' CBT to make its core concepts more available to higher numbers of people than was previously the case.

In children and young people's mental health services, LICBT is relatively new to the scene. Readers will learn of the many applications of LICBT for children and young people experiencing mental health problems. Some of these applications are well established and have been embraced by the children and young people's mental health programme in England while others show promise through emerging research. The aim of this book is to provide readers with working, actionable knowledge of a broad range of interventions from the established and emerging evidence base.

Mental health problems in children and young people

Although the majority of children grow up psychologically well, surveys indicate that more children and young people experience problems with their mental health than was the case 40+ years ago. This may be down to the way we live now compared to several decades ago and how this impacts children's experience of growing up. Rates of mental health problems in children and young people in the UK rose over the period from 1974 to 1999, particularly conduct and emotional disorders (Collishaw, Maughan, Goodman, & Pickles, 2004). More recent surveys indicate that emotional disorders have become more common in 5- to 15-year-olds: up from 4.3% in 1999 and 3.9% in 2004, to 5.8% by 2017 in the UK. The increase since 2004 in emotional disorders is evident in both boys and girls (NHS Digital, 2018).

The survey published by NHS Digital found that 1 in 12 (8.1%) 5- to 19-year-olds had an emotional disorder, with rates higher in girls (10.0%) than boys (6.2%). Anxiety disorders (7.2%) were more common than depressive disorders (2.1%). Approximately 1 in 20 (4.6%) 5- to 19-year-olds had a behavioural disorder, with rates higher in boys (5.8%) than girls (3.4%). A follow-up survey (Health and Social Care Information Centre, 2020) indicated that the incidence of probable mental health disorder at any given time has increased from one in nine (10.8%) to one in six (16%) in children aged 5–16 years.

In children, mental health disorders have a damaging effect on individual and socioeconomic factors and can have a significant negative impact on healthy transition into adulthood. Approximately 50% of mental illness in adulthood (excluding dementia) starts before the age of 15 and 75% by age 18 (The Dunedin Study, n.d.).

The Children and Young People's Improving Access to Psychological Therapies (CYP IAPT) programme commissioned by Health Education England has played a leading role in improving access to psychological treatments through workforce development since it began in 2011. In recent years, 'CYP-IAPT' has been formally disbanded and transitioned into an expected standard of delivery of Children and Young People's Mental Health (CYP MH) services. Despite promising evidence of the programme's many benefits, significant wait times remained and since 2017 the programme changed its aim from workforce transformation to workforce expansion, with the aim of training 1700 new psychological practitioners by 2021. There are now three training streams (1) a LI workforce (children's well-being practitioners), (2) an education-based workforce (education mental health practitioners, and (3) a high intensity workforce (based on the original curriculum which includes training in CBT, systemic family therapy, interpersonal therapy for depression in adolescents, and evidence-based parent training). As a result, practitioners in children and young people's services are increasingly being trained in the delivery of a range of LI interventions to help target mild-to-moderate anxiety, depression, and conduct problems. For more details on the children and young people's mental health training initiative commissioned by Health Education England, see Chapter 22.

Historical context

The concept of LICBT has grown in importance over the past decade in response to the need to provide efficient, effective interventions that can meet the growing demand for mental health treatment. Such interventions are at the heart of the adult IAPT programme in England (Clark, 2018) and to the transformation of children and young people's mental health services in England (Shafran, Fonagy, Pugh, & Myles, 2014), but are also central to addressing the global need to access effective interventions across the age range and contexts (Michelson et al., 2020). In England, due partly to the IAPT programme's structure, such interventions are frequently the first level of intervention provided to adults with depression and specific forms of anxiety who are then 'stepped up' to a higher 'dose' of treatment if there is an insufficient response to LI interventions. LI interventions are designed to require less therapeutic input than conventional treatment and therefore considered 'LI' from the provider's perspective. Such treatments were building on a pre-existing, established evidence base of brief CBT interventions, such as four sessions of problem-solving for emotional disorders provided over 6 weeks in primary care (Catalan et al., 1991), self-help interventions for anxiety and depression (Marks et al., 2003), and abbreviated versions of full CBT protocols (Cape, Whittington, Buszewicz, Wallace, & Underwood, 2010; Clark et al., 1999). In this programme, high intensity therapy refers to traditional CBT delivered by a qualified mental health practitioner, face-to-face, typically weekly for 12–20 sessions.

LICBT: the concept and definition

There is some confusion in the terminology used to describe different forms of CBT, in particular LICBT. Such confusion has implications for research, clinical practice, and service organization. Shafran, Myles-Hooton, Bennett, and Ost (2021) aimed to describe the key components of LICBT in comparison to brief traditional high intensity CBT. The authors proposed that LICBT (1) utilizes self-help materials, (2) is 6 hours or less of contact time with each contact being typically 30 minutes or less, and (3) any input (i.e. support or guidance) can be provided by trained practitioners or supporters. These components distinguish the intervention from brief traditional high intensity CBT which (1) is based on the standard evidence-based CBT treatment, with therapy contact time 50% or less than the full CBT intervention; and (2) is usually delivered by someone with a core mental health professional qualification or equivalent. Brief CBT can refer to either LICBT and/or brief high intensity CBT. The authors aimed to make the distinction between these different forms of intervention to stimulate debate and help consistent and appropriate categorization for future research and practice.

Table 1.1 compares and contrasts the nature of brief high intensity CBT interventions with LICBT to clarify differences and pave the way for a consensus for clinical and research purposes. Bennett-Levy, Richards, Farrand, Christensen, and Griffiths (2010) considered the central components of LI interventions to comprise a reduction in time spent with patients, use of specifically trained practitioners, use of CBT resources whose content is 'less intense' such as self-help books, and improved access to early intervention and preventative CBT components. The 'intensity' of psychological treatments was considered only as 'time to deliver' in the meta-analysis of van Stratten, Hill, Richards, and Cuijpers (2014). The comparison in Table 1.1 draws heavily on previous definitions but is also integrated with descriptions from other sources and, where specified, research data.

Table 1.1 A comparison of LICBT and brief traditional high intensity CBT

	LICBT	Brief traditional high intensity CBT
Who delivers the intervention?	Any input is usually provided by practitioners or supporters who have been specifically trained to deliver the intervention. There is often no input (e.g. unguided self-help books, technology-based programmes)	Input is usually provided by mental health workers with a core professional qualification or equivalent (e.g. accredited CBT practitioners)
Who is it suitable for?	Widely used to address anxiety and depression across the age range and behavioural problems in children (e.g., Bennett et al., 2019; Cuijpers, Donker, van Stratten, Li, & Andersson, 2010). Evidence supports its use for cases of all severity (Bower et al., 2013; Karyotaki et al., 2018). Typically not advocated where there are significant risk issues	Typically used widely for disorders where longer traditional CBT would be appropriate
What is delivered?	Interventions are based on the principles of generic CBT to enable individuals to learn specific techniques (e.g. graded exposure, cognitive restructuring, problem-solving) with the goal of alleviating emotional distress and improving functioning. Between-session reading and exercises are central	Intervention is an abbreviated version of full CBT, supplemented with provision of between-session materials and exercises
Where—is it delivered?	When guidance is provided to support the self-help materials, it is typically done via telephone, face-to-face, video facility, email, texts, or online support/the internet	Traditionally provided face-to-face or via video facility and less often via email/text
When is it delivered?	Typically as first treatment intervention	Can be first treatment intervention or, in countries with 'stepped care', provided after insufficient response to first treatment intervention and/or full therapy is indicated due to complexity such as suicidality
Why is it delivered?	To deliver least burdensome intervention, have high-volume caseloads with rapid turnover and meet demand; based on principles of clinical and cost-effectiveness and appropriate 'dose' of intervention	Improving cost-effectiveness and aiming to provide appropriate 'dose' of intervention
How is it delivered?	A health technology such as self-help books or technology-based intervention is used	Between-session materials and exercises are advocated
How long is therapy?	Any input is typically 6 hours or less of contact, often delivered in 20–30-minute sessions	Therapy contact time is typically 50% or less than the full CBT intervention, usually delivered in 50–60-minute sessions
If not recovered, then what?	Referral to brief or full high intensity therapy	Referral to full therapy or specialist service

Proposed definition of LICBT

Based on Table 1.1, Shafran et al (2022) proposed a definition of LI CBT that (1) utilizes self-help materials, (2) is 6 hours or less of contact time with each contact being typically 30 minutes or less, and (3) any input (support or guidance) can be provided by trained practitioners or supporters. They suggested that brief high intensity CBT (1) be based on the standard evidence-based CBT treatment, with therapy contact time 50% or less than the full CBT intervention; and (2) is usually delivered by someone with a core mental health professional qualification or equivalent. Consequently, brief CBT can refer to either LICBT and/or brief high intensity CBT with therapy contact time 50% or less than the full CBT intervention but we recommend that a distinction is drawn between the different forms for clarity.

Chapter summary

Children and young people's mental health services are being revolutionized in England. As with adult IAPT, it is hoped that many other countries will follow. Resources are not infinite but there is increasing global recognition of the evidence base for LI interventions that can significantly improve the mental well-being of children and young people at scale. LICBT provides the opportunity to improve access to mental health services, and to intervene early in an attempt to pre-empt mental health difficulties continuing into adulthood. As readers will find as they work their way through the book, many of these evidence-based interventions and new technologies offer an opportunity to widen access to counter anxiety, depression, and conduct problems in children and young people. Readers may be drawn to chapters that are immediately relevant to their area of work and may be inspired by other chapters with a focus on new developments in LICBT approaches. There is still no international agreement on what constitutes LICBT and some chapters may seem to fit more under the term brief CBT.

References

Bennett, S. D., Cuijpers, P., Ebert, D. D., McKenzie Smith, M., Coughtrey, A. E., Heyman, I., . . ., & Shafran, R. (2019). Practitioner review: Unguided and guided self-help interventions for common mental health disorders in children and adolescents: A systematic review and meta-analysis. *Journal of Child Psychology and Psychiatry*, *60*(8), 828–847.

Bennett-Levy, J., Richards, D., Farrand, P., Christensen, H., & Griffiths, K. (Eds.). (2010). *Oxford guide to low intensity CBT interventions*. New York: Oxford University Press.

Bower, P., Kontopantelis, E., Sutton, A., Kendrick, T., Richards, D. A., Gilbody, S., . . ., & Liu, E. T. H. (2013). Influence of initial severity of depression on effectiveness of low intensity interventions: Meta-analysis of individual patient data. *BMJ*, *346*, f540.

Cape, J., Whittington, C., Buszewicz, M., Wallace, P., & Underwood, L. (2010). Brief psychological therapies for anxiety and depression in primary care: Meta-analysis and meta-regression. *BMC Medicine*, *8*(1), 38.

Catalan, J. A., Gath, D. H., Anastasiades, P., Bond, S. A. K., Day, A., & Hall, L. (1991). Evaluation of a brief psychological treatment for emotional disorders in primary care. *Psychological Medicine*, *21*(4), 1013–1018.

Clark, D. M. (2018). Realizing the mass public benefit of evidence-based psychological therapies: The IAPT program. *Annual Review of Clinical Psychology*, *14*(1), 159–183.

Clark, D. M., Salkovskis, P. M., Hackmann, A., Wells, A., Ludgate, J., & Gelder, M. (1999). Brief cognitive therapy for panic disorder: A randomized controlled trial. *Journal of Consulting and Clinical Psychology*, *67*(4), 583–589.

Collishaw, S., Maughan, B., Goodman, R., & Pickles, A. (2004). Time trends in adolescent mental health. *Journal of Child Psychology and Psychiatry*, *45*(8), 1350–1362.

Cuijpers, P., Donker, T., van Stratten, A., Li, J., & Andersson, G. (2010). Is guided self-help as effective as face-to-face psychotherapy for depression and anxiety disorders? A systematic review and meta-analysis of comparative outcome studies. *Psychological Medicine*, *40*(12), 1943–1957.

Health and Social Care Information Centre. (2020). *Mental health of children and young people in England,2020: Wave 1 follow up to the 2017 survey*. London: NHS Digital.

Karyotaki, E., Ebert, D. D., Donkin, L., Riper, H., Twisk, J., Burger, S., . . ., & Cuijpers, P. (2018). Do guided internet-based interventions result in clinically relevant changes for patients with depression? An individual participant data meta-analysis. *Clinical Psychology Review*, *63*, 80–92.

Marks, I. M., Mataix-Cols, D., Kenwright, M., Cameron, R., Hirsch, S., & Gega, L. (2003). Pragmatic evaluation of computer-aided self-help for anxiety and depression. *British Journal of Psychiatry*, *183*(1), 57–65.

Michelson, D., Malik, K., Krishna, M., Sharma, R., Mathur, S., Bhat, B., . . ., & Patel, V. (2020). Development of a transdiagnostic, low-intensity, psychological intervention for common adolescent mental health problems in Indian secondary schools. *Behaviour Research and Therapy*, *130*, 103439.

NHS Digital. (2018). *Mental health of children and young people in England, 2017 [PAS]*. London: NHS Digital.

Shafran, R., Fonagy, P., Pugh, K., & Myles, P. (2014). Transformation of mental health services for children and young people in England. In R. S. Beidas, and P. C. Kendall (Eds.), *Dissemination and implementation of evidence-based practices in child and adolescent mental health* (pp. 158–178). New York: Oxford University Press.

Shafran, R., Myles-Hooton, P., Bennett, S., & Ost, L. G. (2021). The concept and definition of low intensity cognitive behaviour therapy. *Behaviour Research and Therapy*, *138*, 103803.

The Dunedin Study. (n.d.). Dunedin Multidisciplinary Health & Development Research Unit. Retrieved 5 June 2021 from https://dunedinstudy.otago.ac.nz/

van Stratten, A., Hill, J. J., Richards, D. A., & Cuijpers, P. (2014). Stepped care treatment delivery for depression: A systematic review and meta-analysis. *Psychological Medicine*, *45*(2), 231–246.

2

Low intensity therapy: a parent's perspective

Lauran O'Neill

Learning objectives

- To understand what receiving a low intensity intervention may be like for a parent.
- To understand a parent's view of the importance of providing low intensity interventions.
- To highlight the importance of clear goals and session-by-session measurement.

Introduction

My daughter is 8 years old, the eldest of two siblings, and has a physical illness for which she needed a procedure. She didn't sleep very well because of anxiety, was picking her skin, and was very anxious about going into hospital. She was in social skills classes at school because she could be quite controlling with friends and she needed quite a lot of preparation for things. We were becoming increasingly frustrated with her because we didn't know what was wrong and so she would get in trouble quite a lot. From our perspective, we gave her every opportunity and she was making a choice not to enjoy herself. We thought that she was being spoiled and rude. I felt constantly frustrated with her and disappointed that she wasn't taking up opportunities or just having fun as a child, the way that a child should.

We completed a questionnaire about her emotions and behaviours when we came to the hospital for another appointment. The results said that she scored highly for anxiety. We always thought she wasn't a particularly happy child but to actually have those concrete results was really interesting for us. We were offered six sessions of low intensity (LI) therapy, and I was over the moon with this. If someone had offered me two sessions with some helpful tips, I probably would have taken it too because private therapy is so expensive. For a National Health Service referral, the general practitioner needs to know so much detail and I don't think my daughter would have met the thresholds for child and adolescent mental health services. There are such long waiting lists too. So being offered six sessions straight away felt like a luxury. We probably wouldn't have done anything about the difficulties had it not been for this.

For me, six sessions were better than nothing and, at that point, we weren't in the mental health system and we didn't know whether six sessions was a short or long amount of therapy time.

My experiences of LI intervention

We had six face-to-face sessions of guided self-help in the hospital. One of the first things to change was my daughter's sleep. At the start of therapy, all the lights had to be on and the doors open. I had to sit on my bed where she could see me from her bedroom and sometimes it would take her 4 hours to go off to sleep. That changed almost overnight, which changed our whole household. She talked about the fear she had and built a ladder with the scariest point at the top, which for her was to sleep in the dark in her room with the door closed. She was so motivated that she went faster than the therapist suggested. At points she was jumping three steps up and she was so excited by it. It was amazing. Within the space of 7 days, she went to sleep in a dark room, with the door closed, and was asleep within about 20 minutes. I think because we had such clear goals at the beginning, we knew what we were working towards and it was obvious that she had achieved the three targets. Having that final endpoint to work towards really helped.

What is LI therapy like to experience as a parent?

Even though it is called LI therapy, I still found it intensive because you dig deeply into things quite quickly. Within the first week we were talking about our family and the ways that we communicate with each other. For us, a family that's normally quite private, it was very intimate and so it felt intense. You have to get behind it fully and you do have to invest fully in it—no one is there to fix your problems for you. There were tasks that were set each session and, particularly at the beginning, we were doing them every single night.

The fact that you've taken a step to talk to someone about your child means that you think about things more consciously. Rather than getting through every day and then just going to sleep and then getting through the next day, by stopping and appraising where you are and working out where you want to be, you can make a big change.

What are the benefits of stepped care?

My daughter had more therapy after the LI therapy, focused specifically on anxiety about a specific procedure in hospital. Having the LI therapy first helped because my daughter and I got used to talking about the difficulties and our family. It gives you practice and you learn what to expect from therapy. You learn that you have very limited time in those meetings so it is really important to prepare beforehand. You also learn what the therapist wants you to talk about and that helps you to be more structured with what you are saying. Suddenly, when you stop and you explain your life to someone, you can actually do a lot of therapy yourself. You take a step back and see things you didn't see before.

What would be helpful for LI therapists to know when they're working with young people and families?

It is quite daunting to go into these situations and meet with people you've never met before. It's a short space of time where you have to trust each other so quickly. I think it is important that families know they won't be judged and the therapists know that parenting and life are stressful and that it's okay that everything is not okay. Not loving every aspect of mothering doesn't mean you don't love to be a mother.

It is also really important that therapists are clear at the beginning about what this therapy might be like. For example, that it will be 2 months of hard work and it will involve lots of you looking into how things are, which might be upsetting.

One of the most helpful things for us was setting really concrete goals, like sleeping with the door closed with the lights off. It meant my daughter always knew what she was aiming for.

Chapter summary

I think the mindset of many schools and mental health services is that children have to be very poorly before they get any input for emotional or behavioural problems. If they don't meet a certain threshold for symptoms, you're told from the offset there's nothing for you. It's crazy that you have to reach such a damaging level before you can access help. Having LI therapy as a preventative or first step is really important. We heard all the time that our daughter was 'good as gold, just quiet in the corner'. Six weeks of LI therapy gave us the strategies to help her anxiety, and through this we learnt that she had symptoms of autism. She then had an autism assessment and now she'll get more resources and help. It all started with 6 weeks of LI therapy and that's brought our family so many benefits.

3

Efficacy of low intensity interventions for mental health problems in children and young people

The evidence

Sophie D. Bennett

Learning objectives

- To understand the current state of the evidence for low intensity interventions in children and young people.
- To be aware of the limitations of the current evidence base.
- To consider who low intensity interventions may be suitable for according to research evidence.

Introduction

There is an increasing evidence base for the use of low intensity (LI) interventions in children and young people. A meta-analysis, pulling together the results of existing studies of self-help for children and young people (Bennett et al., 2019), found that self-help (both guided and unguided) was associated with significant medium-to-large effects on symptoms of anxiety, depression, and disruptive behaviour in children and young people. Larger effect sizes indicate bigger differences between groups, so a medium-to-large effect size suggests that there is a 'medium-to-large sized' difference between scores for the LI intervention groups and the control groups. This suggests that the LI intervention works better than the control intervention. This chapter considers the results of the 50 studies included in this meta-analysis. 'Self-help' is used to mean both clinician-guided and self-guided (or 'unguided') interventions.

Results from meta-analysis of self-help

LI therapies were significantly more effective than no intervention and slightly less effective than traditional higher intensity treatments such as standard face-to-face treatment. In addition, the overall effect size for self-help in comparison to alternative treatments was very small and corresponded to a 'number needed to treat' of ten. This means that ten patients would have to be treated with standard higher intensity face-to-face treatments for one patient to have better outcomes from higher intensity treatments compared to a LI self-help treatment. This difference is very small, especially when the costs of each intervention are considered; many more patients can feasibly be treated with LI treatments compared to standard treatments. The review also found that families were happy with the content and outcomes of the LI treatments.

These potential findings of near equivalence for LI therapies compared to higher intensity interventions are in agreement with a number of previous reviews across mental health disorders in adults. Some have found that the interventions have comparable effect sizes (Cuijpers, Donker, van Straten, Li, & Andersson, 2010; Perkins, Murphy, Schmidt, & Williams, 2009; Priemer & Talbot, 2013). Other reviews have found that although LI interventions are more effective than no intervention, they may be less effective than traditional higher intensity face-to-face therapy (Hirai & Clum, 2006; Mayo-Wilson & Montgomery, 2013).

Considering the different diagnoses or difficulties, an overall medium effect size was found for the 12 depression studies that compared self-help against an inactive control group such as a waiting list. There was a medium-to-large overall effect size for 13 anxiety studies comparing against an inactive control group; all but one of the anxiety studies included children who met full diagnostic criteria and all but one included guidance. The 16 interventions focused on disruptive behaviour demonstrated an overall medium effect size, although the effect was not significant when only studies with low risk of bias (i.e. studies conducted in a way that minimized bias and increased the validity of the results) were considered.

These findings, coupled with ease of accessibility, particularly for communities living a distance from a clinic, suggest that self-help could be a viable option for treatment for common childhood mental health disorders. Given the review found that LI interventions were statistically slightly less efficacious than higher intensity interventions, self-help may be particularly useful if used in a stepped care model where those who do not respond are then offered face-to-face treatment. This could (1) prevent overtreatment for children and young people who might benefit from LI support and (2) reduce waiting times for others by reserving high intensity interventions for those who do not benefit from LI interventions (see Chapter 21).

What characteristics of interventions might work best?

Overall, in studies comparing self-help against control groups, the presence of guidance was associated with better outcome. This finding was significant when disruptive behaviour interventions were considered alone. The same pattern was true in depression studies but the result was not significant. As almost all anxiety studies included guidance, it is not possible to assess whether this is true for anxiety interventions. This overall result is consistent with findings of many reviews of self-help that demonstrate superior effect sizes for greater amounts of therapist contact (e.g. Gellatly et al., 2007—a review of self-help for depression; Lewis, Pearce, & Bisson, 2012—a review of self-help for anxiety disorders; O'Brien & Daley, 2011—self-help for childhood behaviour disorders; Pearcy, Anderson, Egan, & Rees, 2016—a review of self-help for obsessive–compulsive disorder; van Boeijen et al., 2005—self-help for anxiety). Previous research has indicated that increased therapist contact may also be associated with improved acceptability of the intervention (O'Brien & Daly, 2011) and there was some support for this from the 50 studies included in the review. The non-significant difference between studies of the treatment of depression with and without guidance may warrant further investigation. Previous reviews have suggested that the level of therapist contact required may vary according to diagnosis (Newman, Erickson, Przeworski, & Dzus, 2003). It may also vary according to the format of interventions; self-guided single-session treatments show promise (Schleider & Weisz, 2017; see Chapter 23).

Other reviews of the type, rather than amount, of therapist contact suggest that while some therapist contact is important, this does not need to be in the form of 'guidance'; 'non-guidance' contact, such as emails to encourage treatment adherence, are also effective (Talbot, 2012). Many studies were not clear regarding the amount of therapeutic 'guidance' versus non-therapeutic 'encouragement' given and so this was not analysed within our review. However, the meta-analysis did not find any effect of the format of guidance given (i.e. telephone calls, face-to-face, email, or mixed guidance), or of the amount of training of the therapists. There was some evidence for greater effect sizes for computerized interventions compared to bibliotherapy or other types of self-help. However, heterogeneity was high for many of the comparisons. Heterogeneity is a measure of how varied the outcomes of different studies are; high heterogeneity means that the results of the different studies that have been analysed together are very different to each other. This means that the findings from some of these analyses may not be reliable.

Who is it suitable for?

Few patient characteristics appeared to make significant differences to the effect size of self-help. There was a significant effect of age on effect size for the studies comparing against face-to-face treatment, with studies of older children and young people demonstrating greater effect sizes than those of younger children (i.e. self-help appeared to be more effective in older children compared to younger children). Importantly, as in adult studies (Karyotaki et al., 2018), there was no evidence that interventions were only effective in those with mild–moderate difficulties, despite evidence-based guidance commonly only recommending them for this group.

What are the gaps in the literature?

There were relatively few studies with low risk of bias and most studies were relatively small. It is therefore possible that studies were simply not big enough to detect differences between self-help and face-to-face treatments. In addition, there was significant publication bias indicating that studies that did not find self-help worked better than an inactive control may not have been published. Publication bias is often found in studies of psychological interventions (Driessen, Hollon, Bockting, Cuijpers, & Turner, 2015) and may have led to an overestimation of the effect of self-help against control groups.

Overall, additional studies are needed to compare guided self-help treatments against standard face-to-face treatments across anxiety, depression, and disruptive behaviour. Direct comparisons of different methods of self-help (e.g. bibliotherapy compared to computerized treatments) would be helpful. Further research investigating the use of self-help and guided self-help interventions in young people who are under-represented by the current research, such as those with intellectual and developmental disabilities and those from low- and middle-income countries, is warranted. The question regarding who LI interventions are suitable for remains unanswered. Individual patient meta-analyses, whereby the results from individual participants in studies are analysed rather than groups of participants, would help us understand whether LI interventions are only suitable for mild–moderate difficulties, or whether they could be used for more severe symptoms. Research into personalization, investigating exactly which patients benefit from which intensity therapies would be particularly useful. To date, there have been very few trials of stepped care (see Chapter 21), despite many guidelines recommending this model. Stepped care approaches across disorders need further investigation.

Finally, additional research is needed to investigate uptake of, and engagement with, self-help materials. In adults, reviews have found that this can vary significantly between trials. Routine collection of data from practice would support research into how these interventions can be integrated into routine care (see Chapter 8).

Chapter summary

- Self-help can increase access to therapy to meet a growing unmet need.
- Self-help is efficacious in treating common childhood mental health disorders.
- Guided self-help may be more efficacious than self-guided self-help, but this needs further research.
- Self-help interventions for this population may be slightly less effective than traditional higher intensity face-to-face treatments.

Recommended reading

Bennett, S. D., Cuijpers, P., Ebert, D. D., McKenzie Smith, M., Coughtrey, A. E., Heyman, I., . . ., & Shafran, R. (2019). Practitioner review: Unguided and guided self-help interventions for common mental health disorders in children and adolescents: A systematic review and meta-analysis. *Journal of Child Psychology and Psychiatry*, *60*(8), 828–847.

Karyotaki, E., Ebert, D. D., Donkin, L., Riper, H., Twisk, J., Burger, S., . . . & Geraedts, A. (2018). Do guided internet-based interventions result in clinically relevant changes for patients with depression? An individual participant data meta-analysis. *Clinical Psychology Review*, *63*, 80–92.

References

Bennett, S. D., Cuijpers, P., Ebert, D. D., McKenzie Smith, M., Coughtrey, A. E., Heyman, I., . . ., & Shafran, R. (2019). Practitioner review: Unguided and guided self-help interventions for common mental health disorders in children and adolescents: A systematic review and meta-analysis. *Journal of Child Psychology and Psychiatry, and Allied Disciplines*, *60*(8), 828–847.

Cuijpers, P., Donker, T., van Straten, A., Li, J., & Andersson, G. (2010). Is guided self-help as effective as face-to-face psychotherapy for depression and anxiety disorders? A systematic review and meta-analysis of comparative outcome studies. *Psychological Medicine*, *40*(12), 1943–1957.

Driessen, E., Hollon, S. D., Bockting, C. L., Cuijpers, P., & Turner, E. H. (2015). Does publication bias inflate the apparent efficacy of psychological treatment for major depressive disorder? A systematic review and meta-analysis of US National Institutes of Health-funded trials. *PLoS One*, *10*(9), e0137864.

Fleming, T., Bavin, L., Lucassen, M., Stasiak, K., Hopkins, S., & Merry, S. (2018). Beyond the trial: Systematic review of real-world uptake and engagement with digital self-help interventions for depression, low mood, or anxiety. *Journal of Medical Internet Research*, *20*(6), e199.

Gellatly, J., Bower, P., Hennessy, S., Richards, D., Gilbody, S., & Lovell, K. (2007). What makes self-help interventions effective in the management of depressive symptoms? Meta-analysis and meta-regression. *Psychological Medicine*, *37*(9) 1217–1228.

Hirai, M., & Clum, G. A. (2006). A meta-analytic study of self-help interventions for anxiety problems. *Behavior Therapy*, *37*(2), 99–111.

Karyotaki, E., Ebert, D. D., Donkin, L., Riper, H., Twisk, J., Burger, S., . . ., & Geraedts, A. (2018). Do guided internet-based interventions result in clinically relevant changes for patients with depression? An individual participant data meta-analysis. *Clinical Psychology Review*, *63*, 80–92.

Lewis, C., Pearce, J., & Bisson, J. I. (2012). Efficacy, cost-effectiveness and acceptability of self-help interventions for anxiety disorders: Systematic review. *British Journal of Psychiatry*, *200*(1), 15–21.

Mayo-Wilson, E., & Montgomery, P. (2013). Media-delivered cognitive behavioural therapy and behavioural therapy (self-help) for anxiety disorders in adults. *Cochrane Database of Systematic Reviews*, *9*, CD005330.

Newman, M. G., Erickson, T., Przeworski, A., & Dzus, E. (2003). Self-help and minimal-contact therapies for anxiety disorders: Is human contact necessary for therapeutic efficacy? *Journal of Clinical Psychology*, *59*(3), 251–274.

O'Brien, M., & Daley, D. (2011). Self-help parenting interventions for childhood behaviour disorders: A review of the evidence. *Child: Care, Health and Development*, *37*(5), 623–637.

Pearcy, C. P., Anderson, R. A., Egan, S. J., & Rees, C. S. (2016). A systematic review and meta-analysis of self-help therapeutic interventions for obsessive–compulsive disorder: Is therapeutic contact key to overall improvement? *Journal of Behavior Therapy and Experimental Psychiatry*, *51*, 74–83.

Perkins, S. J., Murphy, R., Schmidt, U., & Williams, C. (2006). Self-help and guided self-help for eating disorders. *Cochrane Database of Systematic Reviews*, *3*, CD004191.

Priemer, M., & Talbot, F. (2013). CBT guided self-help compares favourably to gold standard therapist-administered CBT and shows unique benefits over traditional treatment. *Behaviour Change, 30*(4), 227–240.

Schleider, J. L., & Weisz, J. R. (2017). Little treatments, promising effects? Meta-analysis of single-session interventions for youth psychiatric problems. *Journal of the American Academy of Child & Adolescent Psychiatry, 56*(2), 107–115.

Talbot, F. (2012). Client contact in self-help therapy for anxiety and depression: Necessary but can take a variety of forms beside therapist contact. *Behaviour Change, 29*(2), 63–76.

van Boeijen, C. A., van Oppen, P., van Balkom, A. J., Visser, S., Kempe, P. T., Blankenstein, N., & van Dyck, R. (2005). Treatment of anxiety disorders in primary care practice: A randomised controlled trial. *British Journal of General Practice, 55*(519), 763–769.

4

Prevention and early intervention in children and young people

Jenna Sung and Jessica L. Schleider

Learning objectives

- To define and overview the potential utility of low intensity (LI) interventions in preventing child mental health problems.
- To identify the shared goals across LI and prevention-focused programming, along with the number of practical benefits LI prevention programmes confer.
- To clarify the state of knowledge and limitations of existing LI prevention programmes designed for promoting youth mental health and preventing psychopathology.

Introduction: the importance of prevention and early intervention

Half of all mental illnesses start by 14 years of age, but most cases go undetected and are often left untreated (World Health Organization, 2019). When left untreated, childhood-onset mental health difficulties can predict lifelong challenges, including deterioration in physical health, lower educational attainment and achievement, and more days lost at work upon reaching adulthood. The influx of mental health problems during pre- and early adolescence is no coincidence. Early adolescence is a developmental stage characterized by rapid physical, emotional, and social changes. During this period of life, youth face a host of concurrent physical, emotional, and social changes; they also develop foundational cognitive processes and adopt behaviours that may put them at risk or protect them against mental health problems. Thus, intervening prior to and during early adolescence is critical to promoting well-being across the lifespan, reducing risk for psychiatric comorbidities (Copeland, Angold, Shanahan, & Costello, 2014), and decreasing societal costs associated with psychiatric conditions (Beecham, 2014; Bodden, Dirksen, & Bögels, 2008). Prevention efforts at an early age are the key to fostering positive outcomes at the individual (youth), family, and societal levels.

While it can feel more pressing to prioritize the treatment of populations *already experiencing clinical distress*, it is equally as important to invest in programmes that may *prevent* mental illnesses in vulnerable children. For example, depression is one of the most common disorders and the leading cause of disability (Friedrich, 2017; Reddy, 2010). Once developed, depression is very difficult to treat. Despite the efforts and the number of interventions aimed at treating depression, mean effect sizes for interventions targeting depression in children and adolescence have actually *decreased* in recent decades (Weisz et al., 2019). Thus, prevention efforts may be particularly important in decreasing the prevalence and burden of depression.

Prevention efforts (including low intensity (LI) and higher intensity programming) have received considerable attention in the research literature on child mental health. Mrazek and Haggerty (1994) identified three types of prevention programmes: universal, selective, and indicated. *Universal prevention* efforts aim to prevent new incidences of mental health disorders by directing interventions at the entire population. An example of a universal prevention programme may be a school-based emotion regulation programme offered to all students regardless of their current mental health status. This approach has advantages of being less stigmatizing since it does not require labelling and it takes the format of large groups. *Selective prevention* programmes aim to prevent new episodes of mental disorders by selecting for populations at risk for the disorder. Some examples of risk factors for various mental health difficulties are genetic vulnerability, history of abuse, or recent trauma. Thus, a child anxiety prevention programme targeting parents who report a personal history of anxiety disorder would fit this category, as parental anxiety is a known risk factor for anxiety disorders in offspring. *Indicated prevention* programmes aim to prevent new episodes of a mental disorder by directing interventions for those already showing subclinical symptoms. Thus, an indicated prevention programme might target clinically referred individuals who previously reported elevated mental health problems. While programmes with this approach tend to be more resource intensive, it is often more cost-effective as it selects a sample at the greatest risk.

Though there is an inherent challenge to demonstrating that a negative event (e.g. an increase in mental health problems) has in fact been avoided, several meta-analytic reviews have shown the positive effects of prevention programmes for social, behavioural, and psychological problems in children and adolescents. Durlak and Wells (1997) conducted a meta-analysis analysing primary prevention programmes using externalizing/internalizing symptoms, academic achievement, sociometric status, and cognitive and physiological processes as outcomes of interest. Compared to control conditions (including attentional placebos, no-treatment groups, and 'waiting list' groups), these prevention programmes showed a mean effect size of $d = 0.35$ (a small to medium effect) for environmental-centred programmes (e.g. interventions involving modifications to school environments); $d = 0.87$ (a large effect) for programmes designed to boost coping skills and supports specifically during a stressful life transition (e.g. during entry to a new school); and $d = 0.24$

(a small effect) for person-centred programmes (e.g. directly promoting mental health). Notably, these primary prevention programmes were generally delivered in *non-clinical settings* by individuals *without formal training* in mental health treatment. The included interventions took place primarily in school settings (72.9%) and were administered by various providers: mental health professionals (29.9%), teachers and parents (20.9%), graduate students (13%), undergraduate students (9%), and a combination of providers (19.2%). Number of sessions or the length of the interventions were not specifically reported in this meta-analysis; nonetheless, results suggest that adverse mental health outcomes may be successfully mitigated in diverse settings, and that highly trained providers may not be integral to their positive impacts on youth psychological outcomes.

Another meta-analysis looked at selective prevention programmes that aimed to reduce the intergenerational transmission of psychopathology (e.g. the development of depressive symptoms in children of parents with a history of depression; Siegenthaler, Munder, & Egger 2012). Across 13 trials, the average number of sessions was 14.3 with the duration of the intervention lasting from 1 month to 1 year. All interventions involved delivery by mental health professionals (e.g. clinical psychologists, master's level therapists, graduate students) and only three studies included lay providers (e.g. social workers, nurses) in their treatment team. All studies examined interventions that were delivered in person. The meta-analysis concluded that selective prevention interventions decreased the risk for mental disorders in children of parents with mental illness by 40%, when compared to control groups.

The role of LI interventions in prevention

Given the importance of early prevention efforts and their demonstrated utility, it is necessary to consider how to prioritize prevention programmes that will maximize the finite resources and time that providers, agencies, and clients have. Demonstrated by the characteristics of the studies included in the meta-analysis, traditional prevention programmes have generally been resource intensive: lengthy, delivered in person, and administered by highly trained mental health professionals. Adopting design features of LI intervention designs might help optimize the cost-effectiveness of prevention programming, helping to boost its brevity, flexibility, and scalability. LI prevention programmes may, for instance, be well-suited for broad administration in low-resource settings, in contrast to higher-intensity prevention programmes requiring weeks or months of face-to-face service provision (e.g. many of the prevention programmes in Siegenthaler and colleagues' meta-analysis). For example, a school may implement an online, self-guided prevention programme to an entire classroom of students simultaneously, or emergency room clinicians might offer a single session of preventative counselling to individuals identified as 'high risk' for substance use or suicidality upon intake. The structure of LI interventions thus directly complements the mission of mental health prevention programming: To reduce overall costs of mental health service provision at the system level, both guided by a public mental health lens. Shifting the design focus towards LI models of prevention programmes is critical to maximize their intended effect.

In fact, LI prevention programmes confer a number of additional benefits for clients when compared to more intensive prevention programmes, which represent the majority of evidence-based options. Offering LI prevention programmes will lower the traditional barriers for participation (e.g. lower costs), which will increase buy-in since clients who are not experiencing clinical levels of psychopathology may not have the motivation to pursue a more resource intensive programme. LI prevention programmes are also more likely to include populations that are most at risk as low-income communities or communities of marginalized identities are more likely to utilize programmes that are less stigmatizing and pose fewer barriers (e.g. online interventions).

State of knowledge for LI prevention programmes

Despite the number of benefits LI approaches offer that can complement the goals of prevention programmes (as discussed in multiple chapters throughout this book), the majority of LI interventions target populations already experiencing elevated or clinically-significant distress. Consolidated reports on LI interventions for prevention efforts specifically are scarce, which may be exacerbated by the varying operational definitions of LI in the psychological literature. For the purposes of this chapter, LI interventions are defined as 'low usage of specialist therapist time or usage in a cost-effective way' (Bennett-Levy, Richards, and Farrand, 2010) with an added goal to improving access. Though the meta-analysis and systematic reviews discussed below are not specifically focused on LI *and* preventive programmes that meet our definition, components of their review offer insight into the broad landscape of this literature.

A recent meta-analysis (Schleider and Weisz, 2017) examined the clinical utility of a particular category of LI mental health programmes, *single-session interventions* (one variety of LI interventions), defined as 'specific, structured programmes that intentionally involve just one visit or encounter with a clinic, provider, or program' (Schleider, Dobias, Sung, & Mullarkey, 2020; see Chapter 23). This meta-analysis identified 37 prevention programmes and 13 treatment interventions for youth, each of which was designed for administration in a single clinical encounter. Of these 37 single-session prevention programmes, 17 were best characterized as indicated prevention, 8 as selective prevention, and 12 as universal prevention programmes. They targeted various problems including difficulties with substance use ($N = 16$), eating behaviours ($N = 2$), depression or mood ($N = 5$), anxiety ($N = 6$), behavioural problems ($N = 5$), or multiple co-occurring problems ($N = 3$). The majority of the prevention programmes were guided by a clinician or lay provider ($N = 30$), as opposed to being designed for self-administration by youths (e.g. computer-based self-help programmes; $N = 7$). It is important to note that the effect sizes did not significantly differ between prevention programmes (indicated prevention $g = 0.25$; selective prevention $g = 0.47$; universal prevention $g = 0.33$) and treatment programmes ($g = 0.41$) in this meta-analysis, suggesting that single-session interventions can significantly benefit youth mental health both for children *with* and *without* clinically significant difficulties.

In the systematic review and meta-analysis of unguided and guided self-help interventions for children and adolescents detailed in Chapter 3 (Bennett et al., 2019), we identified three prevention programmes for depression that may provide a sense of what such programmes might look like. Stice, Rohde, Seeley, and Gau (2008) examined the effectiveness of bibliotherapy (self-help book; *Feeling Good*) as an indicated prevention intervention that provided participants with cognitive behavioural techniques that can combat negative mood often associated with depression. The study evaluated the intervention's ability to reduce the symptoms of depression in high school students who reported elevated levels of depression (>20 on the Center for Epidemiologic Studies—Depression Scale); compared to the assessment-only control, the participants who received the bibliotherapy demonstrated significant improvement in depressive symptoms and were at significantly lower risk for experiencing an onset of major depression at 6-month follow-up, but not at post-test.

Another study found that an online, indicated prevention programme that delivered behavioural parent training for parents of at-risk adolescents had significant small to medium effects on improved discipline style, child behaviour, intentions, and self-efficacy (Irvine, Gelatt, Hammond, & Seeley, 2015). The programme involved four steps: (1) watching a video vignette that was designed to increase self-efficacy and behavioural intention to foster positive responses for parents who have children with behavioural problems; (2) choosing a topic from bedtime, chores, curfew, depression, grades, fighting, friends, smoking, and stealing; (3) walking through parenting choices and given corrective feedback; and (4) making a personalized action plan by choosing up to three skills they want to practise at home (e.g. using 'I' statements, making clear rules). Attempts to create culturally adapted programmes have also been reported. A study evaluated an internet-based programme for Chinese adolescents (Ip et al., 2016). The adaptation involved translations and content modification to reflect situations that are more familiar to Chinese adolescents. The programme was found to be a valid tool that was culturally relevant to the Chinese populations in Hong Kong.

Chapter summary

This chapter summarizes current understandings and applications of LI approaches to preventing youth mental health problems, including universal, selected, and indicated prevention approaches. Overall, emerging research suggests the potential utility of LI approaches to building accessible, effective prevention programmes for youth mental health difficulties. However, to date, research on LI youth-focused *interventions* and youth-focused *prevention* efforts have remained largely separate areas of study, and research on LI prevention programming remains scarcer than research on LI treatments for already-existing psychopathology. The lack of consolidated reports on LI preventive efforts reflects the relative paucity of LI prevention programmes for all youth problem areas. Given how well LI design features lend themselves to the goals of prevention efforts, the field should prioritize the development and testing of LI prevention programmes. Toward this goal, transdiagnostic LI prevention programmes may warrant special attention as these programmes can simultaneously address multiple problem areas (e.g. broad internalizing distress). Lastly, it is important to keep in mind that research on LI prevention programmes shares limitations common to the treatment literature: existing interventions are often tested within relatively homogeneous samples comprised of white, middle-class, and well-educated families. Research on LI prevention programmes should prioritize inclusive recruitment approaches to ensure future programmes are useful and acceptable within diverse and marginalized communities.

References

Beecham, J. (2014). Annual Research Review: Child and adolescent mental health interventions: a review of progress in economic studies across different disorders. In *Journal of Child Psychology and Psychiatry* (Vol. 55, Issue 6, pp. 714–732). https://doi.org/10.1111/jcpp.12216

Bennett, S. D., Cuijpers, P., Ebert, D. D., McKenzie Smith, M., Coughtrey, A. E., Heyman, I., . . ., Shafran, R. (2019). Practitioner review: Unguided and guided self-help interventions for common mental health disorders in children and adolescents: A systematic review and meta-analysis. *Journal of Child Psychology and Psychiatry, and Allied Disciplines*, 60(8), 828–847.

Bennett-Levy, J., Richards, D. A., & Farrand, P. (2010). Low intensity CBT interventions: A revolution in mental health care. In J. Bennett-Levy, D. A. Richards, P. Farrand, H. Christensen, K. Griffiths, B. Kavanagh, . . ., & C. Williams (Eds.), *Oxford guide to low intensity CBT interventions* (pp. 3–18). Oxford: Oxford University Press.

Bodden, D. H., Dirksen, C. D., & Bögels, S. M. (2008). Societal burden of clinically anxious youth referred for treatment: A cost-of-illness study. *Journal of Abnormal Child Psychology*, 36(4), 487–497.

Copeland, W. E., Angold, A., Shanahan, L., & Costello, E. J. (2014). Longitudinal patterns of anxiety from childhood to adulthood: The Great Smoky Mountains Study. *Journal of the American Academy of Child and Adolescent Psychiatry*, 53(1), 21–33.

Durlak, J. A., & Wells, A. M. (1997). Primary prevention mental health programs for children and adolescents: a meta-analytic review. *American Journal of Community Psychology*, 25(2), 115–152.

Friedrich, M. J. (2017). Depression Is the Leading Cause of Disability Around the World. *JAMA: The Journal of the American Medical Association*, 317 (15), 1517.

Ip, P., Chim, D., Chan, K. L., Li, T. M., Ho, F. K., Van Voorhees, B. W., . . ., (2016). Effectiveness of a culturally attuned internet-based depression prevention program for Chinese adolescents: A randomized controlled trial. *Depression and Anxiety*, 33(12), 1123–1131.

Irvine, A. B., Gelatt, V. A., Hammond, M., & Seeley, J. R. (2015). A randomized study of internet parent training accessed from community technology centers. *Prevention Science*, 16(4), 597–608.

Lize, S. E., Iachini, A. L., Tang, W., Tucker, J., Seay, K. D., Clone, S., . . ., & Browne, T. (2017). A meta-analysis of the effectiveness of interactive middle school cannabis prevention programs. *Prevention Science*, 18(1), 50–60.

Mrazek, P. B., & Haggerty, R. J. 1994. *Reducing risks for mental disorders: Frontiers for preventive intervention research*. Washington, DC: National Academies.

Reddy, M. S. (2010). Depression: The Disorder and the Burden. In *Indian Journal of Psychological Medicine* (Vol. 32, Issue 1, pp. 1–2). https://doi.org/10.4103/0253-7176.70510

Robinson, J., Bailey, E., Witt, K., Stefanac, N., Milner, A., Currier, D., . . ., & Hetrick, S. (2018). What works in youth suicide prevention? A systematic review and meta-analysis. *EClinicalMedicine, 4–5*(October), 52–91.

Rohde, P., Stice, E., Shaw, H., & Brière, F. N. (2014). Indicated cognitive behavioral group depression prevention compared to bibliotherapy and brochure control: Acute effects of an effectiveness trial with adolescents. *Journal of Consulting and Clinical Psychology, 82*(1), 65–74.

Schleider, J. L., Dobias, M. L., Sung, J. Y., & Mullarkey, M. C. (2020). Future directions in single-session youth mental health interventions. *Journal of Clinical Child and Adolescent Psychology, 49*(2), 264–278.

Schleider, J. L., & Weisz, J. R. (2017). Little treatments, promising effects? Meta-analysis of single-session interventions for youth psychiatric problems. *Journal of the American Academy of Child and Adolescent Psychiatry, 56*(2), 107–15.

Siegenthaler, E., Munder, T., & Egger, M. (2012). Effect of preventive interventions in mentally ill parents on the mental health of the offspring: Systematic review and meta-analysis. *Journal of the American Academy of Child and Adolescent Psychiatry, 51*(1), 8–17.e8.

Stice, E., Rohde, P., Seeley, J. R., & Gau, J. M. (2008). Brief cognitive-behavioral depression prevention program for high-risk adolescents outperforms two alternative interventions: A randomized efficacy trial. *Journal of Consulting and Clinical Psychology, 76*(4), 595–606.

Stice, E., Shaw, H., & Marti, C. N. (2007). A meta-analytic review of eating disorder prevention programs: Encouraging findings. *Annual Review of Clinical Psychology, 3*, 207–231.

Weisz, J. R., Kuppens, S., Ng, M. Y., Vaughn-Coaxum, R. A., Ugueto, A. M., Eckshtain, D., & Corteselli, K. A. (2019). Are psychotherapies for young people growing stronger? Tracking trends over time for youth anxiety, depression, attention-deficit/hyperactivity disorder, and conduct problems. *Perspectives on Psychological Science, 14*(2), 216–237.

World Health Organization. (2019). *Adolescent and Young Adult Health*. Retrieved from https://www.who.int/news-room/fact-sheets/detail/adolescents-health-risks-and-solutions

5

Low intensity psychological interventions for children and young people: the economic case thus far

Martin Knapp and Gloria Wong

Learning objectives

- To understand what economic evaluation can offer to the mental health field.
- To explore the economic arguments for low intensity psychological interventions for children and young people.
- To examine current cost-effectiveness evidence for low intensity psychological interventions for children and young people based on key research.
- To appreciate the challenges and solutions in building up economic evidence for children and young people and for low intensity psychological interventions.

Introduction: economic arguments for low intensity psychological interventions in children and young people

Cost-effectiveness, or good value for money in producing goods and benefits at an acceptable cost, is intricately linked with funding decisions and service access. It is thus a key rationale for low intensity (LI) psychotherapies, one that is of particular pertinence in relation to children and young people: demand for mental healthcare in this age group is great, and economic impacts of poor mental health are wide and enduring.

Mental disorders are 'the chronic diseases of the young' (Insel & Fenton, 2005), with 75% of mental disorders beginning before adulthood (Fusar-Poli, 2019). Economic impacts are not limited to increased healthcare use, although these can be considerable, but also to life-years lost (with consequences for productivity); higher likelihood of contacts with social care, special education, criminal justice and other public and private services; and lower educational attainment, employment rates, income, and wealth acquisition (Knapp, King, Healey, & Thomas, 2011; Richards & Abbott, 2009).

Economic evidence can help design a mental healthcare system that not only 'optimally improves the future outcomes of children and adolescents' (Skokauskas et al.,

2018), but is also affordable and makes best use of resources available, both now and in the future. Some psychological interventions (perhaps in combination with medication) are beginning to show both clinical effectiveness and cost-effectiveness in children and young people (Beecham, 2014; Knapp et al., 2016; Romeo, Byford, & Knapp, 2005), although major evidence gaps exist. On the other hand, improving access to these interventions, even in high-resource settings, remains a challenge. If psychological interventions are to be made more widely available in a context of scarce resources—and it is abundantly clear from other chapters in this volume that such interventions can contribute significantly to better health and well-being—then some re-engineering of child and adolescent mental health services (CAMHS) is called for, with LI psychological intervention playing a more prominent role (Kazdin, 2019; McDaid et al., 2020).

Many of the service models with embedded LI psychological interventions, such as stepped care and task-shifted interventions, have been designed (perhaps implicitly) to achieve a balance between cost savings and maximum intensity treatment (Bower & Gilbody, 2005). This balance is therefore an hypothesis that should be scientifically tested, which then requires not just calculation of the budget needed and the savings that might accrue, but full economic evaluation (Knapp & Wong, 2020). We discuss what this means in the next section of this chapter. While evidence of clinical non-inferiority compared with standard treatment is now accumulating, as noted in other chapters, the cost-effectiveness of LI alternatives sometimes appears just to be *assumed* on the basis that they involve lower costs. After explaining what economic evaluation entails, we describe a few key examples of economic evaluation of LI psychological interventions in children and young people to illustrate the necessity and usefulness of economic evidence, particularly its relevance in informing policy and practice decisions.

Economic evaluation

When decision-makers are considering a specific intervention, whether targeted on children's mental health needs or in another area, they will want to check not just whether the objectives of the intervention are met—in this case, whether mental illness is prevented, symptoms alleviated, or quality of life enhanced—but also what resources are needed to do so. Economic evaluations ask whether the resources needed to deliver the intervention are *justified* by the outcomes achieved. This also entails looking at whether there might be future savings, for example, because individuals use fewer services.

If the outcomes of one intervention (call it A) are better than the outcomes of a comparator (intervention B), and if A is associated with lower costs than B (in terms of resources needed to deliver it, plus any downstream savings), then A is clearly more attractive than B from an economics standpoint: it is said to be 'cost-effective'. However, if A generates better outcomes but simultaneously has *higher* costs than B, it is not obvious whether those better outcomes justify the extra resources needed to deliver them. In these circumstances, economic evaluation seeks to highlight the trade-off to inform a decision.

The usual way to summarize evidence collected in an economic evaluation to illustrate this trade-off is first to calculate an incremental cost-effectiveness ratio. This ratio is equal to the extra (or incremental) cost associated with one intervention compared to another divided by the extra (incremental) effect or outcome. If, for example, the evaluation is comparing two interventions for the same condition (e.g. anxiety in adolescents), the decision-maker would probably be most interested in how those two interventions compare in terms of symptom alleviation, and what it costs to achieve those improvements.

There are basically three main types of health economics evaluation: they differ in how they conceptualize and measure outcomes, and that is because they address slightly different questions. The measurement of *costs* is similar across all three types of evaluation, but can nevertheless vary in terms of measurement breadth. An essential component is the resources needed to deliver the interventions themselves. The evaluator would ideally also include other resources that individuals use (e.g. health service contacts or support in school settings) and perhaps also wider economic impacts such as consequences for parents' employment patterns. Breadth of cost measurement depends in part on the purpose of a study and in part on availability of data, and of course raises questions about breadth of policy responsibility (Knapp & Wong, 2020).

The example above—looking at treatments of anxiety in adolescents—describes a typical clinical question: which treatment is best for a specific condition? Outcomes are most usefully measured in this context in terms of condition-specific indicators (such as anxiety symptoms); this is usually called a *cost-effectiveness analysis*. How then does the clinical decision-maker decide whether the better outcomes warrant the higher costs? There is no simple way. The decision-maker must simply reach a judgement: the decision as to whether an intervention is cost-effective is partly based on objectively good science (evaluation design, robust outcome and cost measurement, and appropriate analysis) and partly on subjective value judgements. How much does the decision-maker, acting on behalf of the mental health system or society as a whole, value the improvement in outcomes?

Increasingly, decisions of this kind are being scrutinized in a broader context: treatment for anxiety in adolescents uses up therapist time, medications, and so on, but perhaps the funds required to access those resources would be better allocated to treating, say, diabetes. Health system decision-makers need to decide how to allocate their budgets across competing demands. A form of economic evaluation called *cost–utility analysis* can help them: it measures outcomes in a common unit relevant to both (or all) disease areas. The most frequently used generic outcome of this kind measures quality-adjusted life years (QALYs): does an intervention increase years of life and/or improve the quality of those years?

Cost–utility analyses tell *strategic* decision-makers where they will achieve most impact from the resources they manage. QALYs can be measured by completing a tool such as the EuroQol Five Dimensions (EQ-5D) (EuroQol Group, 1990), which uses ratings on a number of health-related domains such as mobility and pain, and then combines them into a single score that conventionally runs from 0 (death) to 1 (perfect health). There are different QALY-generating tools in use, some of them disease specific or age group specific, but they all aim to produce a measure that allows comparison of treatment effects across different diseases and conditions.

In some countries, cost–utility thresholds have been proposed to guide decisions. In England, the National Institute for Health and Care Excellence (NICE) uses a threshold of between £20,000 and £30,000 per QALY: interventions costing less than this are more likely to be recommended for utilization across the National Health Service than interventions above this range. For the latter, NICE argues that the resources (represented by cost) could be better spent somewhere else in the health system. But this threshold is only to provide guidance and not to be a rigid rule: it nevertheless reminds everyone (clinicians, patients, families, taxpayers, and elected politicians) that resources are not limitless, and so difficult choices have to be made (Appleby, Devlin, & Parkin, 2007).

There is an even wider decision-making context, when resources need to be allocated across different areas of public policy, such as healthcare, housing, and education. In this case, the only feasible outcome measures generic enough to cover those different areas are either money (what is the monetary value of the impacts?) or a high-level well-being measure (what level of happiness is achieved from those impacts?). The former has usually been called a *cost–benefit analysis*, but it is extremely difficult to put monetary value on health outcomes, so this type of evaluation is rare, unless perhaps employment gains are among the relevant outcomes (Knapp et al., 2013). Evaluations measuring well-being are also rare but gradually being explored in health services research contexts (Brazier, Rowen, Lloyd, & Karimi, 2019), and would be quite pertinent in the mental health field.

It needs to be emphasized that economic evaluations focus on just one of the criteria that might inform decisions: the *efficiency* with which resources are used. Decision-makers will take other things into consideration, particularly equity: how fairly are health benefits, well-being, and financial contributions spread across the population?

Current economic evidence from key research

Parent-delivered cognitive behavioural therapy for anxiety disorders

Psychological interventions delivered by parents/carers are examples of task-shifted approaches, where there is a lower skills requirement for training for the interventionist (parents in this case), which may involve lower costs than if the intervention is delivered by a paid specialist.

The cost-effectiveness of a brief guided parent/carer-delivered cognitive behavioural therapy (CBT) and solution-focused brief therapy for childhood anxiety disorders has been compared with solution-focused brief therapy (also a LI psychological intervention) in a pragmatic randomized controlled trial (RCT) (see Chapter 10) (Creswell et al., 2017). The two interventions showed similar clinical outcomes (measured using Clinical Global Impressions of Improvement) and economic outcomes (QALYs). The authors considered both treatment costs and wider societal costs, including educational services, travel costs, time off school (for the child), and time off work (for the main parent/carer). Parent-delivered CBT appeared to cost less, although the difference was not significant: both therapies were delivered with 5 hours of therapist contact. Despite the non-significant differences, when both costs and effects were considered jointly in the incremental cost-effectiveness ratio analysis, there was a high likelihood that brief guided parent-delivered CBT was more cost-effective.

The (possibly) lower costs of parent/carer-delivered CBT could be related to reduced need for face-to-face consultations, associated with travel costs and time, as phone contacts were used for the therapist to provide guidance. Further work is needed to confirm any difference, although this highlights how some aspects of a LI psychological intervention (in this case, clinic attendance) may affect its cost-effectiveness (Stallard, 2017). Another point to note here is the lack of direct comparison of each of these LI psychological therapies with standard CAMH interventions that are lengthier, such as CBT, to understand their cost-effectiveness as an alternative to known cost-effective psychological therapies.

Stepped care for anxiety disorders and stress symptoms in children and young people

The economic case for delivering CBT via a stepped care framework for anxiety disorders in children has recently been examined using data from an RCT in Australia and an open trial in the US (Chatterton et al., 2019; Pettit et al., 2017; Rapee et al., 2017; Yeguez, Page, Rey, Silverman, & Pettit, 2020). The Australian study compared a validated best practice programme (Cool Kids anxiety treatment with ten individual sessions) versus stepped care, which involved LI self-help CBT, standard CBT, and individually tailored treatment in 6- to 17-year-olds (see Chapter 21) (Rapee et al., 2017). The US study used mathematical modelling to compare CBT alone versus CBT in stepped care, which involved eight sessions of computer-administered attention bias modification as a first step for children and young people (mean age of sample 9.66 years) (Pettit et al., 2017).

In the Australian study, stepped care showed similar outcomes to those of the best practice model at 12-month follow-up, using less therapist time, and the first two steps showed most treatment gains (Rapee et al., 2017). Costs included medication, service use, and parental lost productivity and outcome was QALYs. Although stepped care was associated with lower cost of intervention delivery, total costs and outcomes did not differ between groups. The authors argued that stepped care is an attractive option for some parents, although care as usual should be compared against various models of stepped care (Chatterton et al., 2019). Using data from the same trial, the group also found that standard face-to-face therapy is associated with a small significant improvement in clinical outcome, but a marked increase in therapist time and treatment cost, compared with LI methods (printed or electronic plus telephone sessions) (Rapee et al., 2020).

The US study showed that approximately 40% of participants opted for higher intensity CBT upon completing the computer-administered attention bias modification. Cost estimates were based on treatment resources used and Medicaid reimbursement. Compared with the hypothetical CBT-alone condition, stepped care halved treatment session time, and achieved cost savings of up to 48%, although that did not include time variables related to the treatment (e.g. time spent completing homework and travelling) (Pettit et al., 2017). The authors concluded that the stepped care generates substantial cost savings compared with standard CBT (Yeguez et al., 2020).

Another study evaluated the cost-effectiveness of a stepped care model for post-traumatic stress symptoms in children aged 3–7 years in an RCT in the US. The stepped care service was trauma-focused CBT involving three therapist-led sessions, 11 parent–child meetings, weekly brief phone support, psychoeducation, and video demonstrations of relaxation and exposure. Standard therapy involved 12 in-office therapist-led sessions (Salloum et al., 2016). Given that there was no difference in treatment efficacy, simple cost comparison (instead of cost-effectiveness analysis) was done: costs were at least 50% lower with stepped care. Costs covered treatment and compensation for missing work, although data on other service use were not collected, and so some potentially important cost implications were missed.

Single-session intervention and generic CAMHS

For LI therapies not linked to a specific protocol, very brief specialist-led sessions and non-specialist delivered sessions are two very different designs for cost-effective CAMHS. To date, there has been no head-to-head comparison between these two approaches. Comparisons have been made with usual/standard specialist care. For single-session intervention, although there was enough previous research to conduct a meta-analysis for youth psychiatric problems (drawing on 50 trials and over 10,000 participants), no information on formal cost-effectiveness could be found (Schleider & Weisz, 2017). The authors nevertheless suggested that given the similar effect sizes for single-session and longer intervention, it could be a cost-effective alternative or adjunct therapy to usual care given its potential to reduce costs and improve access.

The cost-effectiveness of generic CAMHS has been compared with specialist care in young people with eating disorders in the CostED study (Byford et al., 2019) using decision modelling. Using the Children's Global Assessment Scale as the primary outcome, cost-effectiveness analysis showed similar outcomes and costs between the two interventions, although results were not clear-cut and there were differences in participant characteristics in the two groups (Byford et al., 2019).

Challenges

The thin cost-effectiveness evidence available to date is linked with a two-pronged problem: economic evaluations are challenging in CAMHS contexts, and there is still limited evidence on LI psychological interventions.

In CAMHS, because of the often wide and long-lasting economic consequences, accurate cost-effectiveness analyses would necessitate adoption of a societal perspective (including costs from multiple sectors) and include long-term follow-up. Apart from the limits associated with research funding and the feasibility of tracking individuals over long time periods, there is also a major 'double disincentive': spending in one sector (on the intervention) generates returns in *other* sectors mainly in the future, and so cost-effectiveness findings may be considered irrelevant by some policymakers and budget holders who have to make difficult short-term decisions within bounded contexts.

Another challenge with CAHMS in general is in quantifying QALYs. Commonly used tools for measuring and valuating QALYs, such as the EQ-5D suite (https://euroqol.org/) and Short-Form Six Dimensions (SF-6D) (https://www.sheffield.ac.uk/scharr/research/themes/valuing-health), have rarely been validated in children and young people. Although there are versions for children and young people, their sensitivity to changes in mental health issues remains questionable (Brazier et al., 2014). Some of the above-mentioned studies included mental health-specific quality of life measures, such as the Child Health Utility Nine Dimensions (CHU9D) (https://www.sheffield.ac.uk/scharr/sections/heds/mvh/paediatric/about-chu9d), although these inevitably bring the disadvantage of not being *directly* comparable across populations or conditions.

The general lack of economic evidence for LI interventions is a major challenge. Considering that many protocol-based psychological interventions have proven efficient, we cannot simply *assume* that LI variations would be cost-effective compared with these 'best practice' interventions. The essentially complex nature of these interventions also poses challenges of identifying the components for comparison: not knowing whether varying levels of task-shifting, different transitions across steps in stepped care, use of different delivery modalities, or system contexts (such as workforce readiness) are the key drivers for cost-effectiveness means that more trials are needed before decision-makers in CAMHS can be fully informed about their 'best buys'.

Future economic studies should look at less visible economic consequences (e.g. carer impacts in parent-delivered interventions, acceptance, and non-response/disengagement), and rapidly growing new modalities particularly relevant to children and young people, such as internet-based, app-based including chatbot, and game-based interventions; video conferencing; and text-based online counselling, especially with e-mental health flourishing since the COVID-19 pandemic (see Chapters 24 and 27). CAMHS is a rapidly developing field, with interventions having to align with changing needs of children and young people, a challenge that is faced not only in economic evaluation but also clinical effectiveness studies, making it difficult for stakeholders to make informed decisions about resources allocation.

Potential solutions and looking ahead

An obvious response to the lack of economic evidence in LI psychological interventions for children and young people is to set economic evaluations as default (Knapp & Wong, 2020). Awareness of the necessity of economic evidence has already led some countries such as the UK to mandate economic evaluations for clinical guideline development (Knapp & Lemmi, 2016). The World Economic Forum has also recently collaborated with Orygen, Australia's national youth mental health organization, to develop a Global Framework for Youth Mental Health and an accompanying investment framework (McDaid et al., 2020), which emphasized investing in quality data systems, research partnership, and economic evaluation.

It is therefore encouraging to see many cost-effectiveness studies already in the pipeline. These include a pragmatic, non-inferiority RCT (a type of trial testing whether a new intervention is as effective as a proven intervention) comparing effectiveness and cost-effectiveness of single-session interventions with multi-session CBT for specific phobias in children and youth people (Wright et al., 2018); a cluster RCT (randomizing groups rather than individuals) with economic analysis comparing a brief behavioural intervention (two consultations) for sleep problems in children with attention deficit hyperactivity disorder (Sciberras et al., 2017); a school-based RCT investigating effectiveness and cost-effectiveness of LI problem-solving for common adolescent mental health problems in India, comparing interventions delivered by lay counsellors versus problem-solving booklets (Parikh et al., 2019); and, within the Germany ProHEAD consortium, trials investigating the cost-effectiveness of two online interventions for children and young people at risk of depression (a clinician-guided self-management program, iFightDepression®, and a clinician-guided group chat intervention) (Baldofski et al., 2019), and two interventions based on dissonance theory (assuming that inducing a discrepancy between a person's behaviour and beliefs/attitudes could change the latter, as people seek consistency) and CBT principles added onto an internet-based prevention programme for eating disorders (ProYouth) (Bauer et al., 2019).

These research developments are important not only to provide evidence on what might be more affordable alternatives (non-inferiority with lower costs). Given the unique roles of many LI psychological interventions in CAMHS, there are advantages offered by these interventions, such as user acceptability (e.g. internet-based versus face-to-face intervention) and enhanced engagement (e.g. ease of outreaching), when compared with traditional office-based, one-to-one, face-to-face interventions. These features may increase the value for money of these LI interventions. For example, there appears to be a lower rate of attrition, non-adherence, and non-response with group-based parent-delivered interventions (Blair, Topitzes, & Mersky, 2019). Future economic evaluations with direct comparison between LI and standard psychological interventions will provide insights into their benefits beyond saving money.

Chapter summary

Stakeholders are becoming increasingly aware of the need for economic evidence to inform their difficult decisions. With economic evaluation increasingly considered an integral component in CAMH initiatives (e.g. see headspace in Australia; Hilferty et al., 2015), we have an opportunity to significantly speed up the growth of LI psychological interventions to improve access to better health and well-being in equitable, viable, efficient, and sustainable ways.

Recommended reading

Beecham J. (2014). Annual research review: Child and adolescent mental health interventions: A review of progress in economic studies across different disorders. *Journal of Child Psychology and Psychiatry, and Allied Disciplines, 55*(6), 714–732.

Knapp, M., Ardino, V., Brimblecombe, N., Evans-Lacko, S., Iemmi, V., King, D., . . ., & Wilson, J. (2016). *Youth mental health: New economic evidence.* London: London School of Economics and Political Science.

Knapp, M., & Wong, G. (2020). Economics and mental health: The current scenario. *World Psychiatry, 19*(1), 3–14.

Skokauskas, N., Lavelle, T. A., Munir, K., Sampaio, F., Nystrand, C., McCrone, P., . . ., & Belfer, M. (2018). The cost of child and adolescent mental health services. *Lancet Psychiatry, 5*(4), 299–300.

References

Appleby, J., Devlin, N., & Parkin, D. (2007). NICE's cost effectiveness threshold. *BMJ, 335*(7616), 358–359.

Baldofski, S., Kohls, E., Bauer, S., Becker, K., Bilic, S., Eschenbeck, H., . . ., & ProHEAD Consortium (2019). Efficacy and cost-effectiveness of two online interventions for children and adolescents at risk for depression (E.motion trial): Study protocol for a randomized controlled trial within the ProHEAD consortium. *Trials, 20*(1), 53.

Bauer, S., Bilic, S., Reetz, C., Ozer, F., Becker, K., Eschenbeck, H., . . ., & ProHEAD Consortium (2019). Efficacy and cost-effectiveness of Internet-based selective eating disorder prevention: Study protocol for a randomized controlled trial within the ProHEAD Consortium. *Trials, 20*(1), 91.

Beecham, J. (2014). Annual research review: Child and adolescent mental health interventions: A review of progress in economic studies across different disorders. *Journal of Child Psychology and Psychiatry, and Allied Disciplines, 55*(6), 714–732.

Blair, K., Topitzes, J., & Mersky, J. P. (2019). Brief, group-based parent-child interaction therapy: Examination of treatment attrition, non-adherence, and non-response. *Children and Youth Services Review, 106,* 104463.

Bower, P., & Gilbody, S. (2005). Stepped care in psychological therapies: Access, effectiveness and efficiency. Narrative literature review. *British Journal of Psychiatry, 186,* 11–17.

Brazier, J., Connell, J., Papaioannou, D., Mukuria, C., Mulhern, B., Peasgood, T., . . ., & Parry, G. (2014). A systematic review, psychometric analysis and qualitative assessment of generic preference-based measures of health in mental health populations and the estimation of mapping functions from widely used specific measures. *Health Technology Assessment, 18*(34), vii–viii, xiii–xxv, 1–188.

Brazier, J. E., Rowen, D., Lloyd, A., & Karimi, M. (2019). Future directions in valuing benefits for estimating QALYs: Is time up for the EQ-5D? *Value Health, 22*(1), 62–68.

Byford, S., Petkova, H., Stuart, R., Nicholls, D., Simic, M., Ford, T., . . ., & Eisler, I. (2019). *Alternative community-based models of care for young people with anorexia nervosa: The CostED national surveillance study.* Southampton: NIHR Journals Library.

Chatterton, M. L., Rapee, R. M., Catchpool, M., Lyneham, H. J., Wuthrich, V., Hudson, J. L., . . ., & Mihalopoulos, C. (2019). Economic evaluation of stepped care for the management of childhood anxiety disorders: Results from a randomised trial. *Australian and New Zealand Journal of Psychiatry, 53*(7), 673–682.

Creswell, C., Violato, M., Fairbanks, H., White, E., Parkinson, M., Abitabile, G., . . ., & Cooper, P. J. (2017). Clinical outcomes and cost-effectiveness of brief guided parent-delivered cognitive behavioural therapy and solution-focused brief therapy for treatment of childhood anxiety disorders: A randomised controlled trial. *Lancet Psychiatry, 4*(7), 529–539.

EuroQol Group. (1990). EuroQol—a new facility for the measurement of health-related quality of life. *Health Policy, 16*(3), 199–208.

Fusar-Poli, P. (2019). Integrated mental health services for the developmental period (0 to 25 years): A critical review of the evidence. *Frontiers in Psychiatry, 10,* 355.

Hilferty, F., Cassells, R., Muir, K., Duncan, A., Christensen, D., Mitrou, F., . . ., & Katz, I. (2015). *Is Headspace making a difference to young people's lives? Final report of the independent evaluation of the Headspace Program* (SPRC Report 08/2015). Sydney: Social Policy Research Centre, UNSW Australia.

Insel, T. R., & Fenton, W. S. (2005). Psychiatric epidemiology: It's not just about counting anymore. *Archives of General Psychiatry, 62*(6), 590–592.

Kazdin, A. E. (2019). Annual research review: Expanding mental health services through novel models of intervention delivery. *Journal of Child Psychology and Psychiatry, and Allied Disciplines, 60*(4), 455–472.

Knapp, M., Ardino, V., Brimblecombe, N., Evans-Lacko, S., Iemmi, V., King, D., . . ., Wilson, J. (2016). *Youth mental health: New economic evidence.* London: London School of Economics and Political Science.

Knapp, M., King, D., Healey, A., & Thomas, C. (2011). Economic outcomes in adulthood and their associations with antisocial conduct, attention deficit and anxiety problems in childhood. *Journal of Mental Health Policy and Economics, 14*(3), 137–147.

Knapp, M., & Iemmi, V. (2016). Mental health. In R. M. Scheffle (Ed.), *World Scientific handbook of global health economics and public policy,* Vol. 2 (pp. 1–41). Singapore: World Scientific.

Knapp, M., Patel, A., Curran, C., Latimer, E., Catty, J., Becker, T., . . ., & Burns, T. (2013). Supported employment: Cost-effectiveness across six European sites. *World Psychiatry, 12*(1), 60–68.

Knapp, M., & Wong, G. (2020). Economics and mental health: The current scenario. *World Psychiatry, 19*(1), 3–14.

McDaid, D., Hamilton, M., King, D., Park, A., Scopel Hoffman, M., Silva Ribeiro, W., . . ., Evans-Lacko, S. (2020). *An investment framework to build mental capital in young people*. Sydney: Orygen and World Economic Forum.

Parikh, R., Michelson, D., Malik, K., Shinde, S., Weiss, H. A., Hoogendoorn, A., . . ., & Patel, V. (2019). The effectiveness of a low-intensity problem-solving intervention for common adolescent mental health problems in New Delhi, India: Protocol for a school-based, individually randomized controlled trial with an embedded stepped-wedge, cluster randomized controlled recruitment trial. *Trials*, *20*(1), 568.

Pettit, J. W., Rey, Y., Bechor, M., Melendez, R., Vaclavik, D., Buitron, V., . . ., & Silverman, W. K. (2017). Can less be more? Open trial of a stepped care approach for child and adolescent anxiety disorders. *Journal of Anxiety Disorders*, *51*, 7–13.

Rapee, R. M., Lyneham, H. J., Wuthrich, V., Chatterton, M. L., Hudson, J. L., Kangas, M., & Mihalopoulos, C. (2017). Comparison of stepped care delivery against a single, empirically validated cognitive-behavioral therapy program for youth with anxiety: A randomized clinical trial. *Journal of the American Academy of Child and Adolescent Psychiatry*, *56*(10), 841–848.

Rapee, R. M., Lyneham, H. J., Wuthrich, V., Chatterton, M. L., Hudson, J. L., Kangas, M., & Mihalopoulos, C. (2021). Low intensity treatment for clinically anxious youth: A randomised controlled comparison against face-to-face intervention. *European Child & Adolescent Psychiatry*, *30*(7), 1071–1079.

Richards, M., & Abbott, R. (2009). *Childhood mental health and life chances in post-war Britain: Insights from three national birth cohort studies*. London: The Smith Institute.

Romeo, R., Byford, S., & Knapp, M. (2005). Annotation: Economic evaluations of child and adolescent mental health interventions: A systematic review. *Journal of Child Psychology and Psychiatry, and Allied Disciplines*, *46*(9), 919–930.

Salloum, A., Wang, W., Robst, J., Murphy, T. K., Scheeringa, M. S., Cohen, J. A., & Storch, E. A. (2016). Stepped care versus standard trauma-focused cognitive behavioral therapy for young children. *Journal of Child Psychology and Psychiatry, and Allied Disciplines*, *57*(5), 614–622.

Schleider, J. L., & Weisz, J. R. (2017). Little treatments, promising effects? Meta-analysis of single-session interventions for youth psychiatric problems. *Journal of the American Academy of Child and Adolescent Psychiatry*, *56*(2), 107–115.

Sciberras, E., Mulraney, M., Heussler, H., Rinehart, N., Schuster, T., Gold, L., . . ., & Hiscock, H. (2017). Does a brief, behavioural intervention, delivered by paediatricians or psychologists improve sleep problems for children with ADHD? Protocol for a cluster-randomised, translational trial. *BMJ Open*, *7*(4), e014158.

Skokauskas, N., Lavelle, T. A., Munir, K., Sampaio, F., Nystrand, C., McCrone, P., . . ., & Belfer, M. (2018). The cost of child and adolescent mental health services. *Lancet Psychiatry*, *5*(4), 299–300.

Stallard, P. (2017). Low-intensity interventions for anxiety disorders. *Lancet Psychiatry*, *4*(7), 508–509.

Wright, B. D., Cooper, C., Scott, A. J., Tindall, L., Ali, S., Bee, P., . . ., & Wilson, J. (2018). Clinical and cost-effectiveness of one-session treatment (OST) versus multisession cognitive-behavioural therapy (CBT) for specific phobias in children: Protocol for a non-inferiority randomised controlled trial. *BMJ Open*, *8*(8), e025031.

Yeguez, C. E., Page, T. F., Rey, Y., Silverman, W. K., & Pettit, J. W. (2020). A cost analysis of a stepped care treatment approach for anxiety disorders in youth. *Journal of Clinical Child and Adolescent Psychology*, *49*(4), 549–555.

6

Negative effects of low intensity interventions in children and young people

Alexander Rozental

Learning objectives

- To understand the concept of negative effects.
- To comprehend the nature and occurrence of negative effects among children.
- To understand how negative effects can be monitored and averted.
- To recognize why negative effects should be discussed during the informed consent process.

Introduction

Previous chapters have demonstrated that low intensity (LI) interventions are (1) seen by patients to be important (see Chapter 2), (2) effective (see Chapter 3), and (3) may be cost-effective (see Chapter 5). However, just as in medicine, effective psychological treatments may also have side effects. While the evidence for such side effects, or 'negative effects' is limited for LI therapies in children and young people, they are nonetheless important to consider. This chapter looks at the evidence for negative effects in psychological therapies across adults and children in general, before summarizing the evidence in LI treatments and in children and adolescents specifically. The first empirical evidence of negative effects in psychological treatments is thought to have been provided by Bergin (1966) who noticed that a significant number of patients deteriorated when compared to those in the control conditions. This sparked an interest in the so-called deterioration effect (Bergin, 1966, p. 236), referring to one of the two main categories of negative effects, worsening of symptoms (Table 6.1). Since then, several more rigorous studies have confirmed these findings, suggesting that 5–10% of all patients seeking help for common mental disorders deteriorate in treatment (Lambert, 2013). However, these numbers have been shown to be much higher in children, up to 14.3–24.1% in a study by Warren, Nelson, Mondragon, Baldwin, and Burlingame (2010).

Usually, deterioration is conceptualized as a negative outcome that goes beyond measurement error, as determined by the Reliable Change Index (Jacobson & Truax,

Table 6.1 Negative effects of psychological treatments

Category	Definition	Measurement
Deterioration	Symptom change in a negative direction exceeding the measurement error	Self-report measure, e.g. PHQ-9
Non-response	No change in symptom in any direction and within the limits of the measurement error	Self-report measure, e.g. PHQ-9
Unwanted and adverse events	Any type of negative experience occurring during treatment, in addition to symptom change[a]	Self-report measure, checklist, interview, open-ended questions[b] e.g. NEQ

[a] No consensus exists with regard to their definition.

[b] Can involve the perspective of the patient, clinician, or a significant other.

NEQ, Negative Effects Questionnaire; PHQ-9, Patient Health Questionnaire—9 Items.

1991). This means that the deterioration has to be larger than what can be attributed to the unreliability inherent in the self-report measure. The same procedure can be applied with regard to non-response, which might also be considered a negative outcome (Dimidjian & Hollon, 2010). Loerinc et al. (2015) found that around half of adult patients with anxiety disorders are regarded as non-responders, and Warren et al. (2010) revealed an estimate of 31.4–31.6% in children. However, these numbers tend to vary considerably depending on how non-response is defined. Although causality is still being debated, that is, whether it is treatment or other circumstances that is responsible, it is nonetheless safe to conclude that a proportion of all patients end treatment in a worse-off or unchanged condition than before.

The second category of negative effects concerns what might be referred to as unwanted and adverse events (Linden, 2013), such as novel symptoms and feelings of hopelessness. These are more complex to study than deterioration, with no consensus on how to define, assess, or report them (Rozental et al., 2018). A systematic review by Herzog, Lauff, Rief, and Brakemeier (2019) has demonstrated that self-report measures investigating these incidents span across such factors as symptoms, stigma, problems with the quality of therapy, problems with the therapeutic relationship, and hopelessness, among others. Furthermore, different perspectives can be used for examining such instances, which mean that the patient, clinician, and significant others might regard different aspects as negative in treatment (Table 6.1). Because of these issues, the number of patients experiencing unwanted and adverse events diverge in the literature.

Negative effects in LI interventions

The rising popularity of LI interventions has resulted in increased attention with regard to their possible negative effects (Rozental et al., 2014). Of almost three thousand patients in 29 clinical trials receiving internet-based cognitive behaviour therapy (CBT), 5.8% of the patients deteriorated, as compared to 17.4% in waiting-list controls (Rozental, Magnusson, Boettcher, Andersson, & Carlbring, 2017), while 26.8% were classified as non-responders (Rozental, Andersson, & Carlbring, 2019). Similar estimates were also found in a meta-analysis of individual participants in randomized controlled trials that reported results of self-guided internet CBT compared with control conditions in adults with symptoms of depression (Karyotaki et al., 2018). Moreover, 9.3% reported unwanted and adverse events during treatment using open-ended questions (Rozental, Boettcher, Andersson, Schmidt, & Carlbring, 2015), and 50.9% using a self-report measure (Rozental, Kottorp, et al., 2019).

For children, the number of studies reporting negative effects from LI interventions is much smaller than the number of studies with adults (Vigerland et al., 2016), and no systematic review specifically investigating this issue currently exists. Hence, it is unclear whether negative effects might differ from those in adults. Table 6.2 provides a few recent examples of studies where deterioration and unwanted and adverse events have been explored in children and young people who received LI psychological interventions, suggesting that approximately 5% experience them in treatment. These estimates should be interpreted with some caution as they are not derived from routine care, which may affect such factors as which patients are included. Likewise, the studies exclusively deal with internet-based CBT, while other formats such as bibliotherapy were not included. To what extent these numbers differ from high intensity interventions in children is, however, unclear. Lorenz (2020) used an online survey to investigate the rate of unwanted and adverse events

Table 6.2 Examples of studies reporting negative effects in LI interventions for children

Study	Treatment	Negative effect and assessment	Rate
Topooco et al. (2018)	ICBT for adolescent depression	• Deterioration (>30% increase in symptoms) • Unwanted and adverse events (open-ended question), including increased stress due to workload of treatment and feeling worse while processing the content of treatment	3.0%[a] 7.1%
Topooco et al. (2019)	ICBT for adolescent depression	• Deterioration (>30% increase in symptoms)	1.4%[b]
March, Spence, Donovan, and Kenardy (2018)	ICBT for youth anxiety	• Deterioration (Reliable Change Index)	4.5%
Staples et al. (2019)	ICBT	• Deterioration (Reliable Change Index)	1.4–3.6%[c]

ICBT, internet-based cognitive behaviour therapy.

[a] 12% if considering those with missing data to have deteriorated.

[b] 11% if considering those with missing data to have deteriorated.

[c] Research trial and routine care, respectively.

among adolescents having undergone different forms of psychotherapy, suggesting that 41% of the 366 responders had experienced at least one event as negative, with feeling ashamed of receiving treatment being the most common (14%), followed by perceiving treatment as emotionally painful or difficult (11%).

Preventing negative effects

Routine outcome monitoring has been put forward as a promising method for detecting and reducing the number of patients who deteriorate or do not respond (Boswell, Kraus, Miller, & Lambert, 2015). Basically, the idea is to regularly and systematically check symptom levels via self-report measures, such as prior to each session. Patients who are 'off track', that is, deviating from an expected trajectory, can then be identified and helped (see Chapter 8). This has been evaluated with positive results within the UK adult Improving Access to Psychological Therapies programme, lowering the number of deteriorated patients from 11% to 6% (Delgadillo et al., 2018). Similarly, the idea of continuously monitoring patients is also useful for clinicians as studies demonstrate that it is notoriously hard for them to detect deterioration (Hannan et al., 2005).

Whether a similar approach is useful for preventing unwanted and adverse events from occurring is less clear. However, one self-report measure has been developed in order to spot these negative effects, the Negative Effects Questionnaire (Rozental, Kottorp, et al., 2019), which might help clinicians identify those situations in treatment that may otherwise lead to drop-out or poor therapeutic alliance. The self-report measure can be downloaded (http://www.neqscale.com) and includes items such as 'I felt that the issue I was looking for help with got worse'. In addition, it also differentiates between incidents the patient attributes to treatment and other circumstances. It is currently only available as an adult version, but should be suitable also for adolescents. Separate child and parent versions are under development and used in clinical trials.

The informed consent process

Clinicians need to recognize that an efficacious psychological treatment can have both positive and negative outcomes. However, it is just as important for patients to acknowledge both the potential benefits and risks of undergoing treatment. This includes LI interventions, which have the advantage of being more flexible and less time-consuming, but might inadvertently give rise to such negative effects as being stressed out by or feeling worse during treatment. Only then can a patient make an informed decision of undergoing treatment or not. This should preferably be done during the informed consent process, and could, for instance, consist of a short declaration of how many get better by the proposed interventions as well as the rate, albeit small, of those who also experience negative effects. Presently, clinicians seem to be reluctant to raise the issue out of fear that it may impact treatment outcome or the therapeutic alliance (Bystedt, Rozental, Andersson, Boettcher, & Carlbring, 2014), yet no studies have been able to demonstrate that this would be the case.

Conclusion

Negative effects occur in psychological treatments and for LI interventions. However, current research does not demonstrate that they differ in any way. Overall, a small proportion of all patients deteriorate regardless of treatment, but it does appear to occur more often in children than adults. Meanwhile, non-response is quite common in both populations. To regularly and systematically assess symptoms thus seems to be a viable option to lower these rates and get patients back on track in their treatment. Meanwhile, unwanted and adverse events can also arise during treatment, but there is presently no consensus on how to define, assess, or report them. As such, these negative effects can only be captured by specifically probing for their occurrence, such as via a self-report measure. Last but not least, patients should be informed about both the benefits and risks of undergoing treatment.

Chapter summary

- Negative effects consist of deterioration and non-response, typically explored using self-report measures, and unwanted and adverse events, which can be examined via a variety of different means, such as open-ended questions.
- Deterioration occurs among 5–10% of all patients, but with considerably higher rates in children, 14.3–24.1%.
- Deterioration and non-response can be monitored and prevented through the use of routine outcome monitoring, identifying patients who are 'off track'.
- Unwanted and adverse events can be investigated using, for example, the Negative Effects Questionnaire (http://www.neqscale.com), which is free to use and available in 12 languages.
- As part of the informed consent process, patients should get information on both the positive and negative impacts a treatment might have.

Recommended reading

Lambert, M. J. (2010). *Prevention of treatment failure: The use of measuring, monitoring, and feedback in clinical practice*. Washington, DC: American Psychological Association.
Lambert, M. J., & Harmon, K. L. (2018). The merits of implementing routine outcome monitoring in clinical practice. *Clinical Psychology: Science and Practice, 25*(4), e12268.

Rozental, A., Castonguay, L., Dimidjian, S., Lambert, M., Shafran, R., Andersson, G., & Carlbring, P. (2018). Negative effects in psychotherapy: Commentary and recommendations for future research and clinical practice. *BJPsych Open, 4*(4), 307–312.

References

Bergin, A. E. (1966). Some implications of psychotherapy research for therapeutic practice. *Journal of Abnormal Psychology, 71*(4), 235–246.

Boswell, J. F., Kraus, D. R., Miller, S. D., & Lambert, M. J. (2015). Implementing routine outcome monitoring in clinical practice: benefits, challenges, and solutions. *Psychotherapy Research, 25*(1), 6–19.

Bystedt, S., Rozental, A., Andersson, G., Boettcher, J., & Carlbring, P. (2014). Clinicians' perspectives on negative effects of psychological treatments. *Cognitive Behaviour Therapy, 43*(4), 319–331.

Delgadillo, J., de Jong, K., Lucock, M., Lutz, W., Rubel, J., Gilbody, S., . . ., & McMillan, D. (2018). Feedback-informed treatment versus usual psychological treatment for depression and anxiety: A multisite, open-label, cluster randomised controlled trial. *Lancet Psychiatry, 5*(7), 564–572.

Dimidjian, S., & Hollon, S. D. (2010). How would we know if psychotherapy were harmful? *American Psychologist, 65*(1), 21–33.

Hannan, C., Lambert, M. J., Harmon, C., Nielsen, S. L., Smart, D. W., Shimokawa, K., & Sutton, S. W. (2005). A lab test and algorithms for identifying clients at risk for treatment failure. *Journal of Clinical Psychology, 61*(2), 155–163.

Herzog, P., Lauff, S., Rief, W., & Brakemeier, E. L. (2019). Assessing the unwanted: A systematic review of instruments used to assess negative effects of psychotherapy. *Brain and Behavior, 9*(12), e01447.

Jacobson, N. S., & Truax, P. (1991). Clinical significance: A statistical approach to defining meaningful change in psychotherapy research. *Journal of Consulting and Clinical Psychology, 59*(1), 12–19.

Karyotaki, E., Kemmeren, L., Riper, H., Twisk, J., Hoogendoorn, A., Kleiboer, A., . . ., & Cuijpers, P. (2018). Is self-guided internet-based cognitive behavioural therapy (iCBT) harmful? An individual participant data meta-analysis. *Psychological Medicine, 48*(15), 2456–2466.

Lambert, M. J. (2013). Outcome in psychotherapy: The past and important advances. *Psychotherapy, 50*(1), 42–51.

Linden, M. (2013). How to define, find and classify side effects in psychotherapy: From unwanted events to adverse treatment reactions. *Clinical Psychology and Psychotherapy, 20*(4), 286–296.

Loerinc, A. G., Meuret, A. E., Twohig, M. P., Rosenfield, D., Bluett, E. J., & Craske, M. G. (2015). Response rates for CBT for anxiety disorders: Need for standardized criteria. *Clinical Psychology Review, 42*, 72–82.

Lorenz, T. K. (2020). Predictors and impact of psychotherapy side effects in young adults. *Counselling and Psychotherapy Research, 21*(1), 237–243.

March, S., Spence, S. H., Donovan, C. L., & Kenardy, J. A. (2018). Large-scale dissemination of internet-based cognitive behavioral therapy for youth anxiety: Feasibility and acceptability study. *Journal of Medical Internet Research, 20*(7), e234.

Rozental, A., Andersson, G., Boettcher, J., Ebert, D. D., Cuijpers, P., Knaevelsrud, C., . . ., Carlbring, P. (2014). Consensus statement on defining and measuring negative effects of internet interventions. *Internet Interventions, 1*(1), 12–19.

Rozental, A., Andersson, G., & Carlbring, P. (2019). In the absence of effects: An individual patient data meta-analysis of non-response and its predictors in internet-based cognitive behavior therapy. *Frontiers in Psychology, 10*, 589.

Rozental, A., Boettcher, J., Andersson, G., Schmidt, B., & Carlbring, P. (2015). Negative effects of internet interventions: A qualitative content analysis of patients' experiences with treatments delivered online. *Cognitive Behaviour Therapy, 44*(3), 223–236.

Rozental, A., Castonguay, L., Dimidjian, S., Lambert, M., Shafran, R., Andersson, G., & Carlbring, P. (2018). Negative effects in psychotherapy: Commentary and recommendations for future research and clinical practice. *BJPsych Open, 4*(4), 307–312.

Rozental, A., Kottorp, A., Forsstrom, D., Mansson, K., Boettcher, J., Andersson, G., . . ., & Carlbring, P. (2019). The Negative Effects Questionnaire: psychometric properties of an instrument for assessing negative effects in psychological treatments. *Behavioural and Cognitive Psychotherapy, 47*(5), 559–572.

Rozental, A., Magnusson, K., Boettcher, J., Andersson, G., & Carlbring, P. (2017). For better or worse: An individual patient data meta-analysis of deterioration among participants receiving internet-based cognitive behavior therapy. *Journal of Consulting and Clinical Psychology, 85*(2), 160–177.

Staples, L. G., Dear, B. F., Johnson, B., Fogliati, V., Gandy, M., Fogliati, R., . . ., & Titov, N. (2019). Internet-delivered treatment for young adults with anxiety and depression: Evaluation in routine clinical care and comparison with research trial outcomes. *Journal of Affective Disorders, 256,* 103–109.

Topooco, N., Berg, M., Johansson, S., Liljethorn, L., Radvogin, E., Vlaescu, G., . . ., Andersson, G. (2018). Chat- and internet-based cognitive-behavioural therapy in treatment of adolescent depression: Randomised controlled trial. *BJPsych Open, 4*(4), 199–207.

Topooco, N., Bylehn, S., Dahlstrom Nysater, E., Holmlund, J., Lindegaard, J., Johansson, S., . . ., & Andersson, G. (2019). Evaluating the efficacy of internet-delivered cognitive behavioral therapy blended with synchronous chat sessions to treat adolescent depression: Randomized controlled trial. *J Med Internet Res, 21*(11), e13393.

Vigerland, S., Lenhard, F., Bonnert, M., Lalouni, M., Hedman, E., Ahlen, J., . . ., & Ljotsson, B. (2016). Internet-delivered cognitive behavior therapy for children and adolescents: A systematic review and meta-analysis. *Clinical Psychology Review, 50,* 1–10.

Warren, J. S., Nelson, P. L., Mondragon, S. A., Baldwin, S. A., & Burlingame, G. M. (2010). Youth psychotherapy change trajectories and outcomes in usual care: Community mental health versus managed care settings. *Journal of Consulting and Clinical Psychology, 78*(2), 144–155.

SECTION 2
APPLICATIONS

SECTION 2A

HOW TO USE BRIEF AND LOW INTENSITY INTERVENTIONS WITH CHILDREN AND YOUNG PEOPLE

7

Low intensity assessment

Hannah Vickery (née Whitney)

Learning objectives

By the end of this chapter, you should be able to:
- Structure a low intensity assessment session.
- Complete the core components of a low intensity assessment with a child, young person, and family.
- Gather information in an engaging, age-appropriate, and client-centred way.
- Undertake an accurate risk assessment.
- Summarize client difficulties and collaboratively devise problem statements.
- Collaboratively set goals with children, young people, and parents.
- Consider common challenges and possible solutions experienced within low intensity assessments.

Introduction

The variety of organizations which deliver low intensity (LI) interventions for children and young people (CYP) means that assessment processes are sometimes variable. Some CYP may experience a brief 'screening/triage assessment' and others may undergo a more comprehensive child and adolescent mental health service (CAMHS) assessment, before presenting to a LI service. For the purposes of this chapter, the focus is on conducting a LI assessment which serves the primary functions detailed in Box 7.1.

Given that one of the primary functions of assessment is engagement, it is important that practitioners consider what information is already known within the system before the LI assessment. While remaining open and curious are important qualities in any assessment, having notes to check with the family (from reading previous assessment summaries) demonstrates practitioner interest and a recognition that, for some CYP, they may have told their story repeatedly. For example, a practitioner may map out a basic genogram with information detailed within a triage report or referral letter (Figure 7.1). The practitioner can then use this as part of their information gathering; can ask the client questions about who else is important

---

Box 7.1 Functions of a LI assessment

- Engaging the child/adolescent and/or their parent/carer.
- Sharing information about what the client and family can expect from the LICBT assessment process.
- Gathering information about the presenting problem.
- Using shared decision-making to establish the most appropriate intervention for the client and the presenting problem.

---

in their lives and/or who already in the genogram supports the CYP when they're having difficulties.

Such a method enables the gathering of relevant information, promotes collaborative engagement (i.e. encouraging the CYP to draw pets/relationships on to the genogram—this is possible both face-to-face and via remote delivery using a shared whiteboard application), and can also expedite the assessment by saving the duplication of information. The same approach can be taken to routine outcome measures (ROMs); similarly supporting engagement and avoiding repetition (see Chapter 8).

Core components

Within adult LI interventions, assessment sessions typically take approximately 40 minutes; however, with LI interventions in CYP populations, the assessment is more likely to last 1 hour due to the additional considerations of having time with the young person and parent/carer alone. This reflects that evidence-based assessments in working with CYPs should be multisource (e.g. ROMs, behavioural observation, and clinical interview) and multi-informant (e.g. CYP, parent/carer, and school). While a full social and developmental history is outside the scope of a LI assessment, practitioners are expected to have a fundamental set of skills for working with CYP (see examples in Box 7.2 as well as the core and generic competences detailed by Roth, Calder, and Pilling (2008)).

Information gathering

The LI CYP assessment follows a similar structure to adult LI work with the six elements outlined by Richards and Whyte (2011) detailed in Table 7.1. These are child centred, and information should be provided in a developmentally appropriate way (Fuggle, Dunsmuir, & Curry, 2013).

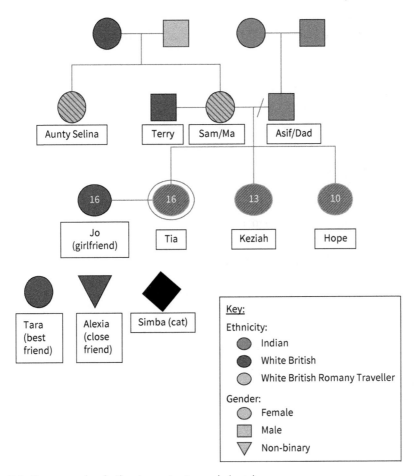

Figure 7.1 Genogram (and other important people/pets).

The initial aspects of the session focus on establishing an early rapport and setting expectations (e.g. length of the session, explaining the limits of confidentiality). Through the use of structured, funnel questioning, moving from general open questions and statements (e.g. 'Tell me what's been difficult for you recently that's led to us meeting today') to requests for more specific information (e.g. 'In what ways does it affect your sleep?'), more facts regarding the problem are gathered. The four 'Ws' detailed in Box 7.3 can be a useful means of eliciting details about the problem.

Through questions regarding the onset and progress of the difficulties, exploration of triggers (e.g. antecedents to moments of high anxiety), and use of the four Ws (Box 7.3), the questions become more focused on the specifics of the difficulties. At the bottom of the funnel, as the nature of the presenting difficulty becomes clearer, the practitioner can check they have covered areas from the FINDIE acronym (Table 7.2).

Box 7.2 Example skills required for all LICBT practitioners working with CYP

- Understanding of childhood development.
- Knowledge of, and ability to recognize symptoms indicative of, neurodevelopmental conditions including attention deficit hyperactivity disorder and autism spectrum disorder.
- Knowledge of legal and ethical frameworks relating to working with CYP.
- Experience of safeguarding training.
- Ability to work with difference (ensuring meaningful consideration of protected characteristics in both assessment and treatment).

Table 7.1 Typical LICBT assessment structure

Introduction	• Introductions: establishing full and preferred names • Brief clear explanation of the practitioner's role • Overview and agree assessment agenda and time available • Confidentiality and informed consent (to treat, to share information, and to record sessions where applicable)

Information gathering: general presentation	• Information gathering:
	  • Family and school/college system (checking content from referral letter/triage details)
	  • Triggers
	  • Onset and progress
	  • Impact
	  • Modifying and maintaining factors
	  • Previous/other current treatment (including medication)
	• Administration of routine outcome measures

Information gathering: risk assessment	• Ideation • Intent • Plans • Actions • Protective factors • Self-harm • Risk to others • Risk from others • Neglect to self and by others
Information gathering: problem formulation	• Emotional symptoms • Behavioural symptoms • Cognitive symptoms • Physical symptoms
Information giving and shared decision-making	• Session summary • Problem statement • Goal setting • Treatment options
Ending the session	• Session summary • Agree next steps and arrange when contact will be made about next appointment (following supervision)

Adapted from Richards and Whyte (2011).

Box 7.3 The four 'W' questions

- What is the problem?
- Where does the problem occur?
- With whom is the problem worse or better?
- When does the problem happen?

Making sense of the problem

After establishing the contextual information mentioned above, attention in the session can then move to explore a recent example of the problem. This should involve eliciting details of the trigger (scenario at the time of the worsened difficulty, e.g. panic attack, episode of worsened mood, or heightened moment of worry) and the Autonomic (physical), Behavioural, Cognitive, and Emotional symptoms experienced. Together, these form the basic cognitive model as detailed by Padesky and Mooney (1990). This exercise begins psychoeducation for the client around the CBT model and can also facilitate the client's better understanding of their difficulties and how their symptoms interact. See Figure 7.2 for a clinical example.

Table 7.2 Clinical example of FINDIE areas and answers

Aspect	Example questions	Clinical example for school-related worries
Frequency	How often do you have those worries?	Every weekday, getting ready for school
Intensity	How strongly do you feel the anxiety that comes with them? 0 is not at all and 10 is unbearable.	Between 5/10 and 10/10 depending on what lessons I have
Number	How many anxious thoughts do you have like that?	Three main worry themes (schoolwork, exams/revision, friendships)—number of worry chains too many to count
Duration	How long do the worries last?	Usually from when I wake until I get into my seat in first lesson—2.5 hours, feels continuous
Impact	How have these worries been affecting your life?	I feel sick and sometimes miss school because of stomach pains, find it hard to get on with family in the mornings, things are becoming 'tense' at home during the week
Exceptions	When do you not have these worries?	Weekend (until Sunday night), holidays, very occasional school days when I feel 'organized'

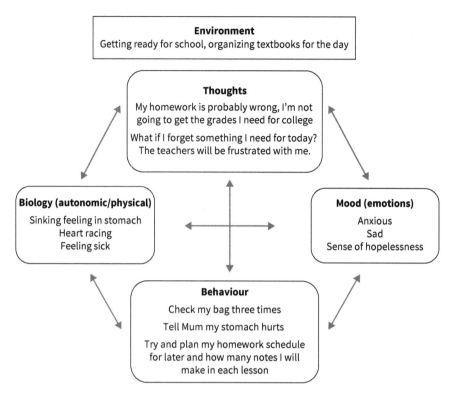

Figure 7.2 Clinical example of the basic cognitive model.

Table 7.3 Clinical example of an ABC chart

Antecedents/Triggers (what happened before)	Behaviour (what happened—as much descriptive detail as possible)	Consequences (what happened after)
I (Mum) asked Luke to get ready for bed at 8pm. Lucy (who is 16) was staying up to watch catch-up TV. Luke wanted to stay up too.	Luke refused to go upstairs, I told him he had to, he shouted at me, he said I love Lucy more than him, he became really distressed and lay in the hallway crying. He wouldn't get up and go and brush his teeth/get changed etc.	I picked him up, carried him upstairs, helped him get ready for bed, cuddled him, read him 2 stories and told him I love him and Lucy equally—I stayed with him until he was asleep at 9.20pm.

In working with behavioural difficulties, or common childhood problems such as disrupted bedtime routines, an alternative mapping of the difficulties is suggested using the principles of functional analysis. In this approach, the assessment looks at triggers (detailed as Antecedents), Behaviour (as in the five areas model), and Consequences; such recording is known as ABC charts; see Table 7.3 for a clinical example.

Risk assessment

Although a LI approach is not indicated for CYP presenting with active risk (e.g. active suicidal ideation, ongoing self-harm behaviour which requires medical attention, domestic violence in the home, and CYP carrying a weapon into school), clients with these experiences may be encountered within assessment sessions, particularly if the service supports self-referral. In addition, as risk is not static, client presentations may have changed since initial referral. Literature suggests that CYP practitioners may avoid asking risk questions unless risk information is raised by the client (O'Reilly, Kiyimba, & Karim, 2016). Risk assessments should be covered at every assessment session and cover the areas detailed in Box 7.4. Risk should be reviewed in brief at subsequent treatment sessions by presenting a summary of the previous risk information and asking if anything has changed. If the client reports any change, each of the areas should again be covered in full.

Risk assessment includes safeguarding: ensuring a child or young person is safe from harm and maltreatment and taking actions to enable all children have the best outcomes (Department for Education, 2018). Inexperienced practitioners may have concerns about conducting risk assessments and the actions that should be taken if

---

Box 7.4 Areas typically examined during a CYP risk assessment

Area of risk

Ideation: suicidal thoughts (important to ask for an example thought—helps establish whether there is active or passive ideation; 'I want to die' vs 'What's the point?')

Intent: active motivation to act (often scaled 0–10 with 0 as zero intention to act on thoughts and 10 certainty that they will)

Plans: specific action plans

Actions: current and past

Protective factors (e.g. social network, engagement with services, family relationships experienced as supportive)

Self-harm

Risk to others (e.g. involvement in fights, carrying of a weapon, aggression towards siblings/parents/carers)

Risk from others (e.g. bullying, cyber-bullying, grooming, physical, emotional or sexual abuse)

Neglect to self (e.g. motivation towards self-hygiene, healthy diet, drug/alcohol use)

Neglect by others (e.g. access to food, clean clothes, warm home, sanitary/hygiene supplies)

a disclosure is made. Practitioners should be reassured that independent risk management is not an expectation of LI practitioners working with CYPs; instead, timely and clear communication of risk information with supervisors and safeguarding leads should be completed in line with service/school risk management protocols. The situation should also be prioritized during the practitioner's next case management supervision (see Chapter 19).

O'Reilly et al. (2016) identify two commonly utilized routes to introducing risk assessments; firstly, to move to detailed questions about risk, when raised by the CYP or family—this requires practitioner flexibility and ensures the session is responsive to what the CYP raises. Making reference to the client's answers to risk-related questions on routine outcome measures (e.g. item 37 on the RCADS; 'I think about death') can introduce the topic of risk to self in this way. Secondly, in other sessions, where the client does not raise any risk content, the practitioner can introduce the next item of the agenda by providing a normalizing rationale for the questions with an emphasis on the importance of keeping the CYP safe (see clinical example in Box 7.5).

Asking questions about suicide does not increase suicidal ideation, in fact the literature suggests it is more likely to decrease suicidality (DeCou & Schumann, 2018). Therefore, practitioners should not express anxiety or apology in introducing a risk assessment and instead are encouraged to introduce it as a routine and important element of understanding how things are for the CYP. Typically, this part of the assessment is completed with the CYP alone unless they request their parent/carer be present; it should be shared with the parent/carer that questions about safety will be covered. See Box 7.5 for an example of how a practitioner might introduce the risk assessment.

Box 7.5 Introducing risk assessment

'Thank you, Kobe, for sharing that with me, that sometimes when you feel really low, you wonder "What's the point?" and "Everyone would be better off if I were dead". It sounds really rough for you when your mood drops like that. I know that we have "risk assessment" down as a topic for later in the session, but I'm thinking it might make most sense to talk about that now. Would that be ok? We will cover three areas; risk to self, risk from others and risk to others.'

'Ok so next on our plan for the session, we have "safety check-in". I talk about this with all children and young people I meet and though some of the questions can seem a bit strange to some people, it is important we cover them all to make sure you're as safe as possible. Does that sound ok? We will ask Mum to leave for this bit unless you would really like her to stay; you tell me.'

The practitioner should ensure their language is developmentally appropriate and this should be rehearsed in teaching/clinical skills supervision. LI practitioners should avoid ambiguous terms such as 'not wanting to be here anymore'; these can imply thoughts of running away as well as suicidal ideation. The agenda item 'risk assessment' can be framed as 'safety check-in' with younger children, for example. Ridge Anderson, Keyes, and Jobes (2016) and Pettit, Buitron, and Green (2018) provide further details regarding assessing risk to self in CYP.

Each area detailed in Table 7.2 should be asked relative to the present and the past. This is important given that previous self-injurious behaviour and previous attempts to end one's life should both inform clinical decision-making around present risk information (Hawton et al., 2012). In instances where a client discloses risk, funnel questioning should be used to elicit the current level of risk and to ensure clear details can be shared in line with service protocols; details regarding the self-injurious behaviour, for example, should be noted clearly as well as access to means of harm (Box 7.6).

Creating problem statements and setting goals

During the latter part of the session, the practitioner should summarize the session and support the CYP and/or parent to establish a problem statement detailing common triggers, symptoms, and the impact of the difficulties. The problem statement (see Box 7.7 for examples) is used to monitor progress, to

---

Box 7.6 Example notes from an assessment of risk to self

Lina reported no suicidal ideation or intent experienced currently or historically. She reported her family, her friends, and her faith (Roman Catholic) as significant protective factors. Lina reported previous self-harm (no actions for past 2 months). She reported previously engaging in scratching with her nails across the inside of her wrists and outside of her forearms, approximately weekly for 2–3 minutes, after incidents of quarrels with friends. She reported one incident of cutting with scissors after such an incident, and that she had cut the outside of her right forearm using kitchen scissors. She reported the cuts had not required medical attention and that the scars are faded. Lina stated that her mother had been aware at the time (Lina informed her) and her mother had since placed sharp knives and scissors in a locked drawer in the kitchen. Lina reported no current thoughts of self-harm, 2/10 intent described, no recent plans or actions, and reports her mother as a protective factor. She also reported that 'it only worked as a release for a short time'.

Box 7.7 Example problem statements

- 'My main problem is feeling irritable all the time and tearful particularly when I have to spend time chatting with people; as a result, I'm finding it difficult to concentrate in school and I don't want to see friends and family.'
- 'I have a really strong fear of dogs, it's worst when I see them outside; I try to avoid walking outside for long and ask Mummy to drive me everywhere. I also can't go to my best friend's house as she has a dog.'
- 'My problem is managing Luke's aggressive behaviour, especially in the mornings before school when I need him to get ready; he screams and kicks and bites me if I ask him to do things. I have started getting ready at 6 am to leave the house by 8.30 am and I regularly shout at him which I hate.'

---

guide the appropriateness and type of LI work, and to inform case management supervision.

From the problem statement, SMART/SMARTER treatment goals (Box 7.8) can be established and the next steps should be outlined. These will typically include discussing possible treatment options, establishing CYP and/or parent/carer preference, and agreeing a time when the practitioner can call the family to confirm the plan following supervision.

Short-term goals (to which the client aims to achieve progress towards within 3–6 months) should be set collaboratively. They should be positively

---

Box 7.8 SMARTER goal setting

- Specific—how clear is the target for change? Would someone who does not know the client be able to see if the goal was being met?
- Measurable—how will the client know when the goal is met?
- Achievable—does the client have access to everything they need in order to make this goal physically and emotionally possible?
- Realistic—how important is it to the client? How much do they want this goal?
- Time-limited—how long will the client work towards this goal?
- Evaluate—how has the client done towards the goal; which of the following Rs is indicated?
- Review/reward—if the goal has not yet been met, consider reviewing the SMART criteria; was something too broad, something missed in terms of realism/measurability? Alternatively, if the goal has been met, be sure to encourage the client to reward themselves.

---

and behaviourally framed (e.g. the addition of a new behaviour/skill rather than the absence of a feeling). Questions such as 'What would be different about your life in terms of what you do or don't do if you were not feeling down/anxious at the moment?' can help clients to think about what change they want to work towards. Utilizing the acronym SMART/SMARTER (Box 7.8) can sometimes be helpful in creating goals that are more meaningful for clients; however, the main ingredients to successful goal-setting is collaboration and relevance for the client. For further guidance on goal-setting and measuring progress to goals, see Law and Jacob's (2015) guide on utilizing goals and goal based outcomes.

Common challenges in LI assessments

Limited time to form a robust therapeutic alliance

The brief nature of LI assessments presents challenges for practitioners in terms of how they form a sound therapeutic relationship at pace (Morrison & Browning, 2018). As Farrand and Williams (2010) highlight, this can lead to criticisms regarding the perceived value that LI places on the relationship between practitioner and client.

Differences in CYP and parent/carer views of the 'problem'

In symptoms of depression, parents have been found to consistently report lower levels than their child's report (Eg, Bilenberg, Costello, & Wesselhoeft, 2018; Orchard et al., 2017). Contrastingly, in anxiety disorders, parents may over-report symptoms, though this varies depending on the age of the child and may be at least partially explained by parent anxiety levels (Niditch & Varela, 2011). In families experiencing behavioural difficulties, CYP may not perceive there to be a problem (van de Meer, Dixon, & Rose, 2008). Parental recognition of their CYP's mental health difficulties is related to a range of factors including the perceived burden, parental attitudes towards help seeking, and perceptions of mental health stigma (Gronholm et al., 2015; Wahlin & Deane, 2012).

Given that children and adolescents often present to services as a result of parent/carer or school concerns, it is not uncommon for the child or young person to be ambivalent towards change. In contrast, as detailed above, when CYP present to services through self-referral, for example, parents/carers may not have shared knowledge/perception of the CYP's difficulties.

Complexity/comorbidity—when to step up

Another challenge experienced in LI assessments is one of unexpected (e.g. not indicated in the referral) complex and comorbid presentations. In trying to establish the onset, presenting difficulties, maintaining factors, and the CYP's goals, the practitioner may experience multiples of each. Alternatively, or additionally, clients may also present with systemic challenges (e.g. young carer for a sibling), risk factors (e.g. historic parental suicide), or neurodevelopmental disorders (e.g. attention deficit hyperactivity disorder or autism spectrum disorder). While comorbid presentations are the norm in CAMHS (Costello, Mustillo, Erkanli, Keeler, & Angold, 2003; Cummings, Caporino, & Kendall, 2014), establishing when a client remains appropriate for LI work and when they should be stepped up can be difficult.

Potential solutions

Insufficient time to form a therapeutic alliance

Practitioner qualities including warmth, empathy, and collaboration all contribute to the formation of a strong therapeutic alliance. Given the time limits of LI assessment, practitioners should focus on how to demonstrate these qualities at every opportunity, including before the session. For example, sending an introductory letter including a biography of the practitioner and a smiling photo, or a brief video file sent by email introducing yourself and how to work the technology if sessions are to be via a remote platform. If the session is face-to-face, the practitioner should ensure they are actively warm and empathic from the initial contact in a waiting room and engage in age-appropriate non-problem discussion as they walk to the clinic space. Cavanagh (2010) also highlights that establishing and managing expectations can be helpful early in sessions to reduce anxiety and to provide clarity. This can be done as part of setting the agenda at the start of the session. Finally, the predominant way to ensure the client engages in the assessment process is to ensure the session is as client centred as possible while remaining committed to the assessment process (Mead & Bower, 2000).

Differences in CYP and parent/carer views of the 'problem'

The use of ROMs to capture different perspectives and to support dialogue between CYP and their parents/carer is wholly appropriate in LI assessments; for example, facilitating a comparison of the scored Revised Child Anxiety and Depression Scale (RCADS; Chorpita, Yim, Moffitt, Umemoto, & Francis, 2000). This should be completed with a normalizing narrative explaining that differences in parent and CYP reports are very typical. In these instances, instead of trying to find a shared problem statement, it may be more beneficial to concentrate on creating a shared goal. When creating a shared goal between child and parent, Jacob, Edbrooke-Childs, Holley, Law, and Wolpert (2015) highlight the importance of ensuring the CYP's voice is appropriately captured. If this is not readily possible, the goal of the person with whom the work will concentrate might be prioritized (e.g. young person if working with the CYP and parent if completing parent-delivered work).

Complexity/comorbidity—when to step up

Following assessment, all clients should be discussed in case management supervision as a priority. The supervisor is responsible for advising when a case should be stepped up for high intensity work. In supervision, the client information including risk assessment, ROMs, and a summary of the clinical interview should be presented. The supervisor should draw on the evidence base and their clinical experience to determine whether the comorbid picture or additional complexities pose likely challenges/interference for LI intervention; these decisions should be made on a case-by-case basis and LI practitioners should remember comorbidity is not, in itself, an exclusion criterion.

Chapter summary

This chapter has provided an overview of a typical structure for a LI assessment session with CYP, detailing its significance as an opportunity for information sharing, information gathering, and, importantly, engaging the CYP in a collaborative working relationship. LI assessments should be evidence based, as well as any subsequent treatment interventions, meaning that as well as being multisource and multi-informant, consideration of the literature detailed in Chapters 8–20 should be borne in mind while conducting assessments.

Recommended reading

Farrand, P., & Williams, C. (2010). Low intensity CBT assessment: In person or by phone. In J. Bennett-Levy, D. A. Richards, P. Farrand, H. Christensen, K. Griffiths, B. Kavanagh, . . ., & C. Williams (Eds.), *Oxford guide to low intensity CBT interventions* (pp. 89–96). Oxford: Oxford University Press.

Fuggle, P., Dunsmuir, S., & Curry, V. (2013). *CBT with children, young people & families*. London: Sage.

Law, D., & Jacob, J. (2015). *Goals and goal-based outcomes (GBOs): Some useful information*. Retrieved from https://www.corc.uk.net/media/1219/goalsandgbos-thirdedition.pdf

Myles, P., & Rushforth, D. (2007). *The complete guide to primary care mental health*. London: Constable and Robinson.

Myles-Hooton, P. (2020). Low intensity CBT assessment. In P. Farrand (Ed.), *Low intensity CBT skills and interventions* (pp. 23–44). London: Sage Publications.

Richards, D., & Whyte, M. (2011). *Reach Out: National programme student materials to support the delivery of training for practitioners delivering low intensity interventions*. London: Rethink.

References

Cavanagh, K. (2010). Turn on, tune in and (don't) drop out: Engagement, adherence, attrition, and alliance with internet-based interventions. In J. Bennett-Levy, D. A. Richards, P. Farrand, H. Christensen, K. Griffiths, B. Kavanagh, . . ., & C. Williams (Eds.), *Oxford guide to low intensity CBT interventions* (pp. 3–18). Oxford: Oxford University Press.

Chorpita, B. F., Yim, L., Moffitt, C., Umemoto, L. A., & Francis, S. E. (2000). Assessment of symptoms of DSM-IV anxiety and depression in children: A revised child anxiety and depression scale. *Behaviour Research and Therapy*, 38(8), 835–855.

Department for Education. (July 2018). *Working together to safeguard children*. https://assets.publishing.service.gov.uk/government/uploads/system/uploads/attachment_data/file/942454/Working_together_to_safeguard_children_inter_agency_guidance.pdf

Fuggle, P., Dunsmuir, S., & Curry, V. (2013). *CBT with children, young people & families*. London: Sage.

Costello, E. J., Mustillo, S., Erkanli, A., Keeler, G., & Angold, A. (2003). Prevalence and development of psychiatric disorders in childhood and adolescence. *Archives of General Psychiatry*, 60(8), 837–844.

Cummings, C. M., Caporino, N. E., & Kendall, P. C. (2014). Comorbidity of anxiety and depression in children and adolescents: 20 years after. *Psychological Bulletin*, 140(3), 816.

DeCou, C. R., & Schumann, M. E. (2018). On the iatrogenic risk of assessing suicidality: A meta-analysis. *Suicide and Life-Threatening Behavior*, 48(5), 531–543.

Eg, J., Bilenberg, N., Costello, E. J., & Wesselhoeft, R. (2018). Self-and parent-reported depressive symptoms rated by the mood and feelings questionnaire. *Psychiatry Research*, 268, 419–425.

Gronholm, P. C., Ford, T., Roberts, R. E., Thornicroft, G., Laurens, K. R., & Evans-Lacko, S. (2015). Mental health service use by young people: The role of caregiver characteristics. *PLoS One*, 10(3), e0120004.

Hawton, K., Bergen, H., Cooper, J., Turnbull, P., Waters, K., Ness, J., & Kapur, N. (2015). Suicide following self-harm: Findings from the multicentre study of self-harm in England, 2000–2012. *Journal of Affective Disorders*, 175, 147–151.

Jacob, J., Edbrooke-Childs, J., Holley, S., Law, D., & Wolpert, M. (2016). Horses for courses? A qualitative exploration of goals formulated in mental health settings by young people, parents, and clinicians. *Clinical Child Psychology and Psychiatry*, 21(2), 208–223.

Law, D., & Jacob, J. (2015). *Goals and goal-based outcomes (GBOs)*. London: CAMHS Press.

Mead, N., & Bower, P. (2000). Patient-centredness: A conceptual framework and review of the empirical literature. *Social Science and Medicine*, 51(7), 1087–1110.

Morrison, J., & Browning, A. (2018). Engagement and assessment within low intensity cognitive behavioural therapy for children and young people presenting with anxiety: Principles and practice. *Journal of Applied Psychology and Social Science*, 4(1), 22–38.

Niditch, L. A., & Varela, R. E. (2011). Mother-child disagreement in reports of child anxiety: Effects of child age and maternal anxiety. *Journal of Anxiety Disorders*, 25(3), 450–454.

Orchard, F., Pass, L., Marshall, T., & Reynolds, S. (2017). Clinical characteristics of adolescents referred for treatment of depressive disorders. *Child and Adolescent Mental Health*, 22(2), 61–68.

O'Reilly, M., Kiyimba, N., & Karim, K. (2016). 'This is a question we have to ask everyone': Asking young people about self-harm and suicide. *Journal of Psychiatric and Mental Health Nursing*, 23(8), 479–488.

Padesky, C. A., & Mooney, K. A. (1990). Clinical tip presenting the cognitive model to clients. *International Cognitive Therapy Newsletter*, 6, 11–12.

Pettit, J. W., Buitron, V., and Green, K. L. (2018). Assessment and management of suicide risk in children and adolescents. *Cognitive and Behavioral Practice*, 25(4), 460–472.

Richards, D., & Whyte, M. (2011). *Reach Out: National programme student materials to support the delivery of training for practitioners delivering low intensity interventions.* London: Rethink.

Ridge Anderson, A., Keyes, G. M., & Jobes, D. A. (2016). Understanding and treating suicidal risk in young children. *Practice Innovations, 1*(1), 3.

Roth, A., Calder, F., & Pilling, S. (2008). *A competence framework for child and adolescent mental health services.* Retrieved from http://www.ucl.ac.uk/CORE

van der Meer, M., Dixon, A., & Rose, D. (2008). Parent and child agreement on reports of problem behaviour obtained from a screening questionnaire, the SDQ. *European Child and Adolescent Psychiatry, 17*(8), 491–497.

Wahlin, T., and Deane, F. (2012). Discrepancies between parent-and adolescent-perceived problem severity and influences on help seeking from mental health services. *Australian and New Zealand Journal of Psychiatry, 46*(6), 553–560.

8

Tools to make low intensity interventions with children and youth more effective

The value of using feedback and outcome tools or routine outcome measures

Duncan Law

Learning objectives

By the end of this chapter, it is hoped that you will:
- Have a better understanding of the value and clinical usefulness of routine outcome measures or feedback and outcome tools.
- Have an overview of the different sorts of tools and how they might help make your practice more effective.
- Reflect on some of the cultural issues around using these tools.
- See the value of client defined, goal-focused tools.
- Understand some of the elements needed to implement the use of feedback and outcome tools in your practice.
- Be interested to use these tools in your own practice.

Feedback and outcome tools

First of all, thank you for pausing at this chapter! It may have been one that you thought you might skip—right? When we think about outcome measures, we tend to think about numbers . . . and who's really interested in numbers anyway? What we are really interested in is doing good work with children and youth, and helping people get better. Well, let me tell you, we're both on the same page (literally and metaphorically!). I'm not a great fan of numbers either, but I do like to do good, collaborative work with children, youth, and their families and that is what this chapter is all about: developing good relationships and doing good work to help people improve their mental well-being. This is important in any mental health intervention, but it is particularly important in low intensity (LI) interventions when time is often limited and you need be adaptive to gather information and generally work more efficiently.

In mental health, when we talk about 'routine outcome measures' we tend to be referring to questionnaires, forms, or checklists, either paper based or digital, that are completed by the young person or by someone who knows them well, such as a parent, caregiver, or teacher. Used meaningfully, these questionnaires can have real value (which we will discuss shortly), but I have an issue with calling them *routine outcome measures*, which is how they tend to be referred to by academics. Let me explain:

- The word '*routine*' suggests something we do without thinking, almost robotically, but these are sophisticated clinical tools—and sophisticated clinical tools should never be used unless it is with a great deal of thought (Law & Wolpert, 2014).
- Second, '*outcome*' suggests we are only interested in the end result: are people better or worse at the end of an intervention? But that is a rather passive stance to take in therapy, we should be interested in how people are doing along the therapy journey. If we get feedback along the way, we have an opportunity to make changes to what we do, to tweak how we work, and improve our chances of helping the young person reach a good outcome (Lambert, 2007).
- Finally, '*measures*' suggests some degree of accuracy in the tool—a bit like a ruler is accurate at measuring length which is a bit misleading when it comes to 'measuring' minds or mental health. When we speak of these tools as measures (which we will do, and this *is* an important part of their function), we need to remember that when we attempt to measure minds, they are not fixed and rigid objects like a stick of wood, but are dynamic and fluid and hard to pin down. So, the 'measurements' we get are likely to have a high degree of inaccuracy—this is fine, as long as we always keep this in mind when we are attempting to track changes in a person's mental health. (Deighton et al., 2014).

My preference is to refer to them as 'feedback tools':

- '*Tools*' are things that help us do good stuff: make chairs, write books, protect the environment, develop vaccines. Tools are not much use on their own, their use depends on the skill of the person using them; skill comes from knowledge (of what the tool's purpose is, and its limitations) and practice (opportunities to learn how to use them well).
- What these particular tools help us to do is to get useful information from our clients about what they might want to change in their lives, and, importantly, how well we are doing at helping them to make those changes: '*feedback*'. This feedback helps us have better conversations with the people we work with. Conversations build relationships and relationships are the foundations of good mental health interventions.

Types of tools

The kinds of feedback tools that are useful in LI interventions fall into three broad categories:

1. Tools that focus on the person's *symptoms and functioning*.
2. Tools that focus on what the client wants to change in their life or their *goals*.
3. Tools that broadly address *satisfaction* with the intervention.

Let's look at some examples of each . . .

Symptom-focused and functioning-focused tools

Now, we are lumping these two types of tools together in this section: tools that track changes in the range of problems a person may be experiencing—in other words, their 'symptoms'—and tools that look at changes in the impact these problems are having on the person's life—how well they are 'functioning'. The reason we tend to put these types of tools together is because we assume that symptoms and functioning are closely related: on the whole, if someone has a lot of symptoms, these are likely to have a bigger impact on their life and affect their functioning, compared with someone who has relatively few, or less severe, symptoms.

The difference between the tools is their focus: some tend to focus more on symptoms, like the Revised Child and Adolescent Anxiety and Depression Scales (RCADS) (Chorpita, Moffitt, & Gray, 2005), or the Beck Youth Inventory (Bose-Deakins & Floyd, 2004), which ask about a wide range of difficulties a child with mental health issues might experience. Others focus more on the *impact* the issues have on functioning or quality of life of the child or youth, like the Outcomes Rating Scale (ORS) (Miller, Duncan, Brown, Sparks, & Claud, 2003), and some focus on both symptoms *and* functioning such as the Strengths and Difficulties Questionnaire (SDQ) (Goodman, Lamping, & Ploubidis, 2010).

So, which are best to use? Should we focus on symptom tools or functioning tools? Well, it depends on what we are interested in, both have their value.

Symptom-focused tools tend to invite the person to look at a list of symptoms and rate which ones they are experiencing. This style of checklist tends to give us lots of information about the types of problems a person is experiencing, and much faster than we might get if we just ask questions as part of a clinical discussion. If used before a first session, this information can be used to build hypotheses about the nature of the difficulties someone might be experiencing and set a 'baseline' measure of a person's difficulties at the start of an intervention. If repeated at the end of an intervention, the ratings can be compared to see what progress (if any) has been made during the course of the work.

Rather than using the tools just at the start and end of the intervention, it is better to use the tools repeatedly (ideally every session). It would not be possible, or helpful, to use very lengthy symptom-focused tools, but some, like the Behavior and Feelings Survey (BFS) (Weisz et al., 2019) are briefer checklists designed to be used during each session. Similarly, the RCADS (Chorpita et al., 2005) has short subscales that can be used to track more specific problem areas such as low mood, panic, etc. In this way, we can monitor progress at each session and use the ratings to facilitate discussions with the person about progress: what is helping, what is not, and what aspect of the intervention (if anything) might be helpful to change.

There are a couple of big downsides to symptom-focused tools:

- First, as the lists of symptoms are predefined by professionals, they sometimes feel irrelevant to the youth we are asking to complete them, as they do not resonate with the person's experience of themselves (Jacob et al., 2018). This can be detrimental to the therapeutic alliance.
- The second, and more serious issue, is that symptom tools have, on the whole, been developed by white, Western academics and tested in largely white, Western communities, and come with a particularly white, Western view of mental health: that symptoms are located in an individual. We need to be particularly mindful that these tools may be less helpful and less relevant to people from Black, Asian, or other minority ethnic groups including those from African, Hispanic, or Asian descent or traditional and indigenous communities (Duncan, Miller, Wampold, & Hubble, 2010; Timimi, 2010).

Tools that focus more on functioning are less prone to these issues because they focus on the impact of the issues (however the issues might be understood). Such tools include the Child Outcome Rating Scale (CORS) (Casey, Patalay, Deighton, Miller, & Wolpert, 2020) which asks about the person's functioning across four domains—school, family, me, everything else—and uses the impact/session-by-session scale of the SDQ (Hall et al., 2015). These are arguably more culturally sensitive than symptom tools but also focus on how the issues are affecting a person's life, which tends to be a more relevant focus for the intervention than symptoms alone.

Goal-focused tools

We could argue that the most useful tools are those that are most relevant to the person seeking help—tools that measure progress on the issues that the person *themselves* most want to work on, in a LI intervention (Law, 2018). This is exactly what goal-focused tools aim to do (Jacob et al., 2018).

Goal-focused tools such as the Goals-Based Outcome (GBO) tool (Law, 2019) or the Top Problems Assessment (TPA) (Weisz et al., 2011) are idiographic, or client-defined, outcome measures that allow the person to define their own focus (goals) for the work. Once set, progress can be tracked on a simple zero to ten (GBO) or zero to four (TPA) scale.

But we mustn't be fooled by goal-focused tools' apparent simplicity. In order to define established goals that the client wants to work towards, we need to use all our therapeutic skills to facilitate a discussion with the client about the changes they want to make in their lives. The task is to facilitate shared decision-making about the focus of the LI work. When young people are actively involved in decisions about their care, the discussion helps the client be more aware of what they want to change. It can help youth feel more involved and motivated to engage (Martin & Feltham, 2020) and lay the foundations of a good therapeutic relationship. Once we have done all this, goal-focused tools offer straightforward and intuitive ways to track and measure progress. The brevity of the measure itself makes these tools very easy to integrate into every session so progress towards goals can be tracked and discussed.

Satisfaction-focused tools

'Satisfaction' is quite a complex mental state. How satisfied we are with a therapeutic encounter will depend on a range of different elements: do we think the therapy is working, is it helping us reach our goals? Do we think what is happening in therapy is important? Do we feel listened to? Do we understand what is being said? All these, and more, go into making up the feeling of being satisfied (or not) with the therapy. So really, satisfaction is an indicator of the quality of relationship between the client and the practitioner and, as stated at the start of this chapter, relationships are the foundations of good therapy. The quality of the therapeutic relationship, is one of the best predictors of change in therapy (Karver, Handelsman, Fields, & Bickman, 2006). So, it is vital we keep an eye on the therapeutic relationship, and satisfaction tools help us do this.

Satisfaction tools can help add to the information we might get from our usual therapeutic conversations with the people we are working with. It is often difficult to give honest, helpful feedback when we are asked directly; we tend to acquiesce. Think about the last time you went out for a meal: at some point in the meal a member of staff is likely to have come over and asked 'How is your meal?' and we generally respond 'Lovely, thank you!' even if the meal is not lovely; culturally, we are primed not to make a fuss. In therapy this issue is even more acute. As practitioners, we are in positions of power; it is even harder to speak truth to power, and harder still if you fear that if you are even a little bit critical, there may be bad and dangerous consequences. This kind of fear is not uncommon for children to feel and particularly those who may have experienced less than optimal parenting and trauma (Fonagy & Allison, 2014).

So, we need to work hard to get honest feedback from our clients. Scott Millar and Barry Duncan have given a great deal of thought to this issue (Hubble, Duncan, &

Miller, 1999). They suggest we need to encourage even small amounts of feedback and really amplify and praise a child who 'dares' to be even a little bit critical. If we can encourage children and youth to share what they do not like about therapy, and about us as therapists, we can change what we do to improve the relationship and be more helpful.

Tools help us open up more channels of communication and show a real intention to listen. One such tool, the Session Rating Scale (SRS) (Duncan et al., 2003), asks the child to rate their satisfaction across four domains: how much the child felt listened to, how important they felt what happened in the session was, how much they liked what the therapist did in the session, and how much they wished they could do something different in the session.

Remember, the main purpose here is to help get *honest* feedback from the people we work with. The best feedback gives us clues about what we aren't doing so well; this gives us information that can help us improve the experience for the client but also gives us valuable learning opportunities to improve ourselves as practitioners.

Used in conjunction with information from goal-focused and satisfaction tools, symptom or functioning tools can provide an excellent backdrop of information to open up more focused, therapeutic discussions with clients, facilitate more effective supervision, and help in our own reflective practice. This makes feedback and outcome tools extremely useful in LI work. Finally, whichever tools we are using, the numbers we get from these tools is not the endpoint. They must always be followed up with a discussion. The numbers we get should be seen as an invitation to a conversation.

Why do we need tools to get good feedback?

I am often asked in workshops on feedback and outcome tools: 'Why do we need questionnaire-based tools, why can't we just ask?' The answer to this question goes back to what we said about tools right at the start of this chapter: tools help us do stuff better. We can, and should, talk to the people we work with about their goals, their symptoms, their functioning, and their experience of interventions. Feedback tools do not replace normal, human, therapeutic conversations but the research evidence suggests that using these tools gives us qualitatively different information from young people, that we don't get from just talking. This additional information, used well and in conjunction with what we get from talking, gives us more to work with and more chance of building a better therapeutic alliance and being more effective practitioners (Bickman, Kelley, Breda, de Andrade, & Riemer, 2011).

In adult mental health settings, where there has been more research done in this area, there is really clear evidence that using feedback tools in addition to normal therapy conversations reduces drop out and can lead to quicker and better intervention outcomes for the people seeking help (Shimokawa, Lambert, & Smart, 2010).

There hasn't been the same amount of research in child and youth services for us to be quite so sure of the impact of feedback tools in LI interventions with children and youth (Bergman et al., 2018), but where there has been research, the effects seem similar to those seen in therapy with adults (Bickman et al., 2011; Cooper, Duncan, Golden, & Toth, 2021). In short: if you use feedback and outcomes tools well, you are likely to be more effective in your interventions.

Alongside improving the efficacy of our interventions, the by-products of using feedback and outcome tools in our practice, are data that allow us to build a better picture of which LI interventions work in real-world child and youth mental health settings. This practice-based evidence adds to the knowledge we have from more controlled research trials and can help to make our services more effective and efficient across the board.

Putting it into practice

It's all very well having great ideas about using feedback and outcome tools in your practice in LI interventions, but there are some things that need to be in place to help you do this:

1. *Training*—although most feedback and outcome tools are relatively straightforward to administer, it is important that good-quality training is in place to help practitioners better understand the intricacies of using these tools, what they can and can't do, and give opportunities to practise using them.
2. *Supervision*—alongside training we need to ensure there are good supervision structures in place where we can reflect on, and improve, how we use the tools, how we integrate them more effectively into practice, and how we better consider the meaning of the information we get back from clients.
3. *Digital support*—finally, we need good data support systems in place that help us score and track the information we get from the tools that make it easy to put data in and, as importantly, help us get data out that show progress (or lack of it) in a visually interesting way that is understandable and engaging to practitioners and youth alike.

It is only when we have all three systems in place that we are really helped to use tools well.

Feedback and reflective practice

Of course, as with all tools, feedback tools only work if we use them well; they are only effective if we use the information we get from them to change our practice in some way.

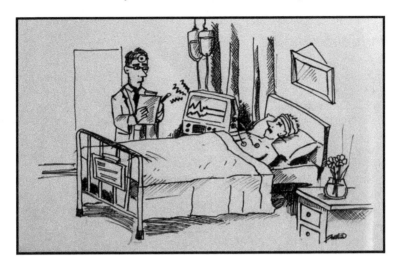

Figure 8.1 Cartoon.

Let's take a look at this cartoon in Figure 8.1, drawn for me by a very talented young person a few years ago, who uses a physical health analogy to make the point. The image shows a conscientious medic who has been using an array of tools to measure the vital signs of their patient. The patient, however, has sadly died—why? Because the doctor only monitored the change and didn't change their treatment based on the (bio)feedback from the patient (in this case, a lowering heart rate, increased blood pressure, and a distinct drop in kidney function). The message in the cartoon is this: there is no point seeking feedback unless we are willing to consider changing our practice based on what we get back. When we talk about the clinically meaningful use of feedback tools, we mean that the tools must be relevant to the client and be used by us as practitioners to change and improve our practice. To do this we need to be open to learning and be helped to improve through good supervision and be in settings where there is effective leadership that creates a psychologically safe culture in which we can reflect and grow.

Chapter summary

We are nearly at the end, and I hope this chapter has helped you reflect on the effective use of feedback and outcome tools in the work you are and will be doing, even better if it has inspired you to use them—and use them better. I hope you feel you have a better understanding of how the meaningful use of feedback and outcomes tools can help you be a better practitioner and help children and youth make important changes in their lives—that's what it's all about—good luck and keep learning!

Recommended reading

For more information and goals and goal-oriented practice go to https://goals-in-therapy.com/ and read Cooper, M., & Law, D. (Eds.). (2018). *Working with goals in psychotherapy and counselling.* Oxford: Oxford University Press.

For lots of useful information on routine outcome measures and feedback and outcome tools visit the Child Outcomes Research Consortium (CORC) website https://www.corc.uk.net/ including links to tools and training videos.

For stimulating ideas on feedback informed practice read Duncan, B. L., Miller, S. D., Wampold, B. E., & Hubble, M. A. (2010). *The heart and soul of change: Delivering what works in therapy.* Washington, DC: American Psychological Association.

For research and ideas on measuring intervention outcomes in youth and lots more besides, visit John Weizs's Lab for Youth Mental Health: https://weiszlab.fas.harvard.edu/measures

References

Bergman, H., Kornør, H., Nikolakopoulou, A., Hanssen-Bauer, K., Soares-Weiser, K., Tollefsen, T. K., & Bjørndal, A. (2018). Client feedback in psychological therapy for children and adolescents with mental health problems. *Cochrane Database of Systematic Reviews, 8,* CD011729.

Bickman, L., Kelley, S. D., Breda, C., de Andrade, A. R., & Riemer, M. (2011). Effects of routine feedback to clinicians on mental health outcomes of youths: Results of a randomized trial. *Psychiatric Services, 62*(12), 1423–1429.

Bose-Deakins, J. E., & Floyd, R. G. (2004). A review of the Beck Youth Inventories of emotional and social impairment. *Journal of School Psychology, 42*(4), 333–340.

Casey, P., Patalay, P., Deighton, J., Miller, S. D., & Wolpert, M. (2020). The Child Outcome Rating Scale: Validating a four-item measure of psychosocial functioning in community and clinic samples of children aged 10–15. *European Child & Adolescent Psychiatry, 29*(8), 1089–1102.

Chorpita, B. F., Moffitt, C. E., & Gray, J. (2005). Psychometric properties of the Revised Child Anxiety and Depression Scale in a clinical sample. *Behaviour Research and Therapy, 43*(3), 309–322.

Cooper, M., Duncan, B., Golden, S., & Toth, K. (2021). Systematic client feedback in therapy for children with psychological difficulties: Pilot cluster randomised controlled trial. *Counselling Psychology Quarterly, 34*(3–4), 21–36.

Deighton, J., Croudace, T., Fonagy, P., Brown, J., Patalay, P., & Wolpert, M. (2014). Measuring mental health and wellbeing outcomes for children and adolescents to inform practice and policy: A review of child self-report measures. *Child and Adolescent Psychiatry and Mental Health, 8*(1), 1–14.

Duncan, B. L., Miller, S. D., Sparks, J., Claud, D., Reynolds, L., Brown, J., & Johnson, L. (2003). The Session Rating Scale: Preliminary psychometric properties of a 'working' alliance measure. *Journal of Brief Therapy, 3*(1), 3–12.

Duncan, B. L., Miller, S. D., Wampold, B. E., & Hubble, M. A. (2010). *The heart and soul of change: Delivering what works in therapy.* Washington, DC: American Psychological Association.

Fonagy, P., & Allison, E. (2014). The role of mentalizing and epistemic trust in the therapeutic relationship. *Psychotherapy, 51*(3), 372–380.

Goodman, A., Lamping, D. L., & Ploubidis, G. B. (2010). When to use broader internalising and externalising subscales instead of the hypothesised five subscales on the Strengths and Difficulties Questionnaire (SDQ): Data from British parents, teachers and children. *Journal of Abnormal Child Psychology, 38*(8), 1179–1191.

Hall, C. L., Moldavsky, M., Taylor, J., Marriott, M., Goodman, R., Sayal, K., & Hollis, C. (2015). Innovations in practice: Piloting electronic session-by-session monitoring in child and adolescent mental health services: A preliminary study. *Child and Adolescent Mental Health, 20*(3), 171–174.

Hubble, M. A., Duncan, B. L., & Miller, S. D. (1999). *The heart & soul of change: What works in therapy.* Washington, DC: American Psychological Association.

Jacob, J., Edbrooke-Childs, J., Lloyd, C., Hayes, D., Whelan, I., Wolpert, M., & Law, D. (2018). Measuring outcomes using goals. In M. Cooper & D. Law (Eds.), *Working with goals in counselling and psychotherapy* (pp. 111–137). Oxford: Oxford University Press.

Karver, M. S., Handelsman, J. B., Fields, S., & Bickman, L. (2006). Meta-analysis of therapeutic relationship variables in youth and family therapy: The evidence for different relationship variables in the child and adolescent treatment outcome literature. *Clinical Psychology Review, 26*(1), 50–65.

Lambert, M. (2007). Presidential address: What we have learned from a decade of research aimed at improving psychotherapy outcome in routine care. *Psychotherapy Research, 17*(1), 1–14.

Law, D. (2018). Goal-oriented practice. In M. Cooper & D. Law (Eds.), *Working with goals in psychotherapy and counselling* (pp. 161–180). Oxford: Oxford University Press.

Law, D. (2019). *The goal-based outcome (GBO) tool: Guidance notes.* London: MindMonkey Associates.

Law, D., & Wolpert, M. (Eds.). (2014). *Guide to using outcomes and feedback tools with children, young people and families.* London: CAMHS Press.

Martin, K., & Feltham, A. (2020). Shared decision-making with young people in mental health services. In L.-M. Brady (Ed.), *Embedding young people's participation in health services: New approaches* (pp. 31–52). Bristol: Policy Press.

Miller, S. D., Duncan, B. L., Brown, J., Sparks, J. A., & Claud, D. A. (2003). The outcome rating scale: A preliminary study of the reliability, validity, and feasibility of a brief visual analog measure. *Journal of brief Therapy, 2*(2), 91–100.

Shimokawa, K., Lambert, M. J., & Smart, D. W. (2010). Enhancing treatment outcome of patients at risk of treatment failure: Meta-analytic and mega-analytic review of a psychotherapy quality assurance system. *Journal of Consulting and Clinical Psychology, 78*(3), 298–311.

Timimi, S. (2010). The McDonaldization of childhood: Children's mental health in neo-liberal market cultures. *Transcultural Psychiatry, 47*(5), 686–706.

Weisz J. R., Chorpita B. F., Frye A., Ng M. Y., Lau N., Bearman S. K., . . ., & Research Network on Youth Mental Health. (2011). Youth top problems: Using idiographic, consumer-guided assessment to identify intervention needs and track change during psychotherapy. *Journal of Consulting and Clinical Psychology, 79*, 369–380.

Weisz, J. R., Vaughn-Coaxum, R. A., Evans, S. C., Thomassin, K., Hersh, J., Ng, M. Y., . . ., & Mair, P. (2019). Efficient monitoring of treatment response during youth psychotherapy: The Behavior and Feelings Survey. *Journal of Clinical Child & Adolescent Psychology, 49*(6), 737–751.

9

Form and function when treating anxiety in youth

Maintaining flexibility within fidelity in low intensity interventions

Margaret E. Crane, Colleen A. Maxwell, Jonathan C. Rabner,
Zuzanna K. Wojcieszak, Lindsay B. Myerberg, and Philip C. Kendall

Learning objectives

- To differentiate function and form within evidence-based interventions.
- To understand a strategy for adapting programmes while maintaining fidelity.
- To guide troubleshooting challenges while maintaining fidelity.

Introduction

Evidence-based interventions (EBIs) have demonstrated beneficial outcomes among children and adolescents (American Psychological Association Task Force on Evidence-Based Practice for Children and Adolescents, 2008). That said, not all manual-based EBIs that demonstrate efficacy in research settings have yielded the same results in community-based settings (Kazak et al., 2010; Kumpfer, Alvarado, Smith, & Bellamy, 2002). An EBI that is found to be efficacious in research but less effective once disseminated into the community may reflect either (1) too rigid adherence to a manualized protocol that does not 'fit' the needs of the individuals receiving the intervention in the community (Sherrill, 2016) or (2) overly loose application (non-adherence) of the programme that compromises fidelity (Elliott & Mihalic, 2004). Perfect adherence to a protocol may be unattainable in any settings given the variety of factors that arise in providing mental health services (e.g. staff turnover, limited practitioner time). What has emerged is a valid tension between following an efficacious manual-based treatment and delivering an intervention that is adapted to the needs of an individual (Kendall & Frank, 2018). This tension often can arise for practitioners with limited therapy experience who are delivering manual-based low intensity interventions.

Intervention adaptations are necessary for widespread application, yet adaptations must be conducted thoughtfully to maintain implementation fidelity (Ijadi-Maghsoodi et al., 2017; McHugh, Murray, & Barlow, 2009). To achieve this balance, we encourage practitioners to operate from a 'flexibility within fidelity' framework (Kendall, Gosch, Furr, & Sood, 2008). Flexibility within fidelity requires that the active ingredients (Campbell et al., 2000) of an EBI are presented, while the 'adaptable periphery' (i.e. precise details or manner in which the intervention is delivered) is tailored to an individual client's needs (Damschroder et al., 2009). This framework allows for modification of the 'form' of a given treatment element (e.g. a structure, an activity), while maintaining the original 'function' of that element (i.e. the purpose, activity, or process by which an outcome is achieved; Hawe, Shiell, & Riley, 2004; Kirk et al., 2019; Wandersman et al., 2008). We note that there is not a one-to-one match between a form (i.e. activity) and function: some activities achieve multiple functions, and a given function may take several forms. Keeping this in mind, we believe, allows service practitioners to preserve the active ingredients of the EBI, while flexibly modifying the adaptable periphery.

Function and form

In this chapter, we use the *Brief Coping Cat* programme (Kendall & Hedtke, 2006) to demonstrate how clinicians can distinguish between the core functions and forms of a treatment manual. *Coping Cat* is a cognitive behavioural therapy programme for youth anxiety (for additional details on the programme, see Podell, Mychailyszyn, Edmunds, Puleo, & Kendall, 2010). There are many versions of Coping Cat, each of which have varying levels of intensity. All Coping Cat versions include the same core cognitive behavioural therapy principles, which can be applied flexibly based on the client's needs. In particular, the examples used during sessions, homework assignments, and exposure tasks are customized to each client. The main differences between the programmes are the number of sessions required and the level of practitioner involvement in teaching skills. Standard Coping Cat is 16 sessions, whereas Brief Coping Cat is eight sessions (Kendall, Crawley, Benjamin, & Mauro, 2013). The computer-assisted version of Coping Cat, *Camp-Cope-A-Lot* (CCAL; Kendall & Khanna, 2020), is 12 sessions long, and is available online. In CCAL, the first six sessions have the client work with a computer to learn relaxation training, cognitive restructuring (e.g. identifying and changing self-talk), and problem-solving skills. In the second six sessions of CCAL, a practitioner implements exposure tasks. Thus, both Brief Coping Cat and CCAL are low intensity interventions. When distinguishing the forms versus functions of Brief Coping Cat, we consider the purpose/goal of each activity or intervention component in each session of the Brief Coping Cat manual. Table 9.1 describes the core functions and forms for each session.

Table 9.1 Function and form of Coping Cat

Session	Function	Form
Overarching (completed in many/all sessions)	Introduce concepts in an order that makes conceptual sense	Divide concepts into eight sessions
	Build therapeutic alliance	Games, positivity, general conversation
	Reinforce/apply therapy concepts through at-home practice	Assign 'Show That I Can' (STIC; i.e. homework) task, STIC task review, completing STIC task in session; suggested STIC task varies by session
	Engage caregiver in treatment process (caregiver modelling, transfer of practitioner, support at home)	Brief meeting with caregiver; phone call with caregiver; email to caregiver; caregiver watching session activities
	Provide the youth and caregivers with information about therapy and interactive activities in an organized way	Client workbook, parent companion workbook
	Use youth's specific worries to decide situations to practise in exposure	Build a fear ladder (i.e. exposure hierarchy) in the manual or using sticky notes; use feelings thermometer or easy/medium/hard to build ladder
	Teach client a way to remember coping skills	FEAR plan: • F step: feeling frightened • E step: expecting bad things to happen • A step: attitudes and actions that can help • R step: results and rewards
Session 1: youth	Build therapeutic alliance	Games, personal facts game
	Set client expectations for programme: • Establish the idea that therapy is collaborative • Assign homework	Ask the client questions; discuss client's goals for therapy; explain that different skills work for different people; 'I'm an expert on anxiety, you're an expert on you'
	Describe connection between thoughts and feelings	Situations–feelings–thoughts worksheet
	Differentiate and label emotions; normalize anxiety	Discuss feelings, feelings charades, label feelings in cartoons; discuss anxiety-provoking situations
Session 1: caregiver meeting	Collaborate with caregivers about treatment expectations	Discuss programme structure; expectations of attendance and homework
	Teach caregivers about therapy concepts	Provide psychoeducation about therapy programme
	Review caregivers' view on behaviours/situations to target in treatment	Ask caregivers about anxiety-provoking situations, and how the client and caregiver respond to those situations

Table 9.1 Continued

Session	Function	Form
Session 2	Make connections between somatic sensations and emotions	How family members react; body drawing of where anxiety is felt; map somatic sensations onto fear ladder
	Understand the function of emotions	Describe fight-or-flight, fire alarm analogy
	Establish connection between thoughts and emotions	Discuss the concept of self-talk (e.g. thought bubbles); discuss self-talk in anxiety-provoking situations (anxious self-talk); differentiate anxious self-talk from coping self-talk
	Practise flexible thinking	Discuss thinking traps; evaluate evidence for the thought; discuss whether a thought is helpful; discuss coping thoughts
Session 3	Teach problem-solving to give the youth more control over their environment	Discuss problem-solving steps; discuss problem-solving for anxious or non-anxious situations
	Differentiate between effort and outcome	Activity (e.g. role play, cartoon strips) to evaluate results with various scenarios that highlight imperfect outcomes; feelings barometer activity
	Teach client to reward self	Review purpose of rewards; make a list of rewards
	Combine coping skills learned so far	Brainstorm how the FEAR plan would be used in anxious situations; coping cards; coping characters
Sessions 4–8	Facilitate an experiential activity in which a client approaches feared situation without engaging in avoidance	Conduct exposure based on client's specific fears (imaginal, *in vivo*, interoceptive); exposures increase in difficulty each session
	Process the exposure with the client	Reward client for completing exposure; review subjective units of distress (SUDS) curve with client; ask the client what aspects of the exposure were easy, what aspects were hard; compare exposure outcome to expectations; plan exposure task for next session
Session 4: youth	Provide framework for exposure work	Review aims/process of exposures (e.g. exposures are gradual, aim is not to remove all anxiety, importance of exposures practice)
	Reinforce therapeutic relationship (e.g. trust, confidentiality, independence) with client	Discuss upcoming caregiver session

(continued)

Table 9.1 Continued

Session	Function	Form
Session 4: caregiver meeting	Educate caregivers about exposure therapy and their role in this part of treatment	Provide information about exposures tasks; ask caregivers about their concerns; offer specific ways caregivers can be involved in exposures
	Plan for exposure work with caregivers	Learn more about the situations in which the client becomes anxious
Session 7	Collaboratively create plan for the remaining course of treatment	Initiate conversation about terminating/continuing therapy; express confidence in the skills gained by both client and caregiver throughout treatment
Session 8	Use an activity to demonstrate the skills learned in treatment	Film commercial; write out a cartoon of treatment progress; share with caregiver; end of therapy celebration (e.g. pizza party)
	Discuss plans and expectations for life and anxiety after treatment ends (i.e. relapse prevention plan)	Conduct session with caregiver and client individually or together; normalize relapse and manage expectations around symptom variation after treatment; brainstorm strategies for preventing relapse; consider how caregivers and client will know when future treatment is needed

Challenges to maintaining fidelity

Clinicians may face challenges to maintaining fidelity, even while being flexible. One challenge facing community clinicians can be a lack of time and resources to adhere to a manual. As reviewed in this chapter, an 'active ingredient' of anxiety treatment is the use of exposure tasks (Peris et al., 2015); however, exposures are rarely implemented by community clinicians (Whiteside, Deacon, Benito, & Stewart, 2016). Does the agency provide the needed time and resources? Indeed, the factors commonly associated with the limited use of exposures are a lack of time to prepare (Becker-Haimes et al., 2017; Farrell, Deacon, Dixon, & Lickel, 2013) and a lack of access to required resources (Ringle et al., 2015). When institutional factors create barriers to treatment fidelity, core functions can be lost.

EBIs are often designed to target a core cluster of disorders (e.g. Coping Cat for anxiety disorders), even with the several comorbidities that are the norm for youth (Kendall et al., 2010; Merikangas et al., 2010). Sometimes, when clinicians attempt to deviate from the protocol to address comorbidities, they may inadvertently stray from fidelity to the core functions.

In the case of Brief Coping Cat, two sessions are 90 minutes long (rather than 50–60 minutes), with the last 30 minutes of the session devoted to working with caregivers. These sessions focus on gaining input about the youth, providing caregivers with tips for managing their youth's anxiety, and offering ways caregivers can reinforce their youth's positive behaviours at home. Caregiver involvement is a core function of this treatment. However, caregiver involvement in care at community clinics may be minimal (Baker-Ericzén, Jenkins, & Haine-Schlagel, 2013; Martinez, Lau, Chorpita, Weisz, & Research Network on Youth Mental Health, 2017). A lack of caregiver involvement can be a barrier to maintaining fidelity, even while being flexible. Lack of caregiver involvement may occur because caregivers have limited time. Such barriers may force clinicians to be flexible in ways that maintain the function of caregiver involvement but seek out an alternate form. For example, rather than meeting with caregivers in sessions, clinicians can give caregivers brief summaries of the skills the youth will practise that week in the form of a letter or telephone call.

Potential solutions

Despite the aforementioned challenges, the use of a function-focused approach offers potential solutions to maximize effectiveness of low intensity EBI for youth (Cho et al., 2019). It can be challenging to both resist distractions that may impede EBI implementation and progress, and to respond appropriately to issues that unpredictably arise (Chorpita, Korathu-Larson, Knowles, & Guan, 2014). An understanding of the core function of an EBI allows clinicians to maintain the 'spirit' of their session while adjusting the form of the intervention to meet immediate needs. First, it is helpful to identify the core function(s) of the activities in each session (Table 9.1). When implementing a new EBI, some clinicians report feeling a pressure to abandon their clinical judgement (Marques et al., 2016), but this is not preferred. In-person training and written manuals that deemphasize the preserving of form to maintain treatment fidelity will reduce this pressure. Training manuals that provide additional handouts or supporting materials to facilitate flexible application are preferred. For example, the Managing and Adapting Practice system includes a searchable online database of treatment recommendations, handouts, and practitioner dashboards to allow practitioners to adjust their treatment plan while maintaining the core functions of EBIs (Southam-Gerow et al., 2014).

Several EBIs provide guidance on how and where to be flexible. For example, the treatment manuals for all Coping Cat programmes provide 'flex' call outs in the prose of the manual. These flex call outs indicate where a practitioner can use flexible methods to achieve a session goal. Even with treatment materials that facilitate flexible application of EBIs, knowledge of the core functions and a strong conceptualization of the client's presenting problem will facilitate flexible implementation. Service practitioners may need to tolerate a degree of uncertainty as they begin to use a new programme. More experienced colleagues can help practitioners develop skills and brainstorm creative solutions (Beidas et al., 2013). We encourage treatment developers to place an emphasis on function over form. For example, framing session goals as core functions and providing worksheets as a potential form. In training events, supervisors can model this approach. Organizations can encourage and reward service practitioners for maintaining flexibility within fidelity through a functions-focused approach.

Case example

To model the form versus function approach, we describe the case of Alex, an 8-year-old child who met diagnostic criteria for social anxiety disorder and attention deficit hyperactivity disorder. Such comorbidity is seen in approximately 10–15% of cases (Merikangas et al., 2010). Alex received Brief Coping Cat within the school setting. Given that Alex received treatment during study hall (i.e. a school period set aside to study or to do homework), the session length had to be adapted to a 20-minute duration (the protocol describes 50–60-minute sessions). Brief Coping Cat addresses psychoeducation over four sessions, but because Alex's sessions were shorter in duration than the typical Brief Coping Cat programme, the number of psychoeducation sessions was expanded to eight sessions. The adaptation did not detract from the content, but it did allow for the programme to address the content within the real-world timeframe. The goal was the mastery of concepts, and the adaption to session duration did not detract from that goal.

Throughout treatment, the brief sessions were well suited to maximize Alex's focus and involvement in treatment: session duration matched with the need to address difficulties with sustained attention. Rewards are part of the programme. In addition to rewarding Alex for completing homework tasks (i.e. 'Show That I Can' (STIC) tasks), the clinician flexibly applied rewards and a sticker chart to track Alex's on-task behaviour. Alex earned a sticker for staying focused on each session activity, typically followed by a short break (e.g. off-topic conversation). When Alex earned a predetermined number of stickers, they earned an end-of-session reward (e.g. playing a game with the practitioner, watching a YouTube video).

Alex's fear of negative evaluation was evident even in the first sessions (e.g. when sharing personal experiences). In response, the practitioner followed the programme (i.e. left time to play a game at the end of each session) but made a minor adaptation. Brief games at the beginning and end of sessions (e.g. tic-tac-toe), as well as occasional physical activities (e.g. playing catch) were used to encourage turn-taking and to model self-disclosure. Additional breaks did not detract from the core functions of treatment, and the additional fun activities likely improved alliance. These activities later served treatment goals because they readily served as examples of differentiating and labelling emotions (session 2) and making connections between somatic sensations and emotions (session 3). Alex had anxiety about reading aloud (fear of failure), so the practitioner initially allowed Alex to complete assignments in the form of drawings (later in treatment, exposure tasks targeted reading in front of an audience). Another example of flexibility within fidelity was the use of cards when constructing the fear hierarchy. Rather than devoting large portions of session time to build a detailed hierarchy (the 'fear ladder'), index cards were used to represent easy/medium/hard situations. New anxiety-provoking situations were added to the deck (the hierarchy) as they came up.

Two Brief Coping Cat sessions include caregivers. Within the school context, an adaptation is needed to maintain the function of caregiver involvement. For Alex's caregivers, brief but regular communication was more feasible than two 30-minute sessions during their work day. Because Alex's caregivers expressed initial scepticism about exposure therapy, communications emphasized the rationale and core functions of treatment where caregivers could be helpful. The practitioner supported Alex's caregivers by sharing outlines of strategies to encourage approach behaviour and behaviour management strategies to reward completion of therapy tasks. The EBI manual was followed, with core strategies included, but they were applied creatively to meet the needs and interests of Alex.

Future research

Following the movement to implement EBIs, our profession moves towards data-supported approaches and away from approaches that are less effective. That said, EBIs are not perfect and can still benefit from additional research findings. Areas in need of examination include further documentation of the core ingredients of a treatment that would be required for flexibility within fidelity (Kendall & Frank, 2018), as well as evaluations of the added value of the form versus function approach to flexibility within fidelity. Relatedly, the Planned Adaptation Model (Lee, Altschul, & Mowbray, 2008) proposes a six-step procedure to guide clinicians through the forms and functions of a given EBI (Jolles, Lengnick-Hall, & Mittman, 2019; Kirk et al., 2019). This chapter identified the forms and functions of Coping Cat, but it followed only two of the six steps in the Planned Adaptation Model (i.e. reviewing existing materials and mapping core functions onto extant theory from the literature). A more rigorous examination of the core functions of EBIs for youth anxiety is warranted (such as by using the Planned Adaption Model). Additionally, future research should examine the effectiveness and necessity of each of the core functions in EBIs. This process may streamline EBIs by testing core functions (Schleider, Dobias, Sung, & Mullarkey, 2019).

From an implementation perspective, research could examine the degree to which training mental health service practitioners to use the core function and form framework improves treatment fidelity and, importantly, youth outcomes. Measures of fidelity could be streamlined to assess for core functions, rather than forms (Gearing et al., 2011). Funding agencies might consider the use of core treatment functions for decisions about reimbursement rates (Powell et al., 2016).

Chapter summary

EBIs are preferred, yet flexibility is needed when implementing EBIs. We recommend maintaining fidelity to EBIs core *functions*, while flexibly adapting the peripheral *forms* (i.e. the way in which a strategy can be implemented). We used the Brief Coping Cat programme for youth anxiety as an example of distinguishing between the core function and peripheral forms of an EBI, and we included a case illustration. Lack of time, limited resources, caregiver involvement, and limited knowledge of EBI core functions remain as threats to implementing EBIs with fidelity. Organizational support, supervision and peer consultation, as well as improved EBI training help ameliorate these challenges.

Recommended reading

Hawe, P., Shiell, A., & Riley, T. (2004). Complex interventions: How 'out of control' can a randomised controlled trial be? *BMJ, 328*(7455), 1561–1563.

Kendall, P. C., & Frank, H. E. (2018). Implementing evidence-based treatment protocols: Flexibility within fidelity. *Clinical Psychology: Science and Practice, 25*(4), e12271.

Kendall, P. C., Gosch, E., Furr, J. M., & Sood, E. (2008). Flexibility within fidelity. *Journal of the American Academy of Child and Adolescent Psychiatry, 47*(9), 987–993.

Wandersman, A., Duffy, J., Flaspohler, P., Noonan, R., Lubell, K., Stillman, L., . . ., & Saul, J. (2008). Bridging the gap between prevention research and practice: The interactive systems framework for dissemination and implementation. *American Journal of Community Psychology, 41*(3–4), 171–181.

References

American Psychological Association Task Force on Evidence-Based Practice with Children and Adolescents. (2008). *Disseminating evidence-based practice for children and adolescents: A systems approach to enhancing care.* Retrieved from https://www.apa.org/practice/resources/evidence/children-report.pdf

Baker-Ericzén, M. J., Jenkins, M. M., & Haine-Schlagel, R. (2013). Therapist, parent, and youth perspectives of treatment barriers to family-focused community outpatient mental health services. *Journal of Child and Family Studies, 22*(6), 854–868.

Becker-Haimes, E. M., Okamura, K. H., Wolk, C. B., Rubin, R., Evans, A. C., & Beidas, R. S. (2017). Predictors of clinician use of exposure therapy in community mental health settings. *Journal of Anxiety Disorders, 49*, 88–94.

Beidas, R. S., Edmunds, J. M., Cannuscio, C. C., Gallagher, M., Downey, M. M., & Kendall, P. C. (2013). Therapists perspectives on the effective elements of consultation following training. *Administration and Policy in Mental Health and Mental Health Services Research, 40*(6), 507–517.

Campbell, M., Fitzpatrick, R., Haines, A., Kinmonth, A. L., Sandercock, P., Spiegelhalter, D., & Tyrer, P. (2000). Framework for design and evaluation of complex interventions to improve health. *BMJ (Clinical Research Ed.), 321*(7262), 694–696.

Cho, E., Wood, P. K., Taylor, E. K., Hausman, E. M., Andrews, J. H., & Hawley, K. M. (2019). Evidence-based treatment strategies in youth mental health services: Results from a national survey of providers. *Administration and Policy in Mental Health and Mental Health Services Research, 46*(1), 71–81.

Chorpita, B. F., Korathu-Larson, P., Knowles, L. M., & Guan, K. (2014). Emergent life events and their impact on service delivery: Should we expect the unexpected? *Professional Psychology: Research and Practice*, 45(5), 387–393.

Damschroder, L. J., Aron, D. C., Keith, R. E., Kirsh, S. R., Alexander, J. A., & Lowery, J. C. (2009). Fostering implementation of health services research findings into practice: Consolidated framework for advancing implementation science. *Implementation Science*, 4(1), 1–15.

Elliott, D. S., & Mihalic, S. (2004). Issues in disseminating and replicating effective prevention programs. *Prevention Science*, 5(1), 47–53.

Farrell, N. R., Deacon, B. J., Dixon, L. J., & Lickel, J. J. (2013). Theory-based training strategies for modifying practitioner concerns about exposure therapy. *Journal of Anxiety Disorders*, 27(8), 781–787.

Gearing, R. E., El-Bassel, N., Ghesquiere, A., Baldwin, S., Gillies, J., & Ngeow, E. (2011). Major ingredients of fidelity: A review and scientific guide to improving quality of intervention research implementation. *Clinical Psychology Review*, 31(1), 79–88.

Hawe, P., Shiell, A., & Riley, T. (2004). Complex interventions: How 'out of control' can a randomised controlled trial be? *British Medical Journal*, 328(7455), 1561–1563.

Ijadi-Maghsoodi, R., Marlotte, L., Garcia, E., Aralis, H., Lester, P., Escudero, P., & Kataoka, S. (2017). Adapting and implementing a school-based resilience-building curriculum among low-income racial and ethnic minority students. *Contemporary School Psychology*, 21(3), 223–239.

Jolles, M. P., Lengnick-Hall, R., & Mittman, B. S. (2019). Core functions and forms of complex health interventions: A patient-centered medical home illustration. *Journal of General Internal Medicine*, 34(6), 1032–1038.

Kazak, A. E., Hoagwood, K., Weisz, J. R., Hood, K., Kratochwill, T. R., Vargas, L. A., & Banez, G. A. (2010). A meta-systems approach to evidence-based practice for children and adolescents. *American Psychologist*, 65(2), 85–97.

Kendall, P. C., Compton, S., Walkup, J., Birmaher, B., Albano, A. M., Sherrill, J., . . ., & Piacentini, J. (2010). Clinical characteristics of anxiety disordered youth. *Journal of Anxiety Disorders*, 24(3), 360–365.

Kendall, P. C., Crawley, S. A., Benjamin, C. L., & Mauro, C. F. (2013). *Brief Coping Cat: Therapist manual for the 8-session workbook*. Ardmore, PA: Workbook Publishing.

Kendall, P. C., & Frank, H. E. (2018). Implementing evidence-based treatment protocols: Flexibility within fidelity. *Clinical Psychology: Science and Practice*, 25(4), e12271.

Kendall, P. C., Gosch, E., Furr, J. M., & Sood, E. (2008). Flexibility within fidelity. *Journal of the American Academy of Child and Adolescent Psychiatry*, 47(9), 987–993.

Kendall, P. C., & Hedtke, K. (2006). *Cognitive-behavioral therapy for anxious children: Therapist manual* (3rd ed.). Ardmore, PA: Workbook Publishing.

Kendall, P. C., & Khanna, M. (2020). *Camp Cope-A-Lot online (online version)*. Ardmore, PA: Workbook Publishing. Retrieved from https://www.copingcatparents.com/Camp_Cope_A_Lot

Kirk, M. A., Haines, E. R., Rokoske, F. S., Powell, B. J., Weinberger, M., Hanson, L. C., & Birken, S. A. (2019). A case study of a theory-based method for identifying and reporting core functions and forms of evidence-based interventions. *Translational Behavioral Medicine*, 34(3), 193–113.

Kumpfer, K. L., Alvarado, R., Smith, P., & Bellamy, N. (2002). Cultural sensitivity and adaptation in family-based prevention interventions. *Prevention Science*, 3(3), 241–246.

Lee, S. J., Altschul, I., & Mowbray, C. T. (2008). Using planned adaptation to implement evidence-based programs with new populations. *American Journal of Community Psychology*, 41(3–4), 290–303.

Marques, L., Dixon, L., Valentine, S. E., Borba, C. P. C., Simon, N. M., & Wiltsey Stirman, S. (2016). Providers' perspectives of factors influencing implementation of evidence-based treatments in a community mental health setting: A qualitative investigation of the training-practice gap. *Psychological Services*, 13(3), 322–331.

Martinez, J. I., Lau, A. S., Chorpita, B. F., Weisz, J. R., & Research Network on Youth Mental Health. (2017). Psychoeducation as a mediator of treatment approach on parent engagement in child psychotherapy for disruptive behavior. *Journal of Clinical Child & Adolescent Psychology*, 46(4), 573–587.

McHugh, R. K., Murray, H. W., & Barlow, D. H. (2009). Balancing fidelity and adaptation in the dissemination of empirically-supported treatments: The promise of transdiagnostic interventions. *Behaviour Research and Therapy*, 47(11), 946–953.

Merikangas, K. R., He, J. P., Burstein, M., Swanson, S. A., Avenevoli, S., Cui, L., . . ., & Swendsen, J. (2010). Lifetime prevalence of mental disorders in US adolescents: Results from the National Comorbidity Survey Replication–Adolescent Supplement (NCS-A). *Journal of the American Academy of Child & Adolescent Psychiatry*, *49*(10), 980–989.

Peris, T. S., Compton, S. N., Kendall, P. C., Birmaher, B., Sherrill, J., March, J., . . ., & Piacentini, J. (2015). Trajectories of change in youth anxiety during cognitive-behavior therapy. *Journal of Consulting and Clinical Psychology*, *83*(2), 239–252.

Podell, J. L., Mychailyszyn, M., Edmunds, J., Puleo, C. M., & Kendall, P. C. (2010). The Coping Cat program for anxious youth: The FEAR plan comes to life. *Cognitive and Behavioral Practice*, *17*(2), 132–141.

Powell, B. J., Beidas, R. S., Rubin, R. M., Stewart, R. E., Wolk, C. B., Matlin, S. L., . . ., & Mandell, D. S. (2016). Applying the policy ecology framework to Philadelphia's behavioral health transformation efforts. *Administration and Policy in Mental Health*, *43*(6), 909–926.

Ringle, V. A., Read, K. L., Edmunds, J. M., Brodman, D. M., Kendall, P. C., Barg, F., & Beidas, R. S. (2015). Barriers to and facilitators in the implementation of cognitive-behavioral therapy for youth anxiety in the community. *Psychiatric Services*, *66*(9), 938–945.

Schleider, J. L., Dobias, M. L., Sung, J. Y., & Mullarkey, M. C. (2019). Future directions in single-session youth mental health interventions. *Journal of Clinical Child & Adolescent Psychology*, *49*(2), 264–278.

Sherrill, J. T. (2016). Adaptive treatment strategies in youth mental health: A commentary on advantages, challenges, and potential directions. *Journal of Clinical Child & Adolescent Psychology*, *45*(4), 522–527.

Southam-Gerow, M. A., Daleiden, E. L., Chorpita, B. F., Bae, C., Mitchell, C., Faye, M., & Alba, M. (2014). MAPping Los Angeles County: Taking an evidence-informed model of mental health care to scale. *Journal of Clinical Child and Adolescent Psychology*, *43*(2), 190–200.

Stirman, S. W., Miller, C. J., Toder, K., & Calloway, A. (2013). Development of a framework and coding system for modifications and adaptations of evidence-based interventions. *Implementation Science*, *8*(1), 65.

Wandersman, A., Duffy, J., Flaspohler, P., Noonan, R., Lubell, K., Stillman, L., . . ., & Saul, J. (2008). Bridging the gap between prevention research and practice: The interactive systems framework for dissemination and implementation. *American Journal of Community Psychology*, *41*(3–4), 171–181.

Whiteside, S. P., Deacon, B. J., Benito, K., & Stewart, E. (2016). Factors associated with practitioners' use of exposure therapy for childhood anxiety disorders. *Journal of Anxiety Disorders*, *40*, 29–36.

SECTION 2B
PROBLEM-SPECIFIC AREAS

10

Low intensity interventions for anxiety disorders in children and adolescents

Cathy Creswell, Chloe Chessell, Claire Hill, and Polly Waite

Learning objectives

- To highlight the need for accessible interventions for anxiety disorders in children and young people.
- To understand the evidence base for low intensity interventions for the treatment of anxiety disorders in children and adolescents.
- To gain an overview of low intensity treatment delivery for childhood anxiety disorders.
- To consider the limits of the evidence base and needs for further development going forward.

Introduction

Anxiety disorders are impairing conditions that are characterized by excessive fear and related behavioural disturbances, most commonly avoidance. They are among the most prevalent mental health disorders in children and young people, with an estimated mean worldwide prevalence of 6.5% (Polanczyk, Salum, Sugaya, Caye, & Rohde, 2015). Anxiety disorders in childhood and adolescence have a significant negative impact on educational, social, and health functioning, create a risk for ongoing anxiety and other mental health disorders in adulthood (Copeland, Angold, Shanahan, & Costello, 2014), and are associated with substantial economic cost (Fineberg et al., 2013), highlighting a need for effective, early intervention. However, only a very small proportion of children and adolescents who could benefit from interventions actually access them. For example, in a recent study, only 2% of children with anxiety disorders identified in the community in England had received cognitive behavioural therapy (CBT; Reardon, Harvey, & Creswell, 2020), despite this being the psychological intervention with the most robust evidence base (James et al., 2013). Similar low rates of service utilization have been found elsewhere in the UK, Australia and the US (Green, McGinnity, Meltzer, Ford, & Goodman, 2005; Lawrence et al., 2015; Merikangas et al., 2011).

One mechanism with potential to increase access to evidence-based interventions is a stepped care model (see Chapter 21) in which low intensity (LI) interventions are delivered initially, with more intensive (/expensive) interventions reserved for those who do not, or can be predicted not to, benefit from the first step treatment (Bower & Gilbody, 2005). Some promising LI approaches for child anxiety problems have been developed and evaluated in recent years, this chapter provides an overview of these, with particular consideration of approaches for preadolescents and adolescents in turn.

LI interventions for preadolescent anxiety disorders

Probably the most extensively evaluated LI approach to treatment for preadolescent anxiety disorders is brief, therapist-guided, parent-led CBT. This approach has been shown to be effective (Cobham, 2012; Rapee, Abbott, & Lyneham, 2006; Thirlwall et al., 2013) and cost-effective compared to another brief psychological intervention (solution-focused therapy) (Creswell et al., 2017).

In Box 10.1 we describe the approach we have used and evaluated in our research group, in which parents are supported by a therapist to work through a book (*Helping Your Child with Fears and Worries*; Creswell & Willetts, 2019) to help them to help their child overcome problems with anxiety (Box 10.1). The most recent version of this treatment consists of six treatment sessions delivered over an 8-week period; four of which are conducted face-to-face (approximately 60 minutes) and two are conducted over the telephone (approximately 20 minutes; giving approximately 4 hours 40 minutes of total therapist contact time). The treatment aims to help parents to support children in gaining exposure to their feared stimuli in order to create opportunities for children to learn new information about their fears, to enhance their confidence and ability to cope in feared situations, and to build child autonomy and independence. The core treatment components include psychoeducation, identification of negative automatic thoughts, exposure to feared stimuli, and problem-solving. Therapists support parents to apply the CBT techniques with their child and to problem-solve any challenges which arise.

Challenges implementing brief, therapist-guided, parent-led CBT

We encourage parents to apply a problem-solving approach to address challenges that are faced in implementing the treatment approach, but some examples of common challenges and possible solutions are shown in Table 10.3.

Box 10.1 Case-based step-by-step description of brief, therapist-guided, parent-led CBT for preadolescent children

Muhammed (7 years old) met diagnostic criteria for separation anxiety disorder and was unable to sleep in his own bed without his parents. An overview of the treatment conducted with Muhammed's parents is outlined below.

- Session 1 (face-to-face): psychoeducation on the development and maintenance of childhood anxiety was shared. For homework, Muhammed's parents were asked to complete a handout on the maintenance of Muhammed's anxiety, looking out for anxious thoughts and behaviours. Treatment goals were developed for Muhammed's parents to discuss with him, including (1) for Muhammed to be able to stay in his bed after his parents have said goodnight, and (2) for Muhammed to be able to sleep on his own, all night, for a week.
- Session 2 (face-to-face): this session focused on helping Muhammed's parents to identify his anxious expectations when he was in anxiety-provoking situations and to hypothesize about what Muhammed would need to learn in order to overcome his separation fears (Table 10.1). An in-session role play was conducted where Muhammed's parents had the opportunity to practise using a curious approach to help Muhammed to notice and share his anxious expectations.

Table 10.1 'What does my child need to learn?'

Goal	What does my child expect will happen?	What does my child need to learn?
For Muhammed to be able to stay in his bed, after his parents have said goodnight	'I won't be able to get to sleep without Mum in the room'	Can Muhammed get to sleep without his mum in his room? How might Muhammed cope in this situation? Will Muhammed cope better than he expects?
For Muhammed to be able to sleep on his own, all night, for a week	'Something bad will happen to me in the night' 'Something bad will happen to Mum in the night'	What actually happens if Muhammed stays in his bed on his own all night? How might Muhammed cope? Will he cope better than he expects?

- Session 3 (face-to-face): a provisional step-by-step plan was developed with Muhammed's parents, to be confirmed with him between sessions (Table 10.2). This step-by-step plan aimed to create opportunities for Muhammed to test out his anxious expectations and allow him to learn the new information that would help him overcome his fears (i.e. that he would be able to get to sleep and it was unlikely that something bad would happen to him) and to increase his perceived ability to cope. The 'ultimate goal' of being able to sleep on his own, all night, for a week was broken down into smaller steps to make it easier for Muhammed to face his fears (and for his parents to help him), and each step was paired with an appropriate reward to encourage

Table 10.2 Muhammed's step-by-step plan

Prediction:	Ultimate goal: 'For Muhammed to be able to sleep on his own, all night, for a week'	Ultimate reward: 'To go to the cinema to see a film that he chooses'
Prediction:	Step 6: 'To be able to go to sleep while mum is downstairs'	Reward: 'To have a friend over for a movie night'
Prediction:	Step 5: 'To be able to go to sleep while mum is in another room upstairs'	Reward: 'To choose the family a takeaway on the weekend'
Prediction:	Step 4: 'To be able to go to sleep while mum is in the room next door'	Reward: 'To be allowed to play computer games, one evening after school'
Prediction:	Step 3: 'To be able to go to sleep while mum is stood outside Muhammed's bedroom door'	Reward: 'Bake cakes with brother'
Prediction:	Step 2: 'To be able to go to sleep, while mum is stood by Muhammed's bedroom door'	Reward: 'Watch a film with mum and dad'
Prediction: 'I won't be able to get to sleep' 'Something bad will happen to me in the night'	Step 1: 'To be able to go to sleep, while mum is sat at the end of Muhammed's bed'	Reward: 'To go to the newsagent after school and choose a small treat (value prespecified)'

Muhammed to give each step a try and to recognize his efforts. Muhammed's parents were encouraged to ask Muhammed to predict what he thought would happen before each step, and to review with Muhammed what he had learned about these predictions after each step.

- Session 4 (telephone): a telephone call was conducted to review how Muhammed had got on with the first step of the step-by-step plan. Muhammed had completed the first step three times and had learned that he was able to get to sleep while his mum sat at the end of his bed. Muhammed's parents agreed to implement the second step of the plan over the next week, to ask Muhammed what he predicted would happen before the step, and to review what he had learned after each step.
- Session 5 (face-to-face): Muhammed's progress on the step-by-step plan was reviewed, and additional steps were added/removed as necessary based on what he had learned from completing the previous step. A structured problem-solving technique was

introduced to Muhammed's parents. This was practised using a relevant problem that Muhammed's parents had encountered during treatment (i.e. motivating Muhammed to engage in the step-by-step plan). Through using the problem-solving technique, Muhammed's parents identified that they would make the step-by-step plan more fun and engaging, by encouraging Muhammed to decorate the step-by-step plan with his favourite cartoon characters. Muhammed's parents were encouraged to use the problem-solving approach to help Muhammed build confidence in his ability to overcome challenges that he faced.

- Session 6 (telephone): a telephone call was conducted to review Muhammed's progress on the step-by-step plan and to see how his parents had got on using the problem-solving technique to support Muhammed to overcome problems. This session also focused on identifying the techniques that Muhammed's parents had found most useful throughout the treatment, and what they were going to continue working on to help Muhammed to continue to make progress in overcoming any remaining or future problems with anxiety.
- Booster session (face-to-face): a booster session was conducted 4 weeks after Muhammed's parents completed the treatment to reinforce the family's progress and to troubleshoot any difficulties. Muhammed had successfully reached his goal of being able to sleep, all night, in his own bed, and had done so for the previous 2 weeks. Muhammed's scores on the relevant routine outcome measures were now in the non-clinical range, and Muhammed's parents felt confident to continue helping Muhammed to achieve his goals.

Technology-enabled treatments for preadolescent anxiety disorders

There is increasing interest in the role that digital solutions could play in the treatment of anxiety disorders in children and adolescents. In response to higher demand

Table 10.3 Common example challenges implementing brief, therapist-guided, parent-led CBT

Challenge	Possible solutions
Child refuses to try a step on the step-by-step plan	• Involve the child in finalizing the step-by-step plan. Ensure the child is motivated to work towards the ultimate goal • Ensure the step is not too difficult for the child. Consider whether the step could be broken down into smaller steps • Remind the child of the reward for having a go at the step • Make the step-by-step plan engaging by incorporating the child's interests
The parent(s) does not have time to implement the treatment techniques at home	• Collaboratively explore with the parent(s) ways to overcome this. For example, setting aside a specific time each week to implement the techniques or involving other parents/caregivers to share the workload

for services, public health services advocate the use of technology to provide health support, advice, and interventions (Department of Health, 2015; European Commission, 2012; NHS England, 2017). The advantages that digital interventions can offer both service users (e.g. greater convenience, increased accessibility) and services themselves (e.g. increased therapist efficiency, cost-effectiveness) make them an attractive offering. LI treatments lend themselves to a digital format as the material can be readily adapted for online presentation as they are highly structured (often manualized) and sequential in nature (Proudfoot et al., 2004), and service users can be appropriately supported through brief telephone or video conferencing sessions. Furthermore, they offer the potential to increase access to evidence-based interventions for child anxiety as they can be effectively delivered by LI psychological therapists (e.g. children's well-being practitioners in the UK).

Online treatments for anxiety disorders in children that have been developed include programmes that involve both children and parents (e.g. Brave in Australia (Spence, Holmes, Donovan, & Kenardy, 2006); BiP Anxiety in Sweden (Vigerland et al., 2016)), and guided parent-led CBT approaches (e.g. Online Support & Intervention for child anxiety (OSI) in the UK (Hill et al., 2022)). These all follow a similar format where the user (child and/or parent) works through a series of modules and is supported remotely by a therapist in applying the CBT techniques. A recent meta-analysis of technology-enabled treatments for child anxiety found that results are encouraging but that more controlled clinical trials (especially in comparison to active treatment conditions) are warranted before these can be offered as a first-line or credible alternative treatment for use in routine clinical practice (Podina, Mogoase, David, Szentagotai, & Dobrean, 2016) (see Chapter 21).

LI interventions for adolescent anxiety disorders

There has been relatively little development and evaluation of brief treatments that are deliverable by non-specialist therapists specifically for adolescent anxiety disorders. In contrast to work with preadolescents, where LI treatments have been developed for adolescents with anxiety disorders this has only been in online formats, which is thought to be likely to have particular appeal for this age group (Grist, Croker, Denne, & Stallard, 2019). Programmes typically involve eight to ten internet sessions, supported by a therapist through regular emails or telephone calls (e.g. BRAVE for Teenagers—ONLINE (Spence et al., 2006); ChilledOut Online (Lyneham et al., 2014)). The content of modules typically focuses on psychoeducation, relaxation (although this is not always included), cognitive restructuring, exposure, problem-solving, and relapse prevention, with homework activities outside of sessions. There is encouraging evidence that this may be effective, both in the short term and at 12-month follow-up, and that young people are generally satisfied with the treatment (Spence et al., 2011; Stjerneklar, Hougaard, McLellan, & Thastum,

2019). However, when delivered to young people referred for treatment in routine practice, positive benefits have been less clear (Waite, Marshall, & Creswell, 2019).

As far as we are aware, there has been no evaluation of treatments (in any delivery format) for adolescent anxiety disorders that are less than eight sessions of a typical clinical session length (i.e. of around an hour) and therefore could be considered 'brief', although there is preliminary evidence for 'intensive' approaches (e.g. six sessions totalling around 20 hours of therapy over 8 days; Chase, Whitton, & Pincus, 2012; Leyfer, Carpenter, & Pincus, 2019). As such, there is no 'go-to' evidence-based brief intervention for adolescent anxiety disorders. However findings from a recent meta-analysis (based on studies of children and adolescents, aged 3–18 years) give some guidance about the core components that should be included in treatment (Whiteside et al., 2020); specifically, more in-session, therapist-assisted exposure was associated with larger treatment effects. There was no apparent effect of stand-alone cognitive strategies on treatment outcome and the inclusion of relaxation appeared to actually have detrimental effects.

In terms of *how* best to deliver exposure to adolescents with anxiety disorders, contemporary models of exposure in adults have led to a number of optimization strategies (Craske et al., 2008) which may be helpful with adolescents although we currently lack evidence for the extent to which they apply in this age group (Plaisted, Waite, Gordon, & Creswell, 2021). Strategies include the clinician and young person identifying a meaningful exposure task and the young person providing their negative prediction about what will occur (with ratings of their belief); designing the activity so that there is as large a mismatch as possible between what the young person predicts and what they experience; encouraging the young person to drop 'safety behaviours'; and conducting exposure tasks in multiple contexts, and then having a discussion about the actual outcome following exposure to consolidate new learning (Craske, Treanor, Conway, Zbozinek, & Vervliet, 2014). Finally, in brief treatments, further exposure or behavioural experiments outside sessions will be crucial. While the evidence does not indicate how parents should be involved in treatment for adolescents to optimize outcomes (Cardy, Waite, Cocks, & Creswell, 2020), it is likely that, for younger adolescents especially, involving parents/carers so that they understand the importance of exposure and how they can facilitate this outside sessions, will be important (Box 10.2).

The future of LI interventions for child and adolescent anxiety disorders

Clearly there is a lot of room for innovation and evaluation of LI treatments for anxiety disorders in children and, particularly, adolescents. To ensure that these treatments are as effective and efficient as they can be, it is critical that developments build on developmentally appropriate theory and evidence, including the growing understanding of components of treatment that are associated with better (e.g. exposure)

Box 10.2 Case-based description of brief CBT for adolescents

Mia (15 years old) had a specific phobia of vomiting (emetophobia), which caused signifi-cant distress and interference in her life. Mia attended six weekly sessions individually in the clinic. Mia's mum also joined the end of sessions as they both felt it would be helpful for her to understand the principles of treatment and to help support her with planned homework activities. To track progress and plan session content, Mia completed questionnaires around her symptoms, overall functioning, and progress with goals prior to each session, and this was reviewed at the beginning of each session.

Sessions began by Mia and her therapist gaining a shared understanding of the problem. This enabled the therapist to provide information to correct misunderstandings about vomiting (psychoeducation) and Mia and her therapist to develop behavioural experiments to test out Mia's beliefs. Mia identified that when she felt nauseous, she believed that she would vomit (100% belief), lose control (80% belief), be 'judged' by others (100% belief), and not be able to cope (90% belief). As a result of this, she spent a lot of time worrying about being sick and planning how she might stop herself being sick or deal with someone else being sick. She was able to identify 'safety behaviours', such as scanning and monitoring her body for any signs of nausea, checking food, carrying a bottle of water with her at all times, and being on the look-out for other people showing signs of illness, as well as possible es-cape routes from situations. She also identified that she avoided eating particular foods, travel, crowded places, using public toilets, and people she perceived to show signs of illness that could be contagious.

Following this, the main focus in sessions was on Mia and her therapist undertaking exposure, through behavioural experiments, to test out her beliefs within the sessions and planning experiments for Mia to do between sessions to increase opportunities for learning. This included experiments that involved Mia exposing herself to situations that she typically avoided, such as eating food from a takeaway or that had reached its 'sell-by' date, exposing herself to vomit by watching videos and listening to audio of people vomiting, and imagining herself vomiting. This was accompanied by drop-ping her safety behaviours, such as not scanning or monitoring her body, carrying a bottle of water, or looking for an escape route (Table 10.4). In addition, the therapist pretended to be sick in the street, using fake vomit, and Mia observed and recorded other peoples' reactions as they passed by. In each experiment, Mia was encouraged to identify her beliefs and give belief ratings before and afterwards. Following each ex-periment, there was a discussion about what she had learned and how she could take this learning forwards. Sessions ended with a plan of further experiments to be con-ducted between sessions as 'homework'. Mia attended a booster session 12 weeks after completing treatment to consolidate her learning, reinforce her progress, troubleshoot any difficulties, and make a plan for dealing with setbacks. At her final assessment, she no longer met diagnostic criteria for her phobia and scores on all self-report measures were in the non-clinical range.

Table 10.4 Mia's Behavioural Experiments Record Sheet

Date	Situation	Prediction What do you think will happen? How would you know if it had? Rate your beliefs (0–100%)	Experiment What will you do to test the prediction? (Remember to drop any safety behaviours)	Outcome What actually happened? Were the predictions correct?	What I learned What did you learn? How likely is it that your predictions will happen in the future? Re-rate your beliefs (0–100%) What can you do to further test your original prediction/s?
02/05	At home	I will be sick (100%) I will lose control (80%) Other people will judge me (stare and frown) (100%) I will not be able to cope (crying and screaming uncontrollably) (90%)	I will eat a yoghurt from the fridge that is past its 'sell-by' date and then I'll go for a walk round the block. I won't check my body for signs that I am going to be sick or keeping swallowing. I won't take a bottle of water with me. I won't keep telling myself 'I'll be ok'.	I wasn't sick and none of the other predictions came true.	I learned that I wasn't sick. Although I felt a bit sick, this was probably just anxiety. I can eat things that are past their 'sell-by' date. I don't need to do anything to stay safe. New ratings: I will be sick (20%) I will lose control (30%) I will be judged (50%) I will not be able to cope (50%) I could test this further by doing other things I avoid, liking having a take-away with friends and seeing what happens.

and worse (e.g. relaxation) treatment outcomes (Whiteside et al., 2020). In addition to face-to-face and online computerized CBT approaches, there is also scope to increase the efficiency of interventions using other technological modalities, such as smartphone or tablet applications (often referred to as mobile health applications, or mHealth apps) and virtual reality programs. More than 10,000 mHealth apps are available that specifically target mental health conditions, such as anxiety, across the lifespan (Torous & Roberts, 2017). However, two meta-analyses of randomized controlled trials of mHealth apps for anxiety disorders did not identify any randomized controlled trials for apps aimed at those under 18 years old (Firth et al., 2017; Podina et al., 2016). Clearly there are lots of mHealth apps available that claim to be helpful in managing child anxiety, but it is important to be cautious in using these with families and to look for the evidence base underpinning them (see Chapters 24 and 27). With regards to virtual reality and applied games, a recent systematic review identified very few studies and these were limited to treating specific phobias (Halldorsson et al., 2021).

Whether intervention innovation is in face-to-face, online, or other formats it will be critical that (1) potential beneficiaries (e.g. children and adolescents, parents, clinicians) are actively involved in their development through co-design to maximize engagement and implementation (Hill et al., 2018; Pennant et al., 2015) and (2) robust evaluation is conducted in the settings in which children and young people with anxiety disorders are accessing support and involving the workforces that are providing it. Clinicians and service providers are encouraged to actively seek evidence of both co-design and robust evaluation when considering novel LI approaches for the treatment of children and young people with anxiety disorders.

Chapter summary

Anxiety disorders in children and young people are common and cause significant short- and potentially long-term impairment. For preadolescent children with anxiety disorders, there is good evidence that brief, therapist-guided, parent-led treatments are effective and cost-effective. There is also promising initial evidence for online interventions for both preadolescents and adolescents. Beyond the trials of online interventions, there has been limited evaluation of LI treatments specifically for adolescents with anxiety disorders, and this is a clear priority for innovation and evaluation; however, the wider literature highlights the potential of exposure-based interventions.

Recommended measures

International Consortium for Health Outcomes Measurement (ICHOM). (2020). *Children and young people with anxiety, depression, OCD and/or PTSD*. Retrieved from https://www.ichom.org/wp-content/uploads/2020/03/PDA_ReferenceGuide_200318-1.pdf

Recommended reading

Andersson, G. (2014). *The internet and CBT: A clinical guide*. Boca Raton, FL: CRC Press.
Creswell, C., Parkinson, M., Thirlwall, K., & Willetts, L. (2019). *Parent-led CBT for child anxiety: Helping parents help their kids*. New York: Guilford Publications.
Creswell, C., Waite, P., & Hudson, J. (2020). Practitioner review: Anxiety disorders in children and young people—assessment and treatment. *Journal of Child Psychology and Psychiatry, 61*(6), 628–643.
Creswell, C., & Willetts, L. (2019). *Helping your child with fears and worries*. London: Robinson.
Rapee, R., Wignall, A., Spence, S., Cobham, V., & Lyneham, H. (2008). *Helping your anxious child*. Oakland, CA: New Harbinger Publications.

References

Bower, P., & Gilbody, S. (2005). Stepped care in psychological therapies: Access, effectiveness and efficiency. Narrative literature review. *British Journal of Psychiatry, 186*(1), 11–17.
Cardy, J. L., Waite, P., Cocks, F., & Creswell, C. (2020). A systematic review of parental involvement in cognitive behavioural therapy for adolescent anxiety disorders. *Clinical Child and Family Psychology Review, 23*(4), 483–509.
Chase, R. M., Whitton, S. W., & Pincus, D. B. (2012). Treatment of adolescent panic disorder: A nonrandomized comparison of intensive versus weekly CBT. *Child & Family Behavior Therapy, 34*(4), 305–323.
Cobham, V. E. (2012). Do anxiety-disordered children need to come into the clinic for efficacious treatment? *Journal of Consulting and Clinical Psychology, 80*(3), 465–476.
Copeland, W. E., Angold, A., Shanahan, L., & Costello, E. J. (2014). Longitudinal patterns of anxiety from childhood to adulthood: The Great Smoky Mountains Study. *Journal of the American Academy of Child & Adolescent Psychiatry, 53*(1), 21–33.
Craske, M., Kircanski, K., Zelikowsky, M., Mystkowski, J., Chowdhury, N., & Baker, A. (2008). Optimizing inhibitory learning during exposure therapy. *Behaviour Research and Therapy, 46*(1), 5–27.
Craske, M., Treanor, M., Conway, C. C., Zbozinek, T., & Vervliet, B. (2014). Maximizing exposure therapy: An inhibitory learning approach. *Behaviour Research and Therapy, 58*, 10–23.
Creswell, C., Violato, M., Fairbanks, H., White, E., Parkinson, M., Abitabile, G., . . ., & Cooper, P. J. (2017). Clinical outcomes and cost-effectiveness of brief guided parent-delivered cognitive behavioural therapy and solution-focused brief therapy for treatment of childhood anxiety disorders: A randomised controlled trial. *Lancet Psychiatry, 4*(7), 529–539.
Creswell, C., & Willetts, L. (2019). *Helping your child with fears and worries: A self-help guide for parents* (2nd ed.). London: Robinson.
Department of Health. (2015). *Future in mind: Promoting, protecting and improving our children and young people's mental health and well-being*. London: Department of Health.
European Commission. (2012). *eHealth action plan 2012–2020: Innovative healthcare for the 21st century*. Brussels: European Commission.
Fineberg, N. A., Haddad, P. M., Carpenter, L., Gannon, B., Sharpe, R., Young, A. H., . . ., & Nutt, D. J. (2013). The size, burden and cost of disorders of the brain in the UK. *Journal of Psychopharmacology, 27*(9), 761–770.

Firth, J., Torous, J., Nicholas, J., Carney, R., Rosenbaum, S., & Sarris, J. (2017). Can smartphone mental health interventions reduce symptoms of anxiety? A meta-analysis of randomized controlled trials. *Journal of Affective Disorders, 218*, 15–22.

Green, H., McGinnity, Á., Meltzer, H., Ford, T., & Goodman, R. (2005). *Mental health of children and young people in Great Britain, 2004*. Basingstoke: Palgrave Macmillan.

Grist, R., Croker, A., Denne, M., & Stallard, P. (2019). Technology delivered interventions for depression and anxiety in children and adolescents: A systematic review and meta-analysis. *Clinical Child and Family Psychology Review, 22*(2), 147–171.

Halldorsson, B., Hill, C., Waite, P., Partridge, K., Freeman, D., & Creswell, C. (2021). Virtual reality and gaming interventions for the treatment of mental health problems in children and young people: The need for rigorous treatment development and clinical evaluation. *Journal of Child Psychology and Psychiatry, 62*(5), 584–605.

Hill, C., Creswell, C., Vigerland, S., Nauta, M. H., March, S., Donovan, C., . . ., & Wozney, L. (2018). Navigating the development and dissemination of internet cognitive behavioral therapy (iCBT) for anxiety disorders in children and young people: A consensus statement with recommendations from the# iCBTLorentz Workshop Group. *Internet Interventions, 12*, 1–10.

Hill, C., Reardon, T., Taylor, L., & Creswell, C. (2022). Online Support and Intervention for Child Anxiety (OSI): Development and Usability Testing. *JMIR Formative Research, 6*(4), e29846.

James, A. C., Reardon, T., Soler, A., James, G., & Creswell, C. (2020). Cognitive behavioural therapy for anxiety disorders in children and adolescents. *Cochrane database of systematic reviews*, (11).

Lawrence, D., Johnson, S., Hafekost, J., Boterhoven de Haan, K., Sawyer, M., Ainley, J., & Zubrick, S. R. (2015). *The mental health of children and adolescents: Report on the second Australian child and adolescent survey of mental health and wellbeing*. Canberra: Department of Health.

Leyfer, O., Carpenter, A., & Pincus, D. (2019). N-methyl-D-aspartate partial agonist enhanced intensive cognitive-behavioral therapy of panic disorder in adolescents. *Child Psychiatry & Human Development, 50*(2), 268–277.

Lyneham, H., McLellan, L., Cunningham, M., Wuthrich, V., Schniering, C., Hudson, J., & Rapee, R. (2014). *ChilledOut Online program*. Sydney: Centre for Emotional Health, Macquarie University.

Merikangas, K. R., He, J.-P., Burstein, M., Swendsen, J., Avenevoli, S., Case, B., . . ., & Olfson, M. (2011). Service utilization for lifetime mental disorders in US adolescents: Results of the National Comorbidity Survey Adolescent Supplement (NCS-A). *Journal of the American Academy of Child & Adolescent Psychiatry, 50*(1), 32–45.

NHS England. (2017). *Next steps on the NHS five year forward view*. Retrieved from https://www.england.nhs.uk/wp-content/uploads/2017/03/NEXT-STEPS-ON-THE-NHS-FIVE-YEAR-FORWARD-VIEW.pdf

Pennant, M. E., Loucas, C. E., Whittington, C., Creswell, C., Fonagy, P., Fuggle, P., . . ., & Kendall, T. (2015). Computerised therapies for anxiety and depression in children and young people: A systematic review and meta-analysis. *Behaviour Research and Therapy, 67*, 1–18.

Plaisted, H., Waite, P., Gordon, K., & Creswell, C. (2021). Optimising exposure for children and adolescents with anxiety, OCD and PTSD: A systematic review. *Clinical Child and Family Psychology Review, 24*(2), 348–369.

Podina, I. R., Mogoase, C., David, D., Szentagotai, A., & Dobrean, A. (2016). A meta-analysis on the efficacy of technology mediated CBT for anxious children and adolescents. *Journal of Rational-Emotive & Cognitive-Behavior Therapy, 34*(1), 31–50.

Polanczyk, G. V., Salum, G. A., Sugaya, L. S., Caye, A., & Rohde, L. A. (2015). Annual research review: A meta-analysis of the worldwide prevalence of mental disorders in children and adolescents. *Journal of Child Psychology and Psychiatry, 56*(3), 345–365.

Proudfoot, J., Ryden, C., Everitt, B., Shapiro, D. A., Goldberg, D., Mann, A., . . ., & Gray, J. A. (2004). Clinical efficacy of computerised cognitive-behavioural therapy for anxiety and depression in primary care: Randomised controlled trial. *British Journal of Psychiatry, 185*(1), 46–54.

Rapee, R. M., Abbott, M. J., & Lyneham, H. J. (2006). Bibliotherapy for children with anxiety disorders using written materials for parents: A randomized controlled trial. *Journal of Consulting and Clinical Psychology, 74*(3), 436–444.

Reardon, T., Harvey, K., & Creswell, C. (2020). Seeking and accessing professional support for child anxiety in a community sample. *European Child & Adolescent Psychiatry, 29*(5), 649–664.

Spence, S., Donovan, C. L., March, S., Gamble, A., Anderson, R. E., Prosser, S., & Kenardy, J. (2011). A randomized controlled trial of online versus clinic-based CBT for adolescent anxiety. *Journal of Consulting and Clinical Psychology, 79*(5), 629–642.

Spence, S., Holmes, J., Donovan, C. L., & Kenardy, J. (2006). *BRAVE for Teenagers—ONLINE: An Internet based program for adolescents with anxie*ty. Brisbane: University of Queensland.

Stjerneklar, S., Hougaard, E., McLellan, L. F., & Thastum, M. (2019). A randomized controlled trial examining the efficacy of an internet-based cognitive behavioral therapy program for adolescents with anxiety disorders. *PloS One, 14*(9), e0222485.

Thirlwall, K., Cooper, P. J., Karalus, J., Voysey, M., Willetts, L., & Creswell, C. (2013). Treatment of child anxiety disorders via guided parent-delivered cognitive–behavioural therapy: Randomised controlled trial. *British Journal of Psychiatry, 203*(6), 436–444.

Torous, J., & Roberts, L. W. (2017). The ethical use of mobile health technology in clinical psychiatry. *Journal of Nervous and Mental Disease, 205*(1), 4–8.

Vigerland, S., Ljótsson, B., Thulin, U., Öst, L.-G., Andersson, G., & Serlachius, E. (2016). Internet-delivered cognitive behavioural therapy for children with anxiety disorders: A randomised controlled trial. *Behaviour Research and Therapy, 76*, 47–56.

Waite, P., Marshall, T., & Creswell, C. (2019). A randomized controlled trial of internet-delivered cognitive behaviour therapy for adolescent anxiety disorders in a routine clinical care setting with and without parent sessions. *Child and Adolescent Mental Health, 24*(3), 242–250.

Whiteside, S. P., Sim, L. A., Morrow, A. S., Farah, W. H., Hilliker, D. R., Murad, M. H., & Wang, Z. (2020). A meta-analysis to guide the enhancement of CBT for childhood anxiety: Exposure over anxiety management. *Clinical Child and Family Psychology Review, 23*(1), 102–121.

11

Brief behavioural activation for treating depressive symptoms in children and adolescents

Julia W. Felton, Morgan S. Anvari, Jessica F. Magidson, and Carl W. Lejuez

Learning objectives

- To describe the prevalence and developmental trends of depressive symptoms across childhood and adolescence.
- To briefly describe common low intensity interventions for children and adolescent depressive symptoms.
- To identify the theoretical context and basic principles of behavioural activation.
- To understand necessary adaptations for delivering behavioural activation to children and adolescents.

Introduction

Depression is a leading cause of disability worldwide, impacting more than 250 million people globally (James et al., 2018), and is one of the most common disorders among young people. Rates of the disorder are relatively low in childhood, but increase precipitously across adolescence, coinciding with other changes that occur during this developmental period, such as greater individuation from parents, increased levels of personal autonomy, and more exposure to stressful events. This developmental course is also marked by the emergence of sex differences in the prevalence of depression. Whereas prior to age 13, boys and girls have similar, low rates of the disorder, by age 18, girls are more than twice as likely as boys to meet clinical criteria for depression (Dalsgaard et al., 2020).

Depression is characterized by a decreased interest and enjoyment in activities (i.e. anhedonia), as well as low mood or, in children, irritability. Subclinical levels of depressive symptomology are relatively common in adolescence, with 25% of girls and 10% of boys reporting at least one symptom of the disorder (Saluja et al., 2004). Depressive symptomology can have a significant and negative impact on children's functioning, and has been linked to increased risk for a myriad of negative outcomes, including academic difficulties (Jaycox et al., 2009), substance use (Henry et al., 1993), and self-harm (Lundh et al., 2011). Moreover, the early emergence of depressive symptoms has been linked to recurrent major depressive disorder in adulthood (Pine et al., 1999).

Evidence base for low intensity interventions for treating depression in youth

Despite the pervasive nature of depression, in the US less than 1% of youth are regularly screened for symptoms of this disorder (Zenlea, Milliren, Mednick, & Rhodes, 2014) and, of these, even fewer go on to receive any form of intervention (Reinert, Nguyen, & Fritze, 2021), let alone evidence-based treatment (Reinert et al., 2021). Low intensity (LI) interventions that are relatively brief may be more easily disseminated and cost-effective than more intensive treatment approaches, suggesting their utility for increasing access to care. A number of brief, targeted interventions have been developed to prevent and treat depressive symptoms among children and adolescents.

For instance, LI cognitive behavioural therapy (CBT) can be delivered individually or in a family format involving parents and/or caregivers. The cognitive component of CBT typically consists of identifying and challenging cognitive distortions and automatic thoughts, whereas the behavioural component typically focuses on scheduling values-based, rewarding activities (i.e. behavioural activation), and increasing coping skills in relevant life domains. While CBT may be delivered as a manualized intervention, research suggests flexibility in intervention delivery may yield the best results in children and adolescents (Weisz, Krumholz, Santucci, Thomassin, & Ng, 2015). CBT interventions for youth yield significant reductions in depressive symptoms post treatment and at follow-up (Oud et al., 2019). In addition to the US, CBT has also been found to effectively reduce depression in youth in low- and middle-income countries (Davaasambuu, Hauwadhanasuk, Matsuo, & Szatmari, 2020). Moreover, computerized CBT may reduce symptoms of depression in adolescents (aged 12–18 years), but findings are inconsistent among children (aged 5–11 years; Pennant et al., 2015). Additionally, there is an emerging evidence base for the effectiveness of single-session interventions, both self-administered and administered by a clinician, aimed at youth depressive symptoms (Sung, Dobias, & Schleider, 2020).

Behavioural activation for children and young people

Behavioural activation (BA) is a component of CBT and also a stand-alone, LI intervention with specific effectiveness for children and young people. BA is straightforward to deliver and has comparable efficacy in reducing depressive symptoms relative to individuals receiving a full course of CBT (Gortner, Gollan, Dobson, &

Jacobson, 1998; Jacobson et al., 1996). BA is based on reinforcement models of de-pression, which suggest that as depressed individuals withdraw from valued activ-ities, they lose opportunities for experiencing positive reinforcement, leading to continued disengagement and sustained depression (i.e. the behavioural cycle).

The most central elements of BA include monitoring activities, identifying activities that are personally meaningful and aligned with one's life values, and scheduling these activities into daily life. By re-engaging with valued activities, individuals increase opportunities for positive reinforcement, thus breaking the behavioural cycle that maintains low mood. These elements are at the core of *Brief BA*, which is a time-limited, LI, manualized version of BA (Lejuez, Hopko, Acierno, Daughters, & Pagoto, 2011). Brief BA has been utilized with young people (aged 12–18) in six to eight sessions with additional booster sessions as needed (Pass, Hodgson, Whitney, & Reynolds, 2018) and is both cost- and time-efficient (Richards et al., 2016). Sessions typically take place weekly or twice a week with 'homework' assigned between meetings. Brief BA utilizes a structured ses-sion format, and clinicians are encouraged to create an agenda at the beginning of each session. Sessions typically focus on time with the youth by themselves; however, clinicians should meet with parents/caregivers regularly to engage them in their child's treatment and progress, especially during the first session. As with other evidence-based interventions, Brief BA also encourages the use of regular assessments of symptomology (see suggested evaluation tools, listed at the end of the chapter) to track intervention progress.

Session 1

The first session of the Brief BA programme is focused on helping the youth and their parent/caregiver understand the symptoms of depression and providing general psychoeducation regarding the behavioural cycles that serve to sustain low mood. We suggest that clinicians introduce these ideas by drawing a dia-gram indicating the bidirectional relations between mood, engagement in valued activities, and positive reinforcement (see Appendix). This is also an opportu-nity to begin discussing what activities the youth values and finds enjoyable (e.g. spending time with friends) versus the types of activities the youth may do that don't align with either their values or their interests (e.g. watching TV all night). It is important to validate for the youth that while the concepts underlying Brief BA and the behavioural cycles that maintain depression are relatively easy to un-derstand, the behavioural cycles can be hard to change. By collaborating in this work together, however, it is possible to break out of these behavioural cycles and create a more rewarding life. Session one closes with the identification of specific and measurable goals that the youth has for treatment. It is important to utilize these goals and the first session broadly to instil hope and set expectations of pos-itive outcomes.

Session 2

In the second session, the interventionist introduces activity monitoring, which requires the youth to record the activities they currently do throughout the day (prior to making any concerted effort to change them). While there are a variety of methods for undertaking monitoring (including paper and pencil diaries, see Appendix A), many adolescents report that they prefer utilizing activity monitoring apps available on smartphones and other electronic devices (Dubad, Winsper, Meyer, Livanou, & Marwaha, 2018). It may be helpful to spend time in the session recording at least 1 day of activities to model this approach for the youth. The interventionist would then help the youth rate each event as enjoyable (i.e. whether the youth thought the activity was fun) and/or important (i.e. whether the activity aligns with the youth's values) on a scale from zero to ten. The session closes by linking these activities to the youth's feelings and further illustrating the relation between mood and behaviour.

Session 3

The third session begins by reviewing the youth's activity log from the previous week. Strategies for encouraging non-compliant clients are exemplified in the case study later in this chapter. It is helpful to ask the youth clarifying questions regarding their behaviours and mood over the past week and to reinforce any effort they made to record their activities. The remainder of the session is spent discussing values. It is possible (indeed, probable) that most children or adolescents may not have spent much time thinking about what they value. In that case, we have found that it can be helpful to use activity sheets that divide values into specific life areas, such as 'family/friends', 'spiritual life', etc. (see Appendix B). Youth are then encouraged to identify values across several domains.

Session 4

This session focuses on identifying specific activities that align with the client's previously identified values. It is important to balance the need to generate as many activities as possible across life areas with the necessity of identifying activities that are realistic and feasible. For instance, the youth may report that they value spending time with their family, but it may not be feasible for the family to go out to dinner together every week. In this case, the interventionist should guide the child to pick a variety of activities, including some that are inexpensive or free and easy to implement.

Session 5

Session 5 is, in many ways, is a continuation of the previous session. The focus is still on identifying valued activities, scheduling them into the youth's upcoming week, and then helping the youth reflect on any changes in their mood. However, in this and subsequent sessions, the interventionist and youth will begin 'putting their heads together' to identify specific barriers to completing activities and determining ways to overcome these obstacles. Some of the most common barriers to completing activities include (1) a lack of necessary resources (transportation, money); (2) a lack of necessary support (from parents, friends); and (3) interference from their symptoms of depression (lack of motivation, fatigue). The interventionist should explore with the youth possible solutions and continue to identify and schedule valued activities into their day taking all of the contextual factors outside of the youth's control into account.

Sessions 6 and beyond

The final sessions of the intervention should focus on continuing to support the youth's activity scheduling and mood monitoring. One helpful tool clinicians can introduce is a contract that the youth would make with a supportive person. The youth is encouraged to discuss with this person the rationale for their treatment and identify specific actions that this individual can take to support the youth in engaging in valued activities.

The interventionist will utilize the remainder of their sessions with the youth to continue to identify valued activities, schedule activities, and monitor the youth's behaviours and subsequent mood. Inevitably, the interventionist will need to engage in collaborative problem-solving with the youth to address barriers to completing scheduled activities and other concerns that may arise. Each of the final sessions should also include a focus on maintaining the progress the youth has made and a discussion regarding how to identify if or when the youth should seek further support. By incorporating relapse prevention throughout the final sessions, the interventionist can support the youth in sustaining change following termination.

Brief BA case example: Sarah

Sarah is a 16-year-old girl who presented for therapy after being diagnosed by her general practitioner with major depressive disorder. She reported an extended period of depressed mood and anhedonia, stating that, although she used to enjoy a number of activities and had a large social network, recently she did not feel like doing anything.

The interventionist began the first session by visually depicting to Sarah how feelings and behaviours can impact one another, creating a seemingly endless loop of withdrawal and depressed mood. The interventionist used an example Sarah gave of getting into a fight with a friend to illustrate how Sarah had subsequently felt sad and decided to skip a party she had been looking forward to. They discussed how Sarah then felt even worse when she heard other kids talking about the party in school the next day and decided that she would rather eat lunch by herself so that she didn't have to listen to her peers discuss what she had missed. The interventionist then had Sarah conduct a thought experiment, where she encouraged Sarah to guess what may have happened if she had chosen to go to the party despite feeling sad about the fight with her friend. They reflected on how engaging in something rewarding, like socializing with friends, may have improved Sarah's mood. The interventionist spent the remainder of the session helping Sarah identify her treatment goals and clarifying how they would measure these achievements. Sarah reported that, by the end of the intervention, she wanted to talk to her friends on the phone twice a week and do something with them in person at least once a week.

During the second session, the interventionist explained the rationale for activity monitoring and helped Sarah identify an app on her phone that she could use to record what she was doing, how important and enjoyable these activities were, and how her mood changed in response to each activity. They agreed that Sarah would monitor her activities for 1 week (until the next session) and that if she forgot to record an event, she would simply add it later or (if that was not possible) start recording again the next day.

In the third session, Sarah reported that she had only completed the activity log on 1 day and had forgotten the rest of the week. The interventionist praised Sarah's efforts and validated how difficult it is to monitor one's behaviour every day. They discussed together what worked well to remember to record the activities on the 1 day she recorded them in her log and brainstormed ideas to help her remember to record activities in the future. They agreed that Sarah would set an alarm on her phone to go off at three different times during the day, reminding her to enter her activities into her phone app. Next, they discussed the concept of personal values. The interventionist explained that 'values are things that you think are really important and guide the things you do. Rather than being something you do or achieve, values are like sign-posts—pointing you in the direction that guides your behaviour, like "being a good student"'. Sarah and the interventionist used a worksheet (see Appendix B) to identify values Sarah held across a variety of domains, as well as specific activities that she could do that were in line with each of the values she identified. For homework, Sarah was asked to continue to practise activity monitoring.

In sessions 4 and 5, Sarah worked with the interventionist to add valued activities into her daily schedule. Despite early successes incorporating new and valued behaviours into her week, Sarah and her interventionist noted that she consistently forgot to engage in scheduled activities over the weekend. Using Socratic questioning, the interventionist uncovered that Sarah often spent the weekends alone with her father while her mother travelled for work. Sarah did not feel that her father supported her treatment and she felt he may ridicule her for engaging in activities she valued (like going to hang out with friends). The interventionist gently probed for additional supportive people in Sarah's life and they agreed that Sarah's aunt would be able to help Sarah accomplish her activities. Together, Sarah and her interventionist discussed creating a contract with her aunt, in which they agreed that Sarah would call her for help, and she would be willing to support Sarah in completing the designated activities, including providing transportation as needed.

The final sessions were spent continuing activity scheduling and problem-solving. Sarah and her interventionist also focused on ending treatment and they scheduled time at the end of the last session to discuss the signs and symptoms of depression that would alert the family that Sarah needed to access further help with Sarah's mother. Finally, the interventionist reviewed the symptom checklist Sarah had completed each week and reflected on the changes in depressive symptoms across the course of the intervention.

Challenges and potential solutions to conducting Brief BA with youth

There are a number of inherent challenges to conducting Brief BA with children and young people. These, and some potential solutions, are shown in Table 11.1.

The future of Brief BA for children and young people

Increasing attention is being paid to testing the efficacy of new and innovative models of delivery of Brief BA. For instance, several digital BA-based applications are now available for mobile phones and computers that help individuals to schedule activities and monitor their mood and behaviour. Digital interventions are both time- and cost-efficient and may be specifically appealing to youth; however, relatively few of these tools have been rigorously tested for efficacy (c.f. Dahne et al., 2019) and many become obsolete given rapidly changing technology.

Other research is examining low-tech models for deploying Brief BA using non-specialists, including medical assistants, nurses, and peer recovery specialists. Given the straightforward and time-limited nature of the intervention, Brief BA may be particularly well suited for dissemination by para-professionals. This approach also increases the number and type of settings where Brief BA can be delivered, including health clinics and schools. Additional lines of inquiry are evaluating the utility of these delivery models for increasing access to care for historically underserved, racial/ethnic minority populations.

Table 11.1 Common challenges and potential solutions to implementing Brief BA with youth

Challenge	Possible solutions
Gaining 'buy-in' from youth	• Review the reinforcement model of depression • Increase focus on youths' values and stated interests • Ensure activities are both pleasant and aligned with youths' values
Instrumental barriers to activity engagement	• Include a mix of activities that range from more expensive to free/inexpensive • Have the youth contract with trusted adults to provide necessary resources for engaging in valued activities (transportation, financial support, etc.)
Concerns regarding appropriateness of activities and the its relation to possible need for parental disclosure	• Ensure alignment between activities and values • Discuss the boundaries around confidentiality and the need to reveal session content to parents at treatment onset • Create a mutually agreeable plan for what the therapist and child will reveal to the parent regarding scheduled activities

Chapter summary

Rates of depression dramatically increase from late childhood through adolescence and are associated with a myriad of negative physical and mental health outcomes. Brief BA is a LI intervention that increases youths' engagement with valued activities and disrupts the behavioural cycles that serve to maintain depressive symptoms. Given the expanding evidence base for innovative models of delivering Brief BA, this approach has the potential to reach children and young people who may be less likely to access traditional mental healthcare.

Recommended assessment tools

- Revised Child Anxiety and Depression Scale (RCADS; Chorpita, Yim, Moffitt, Umemoto, & Francis, 2000).
- Child Depression Inventory (CDI; Kovacs, 1981).

Recommended applications for mood/behaviour tracking

- Moodivate (version 2). https://apps.apple.com/ng/app/moodivate/id1518592206

Appendix A. Conceptual Figure of the Relation Between Activity Level and Mood

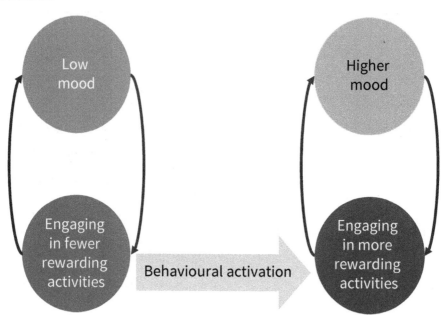

Appendix B. Daily Activity Diary

Time	Activity	Enjoyment (0-10)	Importance (0-10)

Sample completed activity log

Time	Activity	Enjoyment (0-10)	Importance (0-10)
8:00-9:00	Sleep	5	6
9:00–10:00	Facetime friend	6	8
10:00-11:00	Watch TV	4	2
11:00-12:00	Watch TV	2	2
12:00-1:00	Eat lunch	5	5
1:00-2:00	Complete biology homework	4	9
2:00-3:00	Review slides for math test	6	9
3:00-4:00	Talk to mom	9	9
4:00-5:00	Take dog for a walk	8	9
5:00-6:00	Make dinner	5	10
6:00-7:00	Eat dinner with family	8	8
7:00-8:00	Play video games online	9	4
8:00-9:00	Play video games online	6	4
9:00-10:00	Get ready for bed	4	6
10:00-11:00	Sleep	5	6

Appendix C. Life Values Identification Worksheet

Review the life areas in the chart below together:

Physical/psychological well-being
What is important to you about health, exercise, sleep, etc.? What are your mental health goals for this treatment?

Hobbies/Recreation
How do your hobbies contribute to who you are? What passions do you recognize in yourself and in the activities that you enjoy?

Family Relationships
What type of sibling, son/daughter or child do you want to be? What is important to you about family and what qualities make a good family?

Community
What contributions would you like to make to the larger community? Do you enjoy engaging with your community?

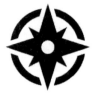

Responsibilities
How do daily responsibilities make you feel accomplished? What role do responsibilities play in your life?

Spirituality
What, if anything, does spirituality mean to you? Are you satisfied with this area of your life?

Education
What are your goals for future education attainment? What kind of student do you want to be?

Social Relationships
What would an ideal friend be like? What do you enjoy and cherish about your friends? How do you engage with friends?

Use the following chart to jot down answers to the questions in the prior chart:

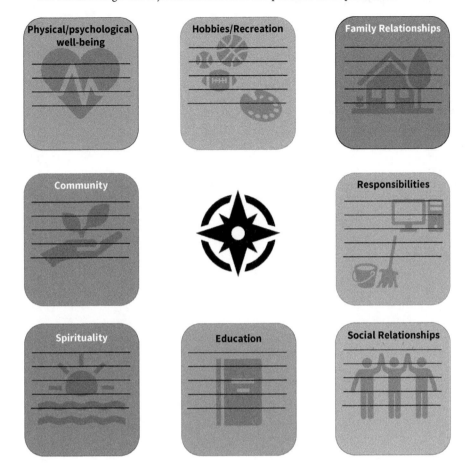

Appendix D. Support Contract

Name a person who can help you do enjoyable / important activities: _____

What is an activity you'd like this person to help you with:

_____

What are the ways this person can help you with this activity:

1. _____

2. _____

3. _____

Recommended reading

Dahne, J., Lejuez, C. W., Kustanowitz, J., Felton, J. W., Diaz, V. A., Player, M. S., & Carpenter, M. J. (2017). Moodivate: A self-help behavioral activation mobile app for utilization in primary care—development and clinical considerations. *International Journal of Psychiatry in Medicine*, *52*(2), 160–175.

Lejuez, C. W., Hopko, D. R., Acierno, R., Daughters, S. B., & Pagoto, S. L. (2011). Ten year revision of the brief behavioral activation treatment for depression: Revised treatment manual. *Behavior Modification*, *35*(2), 111–161.

Martin, F., & Oliver, T. (2019). Behavioral activation for children and adolescents: A systematic review of progress and promise. *European Child & Adolescent Psychiatry*, *28*(4), 427–441.

McCauley, E., Schloredt, K., Gudmundsen, G., Martell, C., & Dimidjian, S. (2011). Expanding behavioral activation to depressed adolescents: Lessons learned in treatment development. *Cognitive and Behavioral Practice*, *18*(3), 371–383.

McCauley, E., Schloredt, K. A., Gudmundsen, G. R., Martell, C. R., & Dimidjian, S. (2016). *Behavioral activation with adolescents: A clinician's guide*. New York: Guilford Publications.

Pass, L., Lejuez, C. W., & Reynolds, S. (2018). Brief behavioural activation (Brief BA) for adolescent depression: A pilot study. *Behavioural and Cognitive Psychotherapy*, *46*(2), 182–194.

Pass, L., Whitney, H., & Reynolds, S. (2016). Brief behavioral activation for adolescent depression: Working with complexity and risk. *Clinical Case Studies*, *15*(5), 360–375.

Reynolds, S., & Pass, L. (2020). *Brief behavioural activation for adolescent depression: A clinician's manual and session-by-session guide*. London: Jessica Kingsley Publishers.

References

Chorpita, B. F., Yim, L., Moffitt, C., Umemoto, L. A., & Francis, S. E. (2000). Assessment of symptoms of DSM-IV anxiety and depression in children: A revised child anxiety and depression scale. *Behaviour Research and Therapy*, *38*(8), 835–855.

Dahne, J., Lejuez, C. W., Diaz, V. A., Player, M. S., Kustanowitz, J., Felton, J. W., & Carpenter, M. J. (2019). Pilot randomized trial of a self-help behavioral activation mobile app for utilization in primary care. *Behavior Therapy*, *50*(4), 817–827.

Dalsgaard, S., Thorsteinsson, E., Trabjerg, B. B., Schullehner, J., Plana-Ripoll, O., Brikell, I., . . ., & Pedersen, C. B. (2020). Incidence rates and cumulative incidences of the full spectrum of diagnosed mental disorders in childhood and adolescence. *JAMA Psychiatry*, *77*(2), 155–164.

Davaasambuu, S., Hauwadhanasuk, T., Matsuo, H., & Szatmari, P. (2020). Effects of interventions to reduce adolescent depression in low-and middle-income countries: A systematic review and meta-analysis. *Journal of Psychiatric Research*, *123*, 201–215.

Dubad, M., Winsper, C., Meyer, C., Livanou, M., & Marwaha, S. (2018). A systematic review of the psychometric properties, usability and clinical impacts of mobile mood-monitoring applications in young people. *Psychological Medicine*, *48*(2), 208–228.

Gortner, E. T., Gollan, J. K., Dobson, K. S., & Jacobson, N. S. (1998). Cognitive–behavioral treatment for depression: Relapse prevention. *Journal of Consulting and Clinical Psychology*, *66*(2), 377–384.

Henry, B., Feehan, M., McGee, R., Stanton, W., Moffitt, T. E., & Silva, P. (1993). The importance of conduct problems and depressive symptoms in predicting adolescent substance use. *Journal of Abnormal Child Psychology*, *21*(5), 469–480.

Jacobson, N. S., Dobson, K. S., Truax, P. A., Addis, M. E., Koerner, K., Gollan, J. K., . . ., & Prince, S. E. (1996). A component analysis of cognitive-behavioral treatment for depression. *Journal of Consulting and Clinical Psychology*, *64*(2), 295.

James, S. L., Abate, D., Abate, K. H., Abay, S. M., Abbafati, C., Abbasi, N., . . ., & Murray, C. J. L. (2018). Global, regional, and national incidence, prevalence, and years lived with disability for 354 diseases

and injuries for 195 countries and territories, 1990–2017: A systematic analysis for the Global
Burden of Disease Study 2017. *Lancet, 392*(10159), 1789–1858.

Jaycox, L. H., Stein, B. D., Paddock, S., Miles, J. N., Chandra, A., Meredith, L. S., . . ., & Burnam, M. A.
(2009). Impact of teen depression on academic, social, and physical functioning. *Pediatrics, 124*(4),
e596–e605.

Kovacs, M. (1981). Rating scales to assess depression in school-aged children. *Acta Paedopsychiatrica,
46*(5–6), 305–315.

Lejuez, C. W., Hopko, D. R., Acierno, R., Daughters, S. B., & Pagoto, S. L. (2011). Ten year revision
of the brief behavioral activation treatment for depression: Revised treatment manual. *Behavior
Modification, 35*(2), 111–161.

Lundh, L.-G., Waangby-Lundh, M., Paaske, M., Ingesson, S., & Bjärehed, J. (2011). Depressive symptoms and deliberate self-harm in a community sample of adolescents: A prospective study. *Depression
Research and Treatment, 2011,* 935871.

Oud, M., De Winter, L., Vermeulen-Smit, E., Bodden, D., Nauta, M., Stone, L., . . ., & Kendall, T. (2019).
Effectiveness of CBT for children and adolescents with depression: A systematic review and meta-
regression analysis. *European Psychiatry, 57,* 33–45.

Pass, L., Hodgson, E., Whitney, H., & Reynolds, S. (2018). Brief behavioral activation treatment for
depressed adolescents delivered by nonspecialist clinicians: A case illustration. *Cognitive and
Behavioral Practice, 25*(2), 208–224.

Pennant, M. E., Loucas, C. E., Whittington, C., Creswell, C., Fonagy, P., Fuggle, P., . . ., & Kendall, T.
(2015). Computerised therapies for anxiety and depression in children and young people: A systematic review and meta-analysis. *Behaviour Research and Therapy, 67,* 1–18.

Pine, D. S., Cohen, E., Cohen, P., & Brook, J. (1999). Adolescent depressive symptoms as predictors of
adult depression: Moodiness or mood disorder? *American Journal of Psychiatry, 156*(1), 133–135.

Reinert, M., Nguyen, T., & Fritze, D. (2021). *The state of mental health in America.* Alexandria,
VA: Mental Health America.

Richards, D. A., Ekers, D., McMillan, D., Taylor, R. S., Byford, S., Warren, F. C., . . ., & Kuyken, W. (2016).
Cost and Outcome of Behavioural Activation versus Cognitive Behavioural Therapy for Depression
(COBRA): A randomised, controlled, non-inferiority trial. *Lancet, 388*(10047), 871–880.

Saluja, G., Iachan, R., Scheidt, P. C., Overpeck, M. D., Sun, W., & Giedd, J. N. (2004). Prevalence of and
risk factors for depressive symptoms among young adolescents. *Archives of Pediatrics & Adolescent
Medicine, 158*(8), 760–765.

Sung, J., Dobias, M. L., & Schleider, J. L. (2020). Single-session interventions: Complementing and
extending evidence-based practice. *Advances in Cognitive Therapy.* Retrieved from: https://www.
academyofct.org/page/AdvancesinCT/Advances-in-Cognitive-Therapy-Newsletter.htm

eisz, J. R., Krumholz, L. S., Santucci, L., Thomassin, K., & Ng, M. Y. (2015). Shrinking the gap between
research and practice: Tailoring and testing youth psychotherapies in clinical care contexts. *Annual
Review of Clinical Psychology, 11,* 139–163.

Zenlea, I. S., Milliren, C. E., Mednick, L., & Rhodes, E. T. (2014). Depression screening in adolescents in
the United States: A national study of ambulatory, office-based practice. *Academic Pediatrics, 14*(2),
186–191.

12

Low intensity interventions for behavioural difficulties

Anna Coughtrey and Sophie D. Bennett

Learning objectives

- To describe the nature and prevalence of behavioural difficulties in children.
- To briefly outline the theories underpinning evidence-based parent programmes for children aged 3–11 years.
- To understand the evidence-base for low intensity parent interventions for prevention and treatment of childhood behavioural difficulties.
- To gain an understanding of which families may benefit from a low intensity parent intervention for common childhood behavioural difficulties.
- To consider what a low intensity evidence-based parent programme may look like in practice.

Introduction

It is normal for young children to experience temper tantrums, whinge, be defiant and non-compliant, to fight with siblings, or to display other problem behaviours such as eating, sleep, and school transition difficulties (Hong, Tillman, & Luby, 2015; Ogundele, 2018). There are many reasons why a child might behave in a way that is seen as challenging by their caregiver(s). Children may be responding and adjusting to a recent traumatic event or adverse childhood experiences, and/or be overwhelmed or dysregulated by their emotions including anger, fear, and anxiety. Such children may have difficulty communicating their needs in appropriate ways. They may seemingly 'act out' simply because they are feeling hungry, tired, frustrated, bored, or overexcited. They may be feeling lonely, unloved, and left out and find that acting with non-compliance and defiance gains them attention. Behaviours in young children are seen as problematic or 'disordered' when the challenging behaviour is beyond what is expected of a child's stage of development, and when the difficulties are severe, persistent, interfere with quality of life, violate societal norms, and cause distress to the child and/or caregiver or another child. Such children are typically not officially diagnosed with oppositional defiant disorder (ODD) or conduct disorder (CD) until they children are over 3–4 years of age (American Psychological Association, 2013; National Institute for Health and Care Excellence [NICE], 2017).

Behavioural difficulties are one of the commonest mental health problems in childhood and reason for referral to services (NICE, 2017; Pilling et al., 2013). Approximately 5–8% of children aged 5–10 years in the UK and the US meet diagnostic criteria for ODD or CD (Green, McGinnity, Meltzer, Ford, & Goodman, 2005; Gutman, Joshi, Parsonage, & Schoon, 2015), and a further 15–20% experience sub-threshold behavioural difficulties that are associated with adverse outcomes in adolescence including increased risk of poor academic achievement, drug and alcohol use, and contact with the criminal justice service (Blair, Leibenluft, & Pine, 2014; Brown, Khan, & Parsonage, 2012; Scott, 2008). Rates are higher in boys than girls (Green et al., 2005; Gutman, Joshi, Parsonage, & Schoon, 2018) and among children from socioeconomically disadvantaged backgrounds (Brown et al., 2012). Other common difficulties associated with behaviour problems include neurodevelopmental conditions such as attention deficit hyperactivity disorder, learning disabilities and language delays, and autism spectrum disorder. Children often present with comorbid behavioural difficulties and recent research has suggested that childhood disruptive behaviour may be best viewed as a multidimensional phenotype rather than distinct subgroups (Bolhuis et al., 2017). The causes of childhood behavioural difficulties are widely accepted as multifactorial (Boden, Fergusson, & Howard, 2010; Brown et al., 2012; NICE, 2017).

Parent training for childhood behavioural difficulties

The recommended intervention for behavioural difficulties in children aged 3–11 years are evidence-based parenting programmes (EBPs) that aim to improve the quality of the parent–child relationship, which is seen as crucial to later pro-social behaviour (NICE, 2017; Scott, Briskman, Woolgar, Humayun, & O'Connor, 2011). Such programmes are typically grounded in cognitive social learning theory (Bandura, 1977) but also draw on theories of coercion (Patterson, Chamberlain & Reid, 1982), attachment (Ainsworth, 1978), parenting style (Baumrind, 1966) and child development (Piaget, 1962). Cognitive social learning theory postulates that children learn behaviours through observation and modelling of significant others (Bandura, 1977). Child behaviour is then inadvertently reinforced through a series of coercive cycles where parental attempts to control or reduce the unwanted child behaviour results in escalation of both parent and child aggression and negative behaviours (Patterson et al., 1982). Such patterns are more likely to develop when parents have an authoritarian and controlling or permissive undemanding parenting style.

Most evidence-based parent training interventions are therefore designed to address parenting practices that have been demonstrated to contribute to the development and maintenance of behavioural difficulties in children aged 3–11 years. As such, parent training interventions are designed to promote authoritative parenting, which is characterized by parental nurturing responsiveness to the child's needs and positive attention for positive behaviours, while clearly communicating limits and boundaries (Baumrind, 1966). Typically these interventions are designed to promote a positive parent–child relationship, through child-directed play methods and focusing parental attention on positive desired behaviour rather than focusing on criticizing unwanted or difficult behaviour, improving communication through clear and consistent descriptions of what the parent wishes the child to do, rather than what not to do, as well as calm and consistent consequences for aggression, and reorganizing family life to prevent trouble and promote success (Leijten et al., 2019; NICE, 2017). Some EBPs are developed specifically based on the developmental cognitive, language, and play stage of the child (e.g. Webster-Stratton, 2016).

Evidence-based parent training interventions for children aged up to 11 years such as the Incredible Years (IY; Webster-Stratton, 2019), Triple P (Sanders, Baker, & Turner, 2012), Helping the Non-Compliant Child (Forehand & McMahon, 1981), and Parent Child Interaction Therapy (Eyberg & Funderburk, 2011) can be delivered in both parent group and individual one-on-one delivery formats in a clinic or home or school. When implemented with fidelity, these programmes have been widely shown to be clinically effective as well as cost-effective in reducing child behaviour problems, promoting positive parenting practices, and improving parental mental health and confidence (Dretzke et al., 2009; Furlong et al., 2012; NICE, 2017; Scott & Gardner, 2015). The evidence base for parent training interventions in children aged 12 years and over is comparatively less well established. Currently, multimodal interventions such as multisystemic therapy are recommended for the treatment of CD and ODD in children aged 12–17 years (NICE, 2017).

It is an alarming fact that despite four decades of research showing the effectiveness of these parenting programmes in reducing child behaviour problems and promoting positive parent–child relationships, they only reach a small fraction of those who could benefit. What stands in the way of increasing the use of parenting programmes to solve one of our most challenging social problems for parents? Barriers to using EBPs include lack of financial resources, resulting in a failure of clinicians to be adequately trained, certified, or supported. In turn, this leads to poor fidelity programme implementation and poor outcomes. Financially constrained agencies search for the 'magic bullet' of a lower-cost intervention that is less comprehensive, requires less training for clinicians to deliver with fidelity, and takes less family or therapist time to complete. Further research is needed to determine the conditions under which shorter EBPs can produce meaningful and sustainable changes and with which populations.

Evidence-base for briefer and lower intensity interventions for preventing childhood behavioural difficulties

Standard EBPs typically involve 10–18 2-hour weekly sessions (Furlong et al., 2013). Most of these interventions have been delivered to high-risk populations and to parents with children diagnosed with ODD or CD. Research with most EBPs has indicated that the longer intervention dosage leads to higher programme outcome effect sizes and more sustainable results. However, shorter and lower intensity prevention interventions may potentially be effective for typical childhood behavioural difficulties, particularly in families that are not at risk for abuse or neglect, do not have high rates of adverse childhood experiences, and/or when such difficulties have not reached the diagnostic threshold for ODD, CD (Sanders, Markie-Dadds, Tully, & Bor, 2000), attention deficit hyperactivity disorder, or other developmental delay. For example, a brief six-session version of the 14- to 18-week IY basic parent programme focusing on positive relationship parenting strategies described on the bottom layers of the IY Parenting Pyramid (i.e. play, coaching, praise, rewards and some limit setting but not timeout, or other discipline consequences, or problem-solving) was evaluated with a control group. Results demonstrated some promising outcomes when used as a universal prevention parenting group intervention in a community setting in Norway. Those receiving the abbreviated IY intervention demonstrated reductions in child behaviour problems and enhancements in positive parenting and parents' sense of competence, which was sustained at 1-year follow-up (Reedtz, Handegård, & Mørch, 2011). This study led to the development of a universal six to ten, 2-hour session parenting programme, called 'Incredible Years Attentive Parenting' for children aged 2–6 years. This programme includes updated video vignettes and covers the basic IY foundational topic sessions of child-directed play, emotion, persistence and social coaching methods, and praise with the addition of strategies to help parents teach children (aged 4–6 years) self-regulation and problem-solving strategies. These latter two topics are added for parents of 4- to 6-year-olds, making the programme eight to ten sessions rather than six sessions for parents of toddlers. Recently, an initial pre-post evaluation demonstrated its effectiveness in a racially diverse US population. Parents who completed the programme in seven to ten sessions reported a significant decrease in conduct problems and an increase in prosocial behaviours in their children (Zhou, Lee, & Ohm, 2021).

A systematic review of self-help interventions for common mental health problems demonstrated that self-help or guided self-help interventions targeting disruptive behaviour were effective, and that the presence of therapist support or guidance may be associated with better outcomes (Bennett et al., 2019). Typically, low intensity (LI) interventions have focused on the use of self-help materials and providing parent books from evidence-based parenting group interventions. For example, parents of 3- to 6-year-olds who read the parent workbook which accompanies the

Helping the Non-Compliant Child therapist manual (*Parenting the Strong-Willed Child*; Forehand & Long, 2002) reported significant decreases in child problem behaviours and found the book useful and easy to implement (Forehand, Merchant, Long, & Garai, 2010). Importantly, the families self-expressed an interest in improving their child's behaviour and children could not be included if they had ever been diagnosed with a mental health disorder. Considering families at greater risk of having a child with behavioural difficulties, Sanders et al. (2000) undertook a study of a ten-session self-directed programme based on the Triple P parent workbook with families with 'at least one adversity factor'(maternal depression, relationship conflict, single-parent household, low gross family income, or low occupational prestige), compared to (1) the parent workbook together with active skills training methods included modelling, role-plays, feedback, and the use of specific homework tasks (standard Triple P); (2) parent workbook, active skills training, partner support and coping skills (enhanced Triple P); or (3) waiting list control. Mothers had to rate their child's behaviour as being in the elevated range on the Eyberg Child Behavior Inventory (ECBI; Eyberg & Ross, 1978) at baseline. At 1-year follow-up there were similar improvements on observational and self-report measures of preschooler disruptive behaviour for enhanced, standard, and self-directed variants of Triple P, although results were not consistent across all outcome measures and the standard and enhanced conditions showed greater reliable improvement on parent-coping disruptive child behaviour (Sanders et al., 2000). There is also evidence that Triple P Online, a self-help web-based adaptation of the original Triple P Positive Parenting Programme encompassing between six and eight self-paced interactive modules each lasting approximately 20 minutes, is effective at reducing child behaviour problems in children demonstrating elevated scores on a standardized measure of behaviour problems (i.e. not necessarily meeting diagnostic criteria for ODD/CD; Baker, Sanders, Turner, & Morawska, 2017; Sanders et al., 2012).

The IY parent book alone has also been compared to the 'basic' IY programme delivered in paediatric primary care by either nurses, or psychologists (Lavigne et al., 2008). Participants were parents of children ages 3–6 years who had ODD. Intervention dosage in the basic IY group was half the usual recommended dosage (2-hour sessions) and was offered either in six 2-hour sessions or 12 1-hour sessions. Results showed significant improvement for all groups, with no overall group differences at 12-month follow-up. However, there was a dose effect, with a reliable, clinically significant gain after *seven and more* therapist-led sessions, compared to no therapist sessions, according to parent reports of behaviour problems, that is, attending seven or more therapist-led sessions was consistently better than self-directed treatment (Lavigne et al., 2008).

Previously, several studies were conducted evaluating the efficacy of a video-based self-administered version of IY basic programme offered in the clinic. In this case, parents of children with ODD were randomly assigned either to (1) an individually self-administered videotape modelling treatment, in which parents watched video vignettes of parenting strategies alone or with their partners using a workbook,

(2) watching the video vignettes in a group with group discussion, (3) a group discussion treatment without video, or (4) to a waiting list control condition. Results indicated the self-administered video-based programme was effective compared to the waiting list control, with fewer parent-reported child behaviour problems and more prosocial behaviours (Webster-Stratton, Kolpacoff, & Hollinsworth, 1988). Greater effects were seen when the video modelling intervention was accompanied by group discussion. This programme delivery was more expensive, as it required a trained group facilitator for the group. The effects of the self-administered delivery method were maintained at 1-year follow-up (Webster-Stratton, Hollinsworth, & Kolpacoff, 1989) but not 3-year follow-up (Webster-Stratton, 1990b). In another study, the addition of two individual in-person consultations with a therapist to the individually self-administered video model resulted in increased parent satisfaction with the individually self-administered intervention compared with the self-administered model without consultation (Webster-Stratton, 1990a). This finding again suggests the importance of some therapist support when offering the self-administered model of learning. However, the individually or self-administered IY programmes were not as effective as the IY model that combined video modelling with therapist-led discussion groups.

In another randomized controlled trial of a home-based IY self-administered basic parent programme (Taylor et al., 2008) parents of children in US 'Head Start' programmes (providing comprehensive early childhood education, health, nutrition, and parent involvement services to low-income children and families) were selected if their children had significant behaviour problems. One group of parents were given computers at home preloaded with the self-administered IY basic parent programme and were instructed how to use it. They also received several home visits with a coach to answer questions. The other randomly selected control parents were given a computer to use at home that did not have the IY basic programme on it. Results suggested that the intervention was effective in working towards parents' identified goals (Taylor et al., 2008). However, analyses indicated no significant differences in observed parenting behaviour between parents in the computer-only condition and those with the computer plus IY programme condition. It seems that a LI, self-administered parenting approach is not sufficient for high-risk populations, who may need the added support of both other parents and a well-trained therapist or IY group leader.

Case example: Emma and Adam

It should be noted that in many cases, such as the example below, the LI intervention for behavioural difficulties is evidence informed, rather than truly evidence based. For example, some services provide individual, LI parenting interventions over a few weeks (as with this example), rather than 18 sessions of 2-hour parent group sessions. There is a need to formally evaluate the impact of these changes on the clinical and cost-effectiveness of the intervention. Similarly, these interventions are increasingly moving online and further research is needed to establish efficacy.

Emma sought help from her GP for support in managing her 5-year-old son Adam's behaviour at home. Emma explained that Adam refused to follow her requests and had daily temper tantrums where he would shout, swear, throw toys, hit furniture, and kick out at her. The behavioural difficulties had started following the birth of Adam's younger sister 3 years previously, when Emma had experienced postnatal depression. Emma described herself as feeling helpless and incompetent when dealing with Adam's behaviour and said that she wished that she could enjoy spending time with her son rather than have daily battles which resulted in her shouting and using empty threats to try and get Adam to follow her requests. She said that she no longer felt confident taking him out of the house as she worried about him having a tantrum in public. No problems were reported at school and Adam's teacher described him as a happy and contented student.

Session 1: psychoeducation and goal setting

The aim of the initial session was to set the stage for sensitive, warm, and nurturing parenting by understanding the multiple factors that contribute to child behaviour. These included Adam's natural temperament, the impact of Emma's own thoughts and behaviour (influenced in part by her own upbringing), and an understanding of the current pattern of moment-to-moment interaction between Emma and Adam which often resulted in an escalation in Adam's challenging behaviour. The therapist and Emma discussed developmentally appropriate child behaviour, and the therapist explained that it is normal for young children to have times when they do not always follow parent's requests, especially after the birth of a sibling and for parents to be frustrated by this. The therapist provided psychoeducation that positive parental attention, non-violent limit setting, and modelling patience, flexibility, and resilience have the biggest impact on improving child behaviour.

The therapist supported Emma to identify her positively phrased treatment goals that would promote prosocial behaviour and positive family relationships rather than focusing on negative behaviour that Emma wanted to eliminate. Collaboratively agreed goals for Emma included (1) for her to be able to effectively implement the instruction for Adam to calmly help tidy his toys away when asked, (2) for Adam and Emma to sit down for 10 minutes three times a week to play together, and (3) for Emma to feel confident to take Adam to the park to play football at the weekend. Emma agreed to monitor Adam's behaviour and her responses over the coming week using the example monitoring sheet (Table 12.1). A home assignment of practice and relevant reading was given.

Table 12.1 Example monitoring sheet

Date/ Time of Day	Situation: What was happening when the behaviour occurred?	Child's Behaviour: What did the child do?	Parent's Response: What did you feel? How did you behave?	Child's Behaviour: What did the child do next?	Comments: Is there anything else that you think contributed to the situation?
Tuesday am	Getting ready to leave for school.	Refused to put shoes on. Messing about playing with Lego.	Shouted. Threatened to put Lego in the bin.	Cried. Put shoes on. Sulked all the way to school.	Tuesday mornings are stressful because I have a weekly meeting with my boss.
Thursday pm	Playing with sister after school before dinner.	Hit sister.	Shouted. Put him in time out.	Ran back into living room and hit sister again.	I was distracted making dinner. He was very tired as he'd been on a school trip all day.

Session 2: the power of child-led play

The therapist explained that child-led play is a powerful part of building strong attachments between family members and promoting warm relationships and that this technique would form the foundation of all future parenting techniques covered in the intervention. The therapist explored Emma's attitude to play and emphasized the opportunity that play gave her for responding to Adam in a way that promoted his feelings of self-worth, competence, and attachment. Emma explained that she had found it hard to find time to play with Adam since his sister was born and he started school, and that she often felt silly when Adam wanted her to engage in imaginative play. The key principles of child-led play were introduced including the opportunity for Emma to give Adam her undivided attention for a short 15-minute period each day, following Adam's interests and imagination rather than using play as an opportunity to teach or correct, avoiding asking questions, and instead being an appreciative audience by describing and commenting on what Adam was doing during play. The therapist explained that Emma's descriptive commenting could be tailored to promote Adam's emotional literacy, for example, by noticing and commenting on the times he felt happy, relaxed, confident, proud, loved, tense, or frustrated and also focusing her attention on the prosocial behaviour that she wanted to see more of, such as Adam allowing his younger sister to join in with some of the play. An in-session role-play practice was used to demonstrate the descriptive commenting technique to Emma and Emma was encouraged to spend 15 minutes each day using descriptive commenting in conjunction with child-led play with Adam. The therapist explained that spending this time together was important even on a 'bad day' as it provided an opportunity for Emma to appreciate Adam's strengths and nurture their positive relationship. Emma was provided with reading material on descriptive commenting and emotion coaching so that she could refer back to these to refresh her memory of the discussion as needed.

Session 3: positive attention, encouragement, and praise

Emma explained that spending 15 minutes using child-led play each day had helped improve their relationship and that she was starting to enjoy being a parent again. To her surprise, she had noticed that Adam had been calmer after playing with her and had fewer angry outbursts. The therapist emphasized the value and importance of continuing to use this technique on a daily basis going forward. The therapist introduced praise as a technique to help Emma to capture the moments where she valued Adam's behaviour (e.g. playing quietly while she was talking on the phone) and to encourage wanted behaviour by focusing on the process not just the final outcome (e.g. praising attempts to tidy up rather than waiting until all the toys were in the box). In order to maximize the effectiveness of praise, Emma and the therapist discussed making praise specific, labelled, and genuine, for example, 'I saw you share your cars with your friend while I was talking on the phone. I felt so proud of you for being so friendly.' The therapist scaffolded Emma to think of a list of possible scenarios where she could use effective praise to give attention to Adam's positive behaviour. Emma was provided with handouts on using praise effectively, to review after the session.

Session 4: rewards and celebrations

Rewards were introduced to help Emma support Adam to engage with homework set by school. Emma said that she had tried using a sticker chart in the past but that it hadn't been successful as Adam often ended up shouting or swearing at her when they were doing homework so she took any stickers he had earned away. The therapist explained that in order to shape behaviour and encourage intrinsic motivation, rewards should emphasize Adam's effort rather than the final outcome and that rewards should never be mixed with punishments or the removal of privileges. Emma and the therapist collaboratively discussed how to set both herself and Adam up for success, for example, by starting with the homework tasks he found most interesting and enjoyable, doing homework at a time when Adam was not tired or hungry, and by making homework as fun as possible. Emma was scaffolded to draw up a list of suitable rewards that could be used in combination with praise to reinforce the progress that Adam was making. For example, 'You've worked so hard on your reading practice this week, you must feel really pleased with the progress you're making. Would you like to choose what we have for dinner tonight so that we can all celebrate how hard you're working?' Emma was provided with handouts on rewards and persistence coaching (i.e. praise and rewards for effort rather than outcome, e.g. being patient, staying calm, concentrating, persisting with something difficult, and trying again).

Session 5: limit setting

Emma and the therapist evaluated both the number and type of commands that she gave to Adam on a daily basis, and identified that, like many parents, Emma was giving many unnecessary commands and prompts to Adam as she was expecting him to refuse to comply. The therapist helped Emma recognize the importance of thinking carefully before giving a command to ensure that it was necessary, and that giving fewer, and more realistic commands about the issues that really mattered would help increase the likelihood of Adam following her requests and provide her with an opportunity to praise him. The therapist introduced the key components of effective commands including giving one single clear, positive, and polite command which clearly detailed the behaviours required and giving the child time to comply. Emma and the therapist discussed ways of rephrasing her common commands to fit these requirements (e.g. 'Put your bricks in the box please' rather than 'Tidy your toys away and come and sit down and eat your tea'). They discussed ways to reduce common power struggles, for example, by focusing on suggestions for what Adam could do rather than commands that left him feeling rigidly prohibited from fun activities (e.g. 'We can't go to the park now because it's time for school, but you can race on your scooter on the way there'). Again, Emma was provided with handouts on 'effective commands' to review after the session.

Session 6: active ignore and review

Emma explained that although Adam's behaviour had improved considerably, he often still whinged and moaned particularly when following her requests (e.g. to tidy up his toys). The therapist introduced the idea of active ignore for these behaviours, with the goal of removing parental attention (and therefore potential reinforcement). The therapist explained that by switching Emma's focus to the alternative behaviours that she wanted to see more of (e.g. tidying away his toys without moaning, putting on his shoes, etc.) she would be creating opportunities for praise and rewards, rather than potentially escalating unwanted behaviours by herself becoming irritated and frustrated. Emma and the therapist discussed how ignore was to be used with a limited number of unwanted behaviours, and was an active process, whereby she would always be on the lookout for an opportunity to re-engage and praise Adam while also ensuring that she was not inadvertently reinforcing the whinging (e.g. by rolling her eyes or looking pointedly at Adam). The therapist explained the importance of consistency with the use of ignore, and prepared her for the fact that sometimes children's behaviour would initially get worse when they did not get the response that they were used to receiving before it got better.

As this was the final session, time was also spent reviewing progress toward goals, with a particular focus on the strategies that Emma had found most useful. Emma was encouraged to keep her notes and handouts together in a folder so that she could easily access them in the future. Possible challenges in the future which may have impacted on Adam's behaviour (e.g. Adam transitioning to a new school year, Emma starting a new job) were discussed and Emma was supported to make a plan to overcome any impact these challenges would have on her ability to continue to implement the techniques that she had learnt over the course of the intervention.

Challenges of implementing brief interventions for behavioural difficulties

Some examples of the common challenges and potential solutions to implementing brief interventions for behavioural difficulties in children are shown in Table 12.2.

The future of LI interventions for behavioural difficulties in children

LI interventions for typical behavioural difficulties in children show promise as a preventive universal parent programme. Further research is needed to develop the evidence base in order to understand how and when such interventions can be most effectively implemented, with whom, and what intervention dosage is needed. Given the widely accepted view that, if left untreated, children with behavioural difficulties are at increased risk of continued emotional, behavioural, and social negative consequences throughout adolescence and into adulthood, future research should focus on the role LI interventions could play in the prevention of disruptive behaviour with a particular focus on long-term follow-up of children and families. More work is needed to understand the impact of such interventions on broader outcomes, such as parental mental health, and to determine whether such interventions can be suitably personalized for children with comorbid physical health conditions or neurodevelopmental disorders. A number of programmes, such as IY and Triple P, are now being delivered remotely online, either with groups of parents and/or individually. IY videos are being streamed and used for IY group leader-led online discussions and setting up online practices. It is possible that future models could adopt a hybrid 'blended' approach through accessing streamed materials and remotely delivered therapeutic support (Erbe, Eichert, Riper, & Ebert, 2017) combined with some 'in-person' group or individual meetings.

Chapter summary

Behavioural difficulties in children are common and sometimes associated with significant short- and long-term difficulties. There is promising initial evidence

Table 12.2 Common challenges and potential solutions to implementing LI parent training interventions for children with behavioural difficulties

Challenge	Possible solutions
The parent(s) believes that the problem lies within the child and that the child should be receiving the intervention rather than the parent	• Allow parent(s) time to explain the difficulties faced by the family and encourage them to identify and name their thoughts and feelings about their child • Take a non-blaming, non-judgemental stance. Explain that the purpose of the intervention is to help parents find what works best for them and their child(ren) and that the parent is viewed as an expert on their child • Focus on parent, child, and family strengths and collaboratively explore how the strategies can help expand and build on these strengths • Instill hope and remind parent(s) that they can change their own thoughts, feelings, and behaviour. Explore the impact that these changes would then have on both the child and the wider family
The parent(s) wants to start with techniques that focus on reducing unwanted behaviour rather than introducing child-led play	• Normalize parent(s) viewpoint. Many will have already heard of or tried the strategies in the intervention. The role of the therapist is to help the parent(s) adjust the strategies so that they are successful in reaching their goals • Use in-session role-plays to demonstrate to the parent(s) the power of child-led play, praise, and rewards • Explain the theoretical background and evidence for improving the parent–child relationship and how this forms the foundation for other strategies covered later in the intervention
The parent(s) struggle to find time to implement the strategies consistently at home	• Understand the barrier(s) faced by the parent(s), e.g. lack of time, other parent/caregiver(s) dismissive of approach • Collaboratively generate practical solutions, e.g. using child-led play when other siblings are at school or napping

that brief and LI interventions including guided self-help and self-administered approaches in clinics or homes are effective in promoting positive parent–child relationships and proactive parental discipline. Further research is needed to understand who these interventions are suitable for (e.g. considering severity of behavioural difficulties and complexity of family circumstances). Research also needs to investigate how to optimize delivery of LI parent self-directed interventions for behavioural difficulties to ensure prevention of future antisocial behaviour into adolescence and beyond.

Recommended measures

- Brief parental self-efficacy scale: https://www.corc.uk.net/media/1279/brief-parental-self-efficacy-scale.pdf
- Child Behaviour Checklist (Achenbach, 1999; Achenbach & Edelbrock, 1983).

- Eyberg Child Behavior Inventory (Eyberg & Ross, 1978; Robinson, Eyberg, & Ross, 1980).

Recommended reading

Forehand, R. L., & Long, N. (2002). *Parenting the strong-willed child* (2nd ed.). New York: McGraw-Hill.
Forehand, R. L., & McMahon, R. J. (1981). *Helping the non-compliant child*. New York: Guilford Press.
Perry, P. (2019). *The book you wish your parents had read (and your children will be glad that you did).* London: Penguin Random House.
Sanders, M. R., Kirby, J. N., Tellegen, C. L., & Day, J. J. (2014). The Triple P-Positive Parenting Program: A systematic review and meta-analysis of a multi-level system of parenting support. *Clinical psychology review, 34*(4), 337–357.
Webster-Stratton, C. (2012). *Collaborating with parents to reduce children's behavior problems: A book for therapists using the Incredible Years programs*. Seattle, WA: Incredible Years Inc.
Webster-Stratton, C. (2019). *The incredible years: A trouble shooting guide for parents of children aged 2–8 years* (3rd ed.). Seattle, WA: Incredible Years Inc.

References

Achenbach, T. M. (1999). The Child Behaviour Checklist and related instruments. In M. E. Maruish (Ed.). *The use of psychological testing for treatment planning and outcomes assessment* (pp. 429–266). Mahwah, NJ: Lawrence Erlbaum Associates Publishers.
Achenbach, T. M., & Edelbrock, C. S. (1983). *Manual for the Child Behaviour Checklist and Revised Child Behaviour Profile*. Burlington, VT: University Associates in Psychiatry.
Ainsworth, M. D. S. (1978). The Bowlby–Ainsworth attachment theory. *Behavioural and Brain Sciences, 1,* 436–438.
American Psychiatric Association. (2013). *Diagnostic and statistical manual of mental disorders* (5th ed.). Arlington, VA: American Psychiatric Association.
Baker, S., Sanders, M. R., Turner, K. M. T., & Morawska, A. (2017). A randomised controlled trial evaluating a low-intensity interactive online parenting intervention, Triple P Online Brief, with parents of children and early onset conduct problems. *Behaviour Research and Therapy, 91,* 78–90.
Bandura, A. (1977). Self-efficacy: Toward a unifying theory of behavioural change. *Psychological Review, 84*(2), 191–215.
Baumrind, D. (1966). Effects of authoritative parental control on child behaviour. *Child Development, 37*(4), 887–907.
Bennett, S. D., Cuijpers, P., Ebert, D. D., McKenzie Smith, M., Coughtrey, A. E., Heyman, I., . . ., & Shafran, R. (2019). Unguided and guided self-help interventions for common mental health disorders in children and adolescents: A systematic review and meta-analysis. *Journal of Child Psychology and Psychiatry, 60*(8), 828–847.
Berkovits, M. D., O'Brien, K. A., Carter, C. G., & Eyberg, S. M. (2010). Early identification and intervention for behaviour problems in primary care: A comparison of two abbreviated versions of parent-child interaction therapy. *Behaviour Therapy, 41*(3), 375–387.
Blair, R. J., Leibenluft, E., & Pine, D. S. (2014). Conduct disorder and callous-unemotional traits in youth. *New England Journal of Medicine, 372*(8), 784–2216.
Boden, J. M., Fergusson, D. M., & Howard, L. J. (2010). Risk factors for conduct disorder and oppositional/defiant disorder: Evidence from a New Zealand birth cohort. *Journal of American Academy of Child and Adolescent Psychiatry, 49*(11), 1125–1133.

Bolhuis, K., Lubke, G. H., ven der Ende, J., Bartels, M., van Beijsterveldt, C. E. M., . . ., & Tiemeier, H. (2017). Disentangling heterogeneity of childhood disruptive behaviour problems into dimensions and subgroups. *Journal of the American Academy of Child and Adolescent Psychiatry, 56*, 687–686.

Brown, E. R., Khan, L., & Parsonage, M. (2012). *A chance to change: Delivering effective parenting programmes to transform lives.* London: Centre for Mental Health.

Dretzke, J., Davenport, C., Frew, E., Barlow, J., Stewart-Brown, S., Bayliss, S., Taylor, R., Sandercock, J. and Hyde, C. (2009). The clinical effectiveness of different parenting programmes for children with conduct problems: A systematic review of randomised controlled trials. *Child and Adolescent Psychiatry and Mental Health, 3*(1), 1–10.

Erbe, D., Eichert, H. C., Riper, H., & Ebert, D. D. (2017). Blending face-to-face and internet-based interventions for the treatment of mental disorders in adults: Systematic review. *Journal of Medical Internet Research, 19*(9), e306.

Eyberg, S. M., & Funderburk, B. W. (2011). *Parent–child interaction therapy protocol.* Gainesville, FL: PCIT International.

Eyberg, S. M., & Ross, A. W. (1978). Assessment of child behaviour problems: The validation of a new inventory. *Journal of Clinical Psychology, 7*(2), 113–116.

Forehand, R. L., & Long, N. (2002). *Parenting the strong-willed child* (2nd ed.). New York: McGraw-Hill.

Forehand, R. L., & McMahon, R. J. (1981). *Helping the non-compliant child.* New York: Guilford Press.

Forehand, R. L., Merchant, M. J., Long, N., & Garai, E. (2010). An examination of parenting the strong-willed child as bibliotherapy for parents. *Behaviour Modification, 34*, 57–76.

Furlong, M., McGilloway, S., Bywater, T., Hutchings, J., Smith, S. M., & Donnelly, M. (2012). Behavioural and cognitive-behavioural group-based parenting programmes for early-onset conduct problems in children aged 3–12 years. *Evidence Based Child Health: A Cochrane Review Journal, 2*, 318–692.

Green, H., McGinnity, A., Meltzer, H., Ford, T., & Goodman, R. (2005). *Mental health of children and young people in Great Britain, 2014.* Basingstoke: Palgrave Macmillan.

Gutman, L. M., Joshi, H., Parsonage, M., & Schoon, I. (2015). *Children of the new century: Mental health findings from the Millennium Cohort Study.* London: Centre for Mental Health.

Gutman, L. M., Joshi, H., Parsonage, M., & Schoon, I. (2018). Gender-specific trajectories of conduct problems from ages 3–11. *Journal of Abnormal Child Psychology, 46*(7), 1467–1480.

Hong, J. S., Tillman, R., & Luby, J. L. (2015). Disruptive behaviour in preschool children: Distinguishing normal misbehaviour from markers of current and later childhood conduct disorder. *Journal of Pediatrics, 166*(3), 723–730.

Lavigne, J. V., Lebailly, S. A., Gouze, K. R., Cicchetti, C., Pochyly, J., Arend, R., . . ., & Binns, H. J. (2008). Treating oppositional defiant disorder in primary care: A comparison of three models. *Journal of Pediatric Psychology, 33*(5), 449–461.

Leijten, P., Gardner, F., Melendez-Torres, G. J., van Aar, J., Hutchings, J., Schulz, S., . . ., & Overbeek, G. (2019). Meta analyses: Key parenting programme components for disruptive child behaviour. *Journal of American Academy of Child and Adolescent Psychiatry, 58*(2), 180–190.

National Institute for Health and Care Excellence. (2017). *Antisocial behaviour and conduct disorders in children and young people: Recognition and management.* London: National Institute for Health and Care Excellence.

Ogundele, M. O. (2018). Behavioural and emotional disorders in childhood: A brief overview for paediatricians. *World Journal of Clinical Pediatrics, 7*(1), 9–26.

Patterson, G. R., Chamberlain, P., & Reid, J. B. (1982). A comparative evaluation of a parent-training programme. *Behaviour Therapy, 13*(5), 638–650.

Piaget, J., & Inhelder, B. (1962). *The psychology of the child.* New York: Basic Books.

Pilling, S., Gould, N., Whittington, C., Taylor, C., Scott, S., & Guideline Development Group. (2013). Recognition, intervention, and management of antisocial behaviour and conduct disorders in children and young people: Summary of NICE-SCIE guidance. *BMJ, 346*, 33–37.

Reedtz, C., Handegård, B. H., & Mørch, W.-T. (2011). Promoting positive parenting practices in primary pare: Outcomes and mechanisms of change in a randomized controlled risk reduction trial. *Scandinavian Journal of Psychology, 52*(2), 131–137.

Robinson, E. A., Eyberg, S. M., & Ross, A. W. (1980). The standardisation of an inventory of child conduct problem behaviours. *Journal of Clinical Child Psychology, 9*(1), 22–28.

Sanders, M. R., Baker, S., & Turner, K. M. (2012). A randomised controlled trial evaluating the efficacy of Triple P Online with parents of children with early-onset conduct problems. *Behaviour Research and Therapy*, *50*(11), 675–684.

Sanders, M. R., Bor, W., & Morawska, A. (2007). Maintenance of treatment gains: A comparison of enhanced, standard, and self-directed Triple P-Positive Parenting Program. *Journal of Abnormal Child Psychology*, *35*(6), 983–998.

Sanders, M. R., Markie-Dadds, C., Tully, L. A., & Bor, W. (2000). The triple P-positive parenting programme: A comparison of enhanced, standard, and self-directed behavioural family intervention for parents of children with early onset conduct problems. *Journal of Consulting and Clinical Psychology*, *68*(4), 624–640.

Sanders, M. R., Markie-Dadds, C., & Turner, K. M. T. (2012). *Practitioner manual for standard Triple P* (2nd ed.). Brisbane: Triple P International.

Scott, S. (2008). An update on interventions for conduct disorder. *Advances in Psychiatric Treatment*, *14*(1), 61–70.

Scott, S., Briskman, J., Woolgar, M., Humayun, S., & O'Connor, T. G. (2011). Attachment in adolescence: Overlap with parenting and unique prediction of behavioural adjustment. *Journal of Child Psychology and Psychiatry*, *52*(10), 1052–1062.

Scott, S., & Gardner, F. (2015). Parenting programs. *Rutter's Child and Adolescent Psychiatry*, 483–495. https://onlinelibrary.wiley.com/doi/abs/10.1002/9781118381953.ch37

Taylor, T. K., Webster-Stratton, C., Feil, E. G., Broadbent, B., Widdop, C. S., & Severson, H. H. (2008). Computer-based intervention with coaching: An example using the Incredible Years programme. *Cognitive Behaviour Therapy*, *37*(4), 233–246.

Webster-Stratton, C. (1990a). Enhancing the effectiveness of self-administered videotape parent training for families with conduct-problem children. *Journal of Abnormal Child Psychology*, *18*(5), 479–492.

Webster-Stratton, C. (1990b). Long-term follow-up of families with young conduct problem children: From preschool to grade school. *Journal of Clinical Child Psychology*, *19*(2), 144–149.

Webster-Stratton, C., Hollinsworth, T., & Kolpacoff, M. (1989). The long-term effectiveness and clinical significance of three cost-effective training programmes for families with conduct-problem children. *Journal of Consulting and Clinical Psychology*, *57*(4), 550–553.

Webster-Stratton, C., Kolpacoff, M., & Hollinsworth, T. (1988). Self-administered videotape therapy for families with conduct problem children: Comparison with two cost-effective treatments and a control group. *Journal of Consulting and Clinical Psychology*, *56*(4), 558–566.

Webster-Stratton, C. (2016). The incredible years: Use of play interventions and coaching for children with externalizing difficulties. In L. A. Reddy, T. M. Files-Hall, & C. E. Schaefer (Eds.), *Empirically based play interventions for children* (pp. 137–158). American Psychological Association. https://doi.org/10.1037/14730-008

Webster-Stratton, C. (2019). *The Incredible Years: A trouble shooting guide for parents of children aged 2–8 years* (3rd ed.). Seattle, WA: Seattle Incredible Years Inc.

Zhou, X., Lee, R. M., & Ohm, J. (2021). Evaluating the feasibility of the Incredible Years attentive parenting programme as universal prevention for racially diverse populations. *Journal of Prevention and Health Promotion*, *2*(1), 32–56.

13

Low intensity interventions for sleep problems in children and adolescents

Dimitri Gavriloff, Felicity Waite, and Colin A. Espie

Learning objectives

- To be able to describe the processes by which sleep is regulated.
- To understand how sleep changes across childhood and adolescence.
- To be able to recommend healthy sleep habits for children and young people and explain their theoretical rationale.
- To be able to implement evidence-based low intensity cognitive behavioural interventions for child and adolescent sleep problems.

Introduction

Sleep plays a foundational role in human development (Ednick et al., 2009) and is associated with a range of active processes crucial to optimal human function. These include those associated with *physical health*, such as facilitating metabolic processes (Van Cauter, Spiegel, Tasali, & Leproult, 2008) and clearance of metabolic waste from the brain (Xie et al., 2013); *cognitive functioning*, such as learning and memory consolidation (Diekelmann & Born, 2010; Stickgold, 2005); and *mental health* including emotional regulation (Palmer & Alfano, 2017). There are two key processes which regulate sleep: (1) the accumulation of sleepiness across periods of wakefulness, known as 'sleep pressure'; and (2) the timing of our circadian rhythm, known as the 'body clock' (Borbély et al., 1982, 2016). Put simply, the longer we maintain wakefulness, the more 'debt' we owe to sleep and the higher pressure there is to fall asleep. Crucially, this pressure to sleep is offset by alertness, mediated by the circadian process. This alertness builds during the biological morning and peaks in the middle of the day, waning as the day and evening progress. It is signals from the external environment, principally cycles of light and dark, but also temperature change, as well as regularity of behavioural patterns that synchronize our circadian rhythm with the world around us. Attempts to sleep when either sleep pressure is insufficient (e.g. following a late afternoon nap) or circadian alertness is too high (e.g. too early in the evening), result in sleep difficulties. Additionally,

sleep can be disrupted by hyperarousal and the activation of the acute stress response, particularly associated with pre-sleep worry and sleep effort (i.e. *trying
to get to sleep*).

Not only do children and adolescents have a need for more sleep than their
parents, but the nature and timing of their sleep is subject to dynamic change
across the developmental trajectory. Very young children will actually spend more
time asleep than awake across a 24-hour period, doing so in relatively brief blocks
throughout the day and night (Coons & Guilleminault, 1984). This begins to consolidate into longer blocks of predominantly nocturnal sleep as the infant's circadian rhythm becomes established by the age of around 3 months (Lodemore,
Petersen, & Wailoo, 1991; Rivkees, 2003). During infancy and toddlerhood, these
higher sleep needs are achieved with earlier nightly sleep onset supplemented by
periods of daytime napping (Henderson, France, Owens, & Blampied, 2010), from
which children generally wean at preschool age (Staton et al., 2020). As children
continue to develop, the number of hours of sleep they need reduces, such that the
10–13 hours needed by most preschoolers reaches a range of between 8 and 10
hours by adolescence (Hirshkowitz et al., 2015; Paruthi et al., 2016) (Table 13.1).
Crucially, however, the timing of the circadian rhythm also begins to delay during
early adolescence (meaning teenagers don't feel sleepy until later at night and then
wake later the next day). The onset of the nocturnal sleep period may be considerably later for many teenagers when compared to those of their parents and younger
siblings (Roenneberg et al., 2007).

Sleep disorders are commonly seen in children and young people (Owens, 2008),
although they are generally underdiagnosed in clinical settings (Meltzer, 2010).
Insomnia disorder, regular and persistent difficulties falling asleep or staying asleep
that affect daytime performance, is by far the most common sleep problem experienced by children, young people, and their parents (Mindell, Li, Sadeh, Kwon,
& Goh, 2015). Importantly, insomnia may present in considerably different ways
across the age range, with children and young people each employing distinctive
strategies for its management. Younger children, for instance, may display bedtime

Table 13.1 Recommended sleep durations by age

Age range	Recommended (hours)	May be appropriate (hours)
Newborn (0–3 months)	14–17	11–19
Infant (4–11 months)	12–15	10–18
Toddler (1–2 years)	11–14	9–16
Preschool (3–5 years)	10–13	8–14
School age (6–13 years)	9–11	7–12
Teen (14–18 years)	8–10	7–11

Data from Hirshkowitz et al. (2015).

resistance, insistence on parental presence at bedtime, calling out for parents to re-settle them at night, and tantrums when left on their own. Conversely, adolescents may try and find other activities (such as using their smartphone, video gaming, or talking with friends) to either pass the time or distract themselves from their diffi-culties with sleep initiation (Hale & Guan, 2015).

Understanding what underpins the presenting problem is a crucial first step in informing optimal treatment approaches. In younger children, sleep problems are often perpetuated by the development of unhelpful sleep-onset associations (Owens, 2008), which typically require the caregiver's involvement in the facilitation of sleep onset (e.g. presence, rocking, patting). The difficulty is that once established, the stimulus and con-text is again required to facilitate sleep re-initiation when the child wakes briefly at night following natural cycling through the different stages of sleep (Honaker & Metzler, 2014). Other important factors that contribute to why some children may take a long time to fall asleep include being put to bed at a time that is incompatible with their own endogenous circadian timings (LeBourgeois, Wright, LeBourgeois, & Jenni, 2013), problems with parental limit setting (Owens, 2008), and absence of consistent bed-time routines (Mindell & Owens, 2015; Mindell & Williamson, 2018). Insomnia can also be associated with poor sleep hygiene practices, such as a child's or young person's use of caffeine (e.g. through soft drinks, energy drinks), inappropriate sleep schedules (e.g. schedules with high night-to-night variability, consistent staying up, or sleeping in late), or use of technology at inappropriate times (e.g. playing video games with friends before bed). Social and environmental factors are also important elements for consid-eration and household light, noise, and temperature can all influence sleep continuity. In adolescents and older children, pre-sleep psychophysiological arousal (i.e. being on edge, alert, worrying, etc.) is likely to play a larger part in the sleep problem, as are dis-ruptions to positive associations between bed and sleep.

The consequences of chronic poor sleep in children and young people are sig-nificant and have been shown to negatively impact a wide range of domains that include behaviour, emotion regulation and mood, neurocognitive function, and educational outcomes (Beebe, 2011; Cook et al., 2020; Miller, 2015; Mindell et al., 2016; Owens, Adolescent Sleep Working Group, & Committee on Adolescence, 2014; Sadeh, Gruber, & Raviv, 2002; Sadeh, Tikotzky, & Kahn, 2014; Williamson, Mindell, Hiscock, & Quach, 2020). Children and adolescents who experience per-sistent difficulties in getting to sleep or in returning to sleep if they wake up during the night are at a much higher risk of developing a range of mental health difficulties, including depression and anxiety (Blank et al., 2015), as well as a higher risk of sui-cidality (Goldstein, Bridge, & Brent, 2008).

Assessment and formulation

Typically, current patterns of sleep and wake are assessed using a sleep diary (Table 13.2), ideally over a 2-week period. The detail of the items included in the diary will vary according to the age of the child but usually include core information on when the child got into bed, how long it took them to fall asleep, how many times they woke during the night, how long in total those awakenings lasted, the time at which they woke in the morning (i.e. and didn't return to sleep), when they got out of bed, and their total sleep time. Additionally, information on pre-bed behaviour such as the timing and structure of bedtime routines, parental involvement in settling or resettling, and any illness or current stressors can be included in the notes of the diary to give context to the data. A full clinical history that includes information on precipitants, sleep history, developmental history, any previous treatment, physical and mental health, daytime sequelae, other sleep symptoms, behavioural assessment of the sleep problem, and impact on the family and the schooling and social relationships of the young person should underpin assessment of the sleep problem. Helping both children and parents explore the nature of the sleep problem and the range of perspectives on it can be a helpful means of encouraging lasting behaviour change. Screening questionnaires designed for use in paediatric populations include the Brief Infant Sleep Questionnaire (0–3 years; Sadeh, 2004), the Children's Sleep Habits Questionnaire (3–12 years; Owens, Spirito, & McGuinn, 2000) and the Sleep Self Report (Owens et al., 2000) for adolescents.

There are several theoretical models of insomnia, originally developed for adults, that can be helpful for conceptualizing sleep problems, particularly in older children and adolescents (Espie, Broomfield, MacMahon, Macphee, & Taylor, 2006; Harvey, 2002). Although also developed in relation to adult sleep, the diathesis–stress, '3 P' model developed by Spielman, Caruso, and Glovinsky (1987) is easily articulated and can be used to effectively illustrate where treatment should be targeted. In this model, sleep problems are understood to develop based upon an individual's *predisposition* to poor sleep (e.g. psychological disposition, neurodevelopmental attributes, genetics, home environment). *Precipitants* (e.g. life-stressors, transitions, developmental milestones, environmental change) may result in acute sleep disturbance. This sleep disturbance is then *perpetuated* by changes to cognitions and behaviours that are typically aimed at short-term mitigation of the problem but have the unintended consequence of keeping things stuck (e.g. parental involvement in settling the child to sleep, daytime worry about sleep, night-to-night variability in sleep patterns). Collaboratively identifying perpetuating factors is a cornerstone of effective assessment.

Setting the scene: healthy sleep practices

A comprehensive approach to the management of sleep problems in children and young people starts with an appreciation of the foundations upon which good sleep is built. Often referred to as 'sleep hygiene' (Hauri, 1977), clinical advice on healthy sleep practices typically focuses on creating an appropriate environment for sleep, and optimizing sleep-promoting behaviours (see Allen, Howlett, Coulombe, &

Table 13.2 Sample sleep diary

Today's date	3/4/22							
1. If your child has napped today, when did they nap and for how long?	1 nap at 1 pm for 1 hour and 30 mins							
2. What time did your child go to bed at night?	7:30 pm							
3. What time did they fall asleep?	7:45 pm							
4. How long did it take them to fall asleep?	15 mins							
5. Did they wake during the night? If so: What time did they wake? What did they do? How did you/partner respond? How long did it take child to resettle?	Yes 9 pm: cried loudly for 5 mins and then resettled herself 11 pm: as above 1 am: crying—gave a bottle (30 mins to resettle)							
6. What time did they wake for the day? What woke them? What did they do?	6 am: woke spontaneously. Came into bed with us, went back to sleep							

Table 13.2 continued'

7. What time did they get out of bed to start the day?	7.15 am						
8. How would you rate the quality of their sleep?	☐ Very poor ☑ Poor ☐ Fair ☐ Good ☐ Very good	☐ Very poor ☐ Poor ☐ Fair ☐ Good ☐ Very good	☐ Very poor ☐ Poor ☐ Fair ☐ Good ☐ Very good	☐ Very poor ☐ Poor ☐ Fair ☐ Good ☐ Very good	☐ Very poor ☐ Poor ☐ Fair ☐ Good ☐ Very good	☐ Very poor ☐ Poor ☐ Fair ☐ Good ☐ Very good	☐ Very poor ☐ Poor ☐ Fair ☐ Good ☐ Very good
10. Comments/notes (if applicable)	Very hot in her room due to weather						

Corkum, 2016, for recommendations and their respective rationales and evidence bases). Rather than a prescriptive list of practices by which parents and their children should passively abide, explanation of the rationale for why these practices are recommended is crucial in promoting successful engagement. This enables young people and caregivers to adapt the strategies when needed, within the spirit of the guideline (e.g. managing bedtimes of multiple children, limited living space). Additionally, it can help to reduce misunderstandings which perpetuate challenging parent–child dynamics (e.g. those experienced by parents unable to wake a child in time for school).

Creating the right environment for sleep

Keep the bedroom dark, quiet, and cool: our circadian evolution has geared humans towards being active and alert during the day and being inactive and to sleep at night. The night-time environment is one that is darker, quieter, and cooler than it is during the day. A useful place to start in terms of setting up a bedroom is by seeking to replicate these external night-time characteristics. Light has a powerful influence over our circadian process and stimulates alertness. Keeping the bedroom dark is, therefore, very important. Use of a night light is fine if it helps the child feel calm (i.e. reduces hyperarousal/anxiety) and aids sleep. If external morning or evening light is an issue, then use of blackout blinds may be sensible. At night, our core body temperature drops by a couple of degrees following its natural circadian rhythm. Keeping the bedroom cool (approximately 18°C), while ensuring that the child has adequate warm and appropriate bedding, allows this to happen and prevents sleep disturbance as a result of being too hot.

    Make the bedroom an oasis for sleep: just as we might associate sitting at the dining table with eating dinner, it is important to ensure that beds and bedrooms are associated with sleep. In an ideal world, this means only using bed for sleep, but in practice, this can be tricky. The association can often become confused if the bedroom is generally used for stimulating things which might interfere with sleep, such as watching television, playing video games, or when the bedroom is used as a place of punishment by caregivers. Furthermore, use of electronic devices has been shown to 'displace' sleep and may even take the place of a healthy bedtime routine. It is often a good idea to gently remove things which interfere with sleep, but important to also find space and time for their use elsewhere so that the child does not feel at a disadvantage. Recommendations will, of course, be tailored to the needs of the individual but might include suggesting that teenagers doing their homework somewhere other than their bedroom or giving children a designated and comfortable place in the house in which to rest and relax undisturbed. Another approach is to frame this with children and young people as a behavioural experiment, where hypotheses may include whether or not removing electronics from the bedroom helps sleep. When unable to get to sleep, having a beanbag or comfortable chair in the room on which to sit and read, rather than lying in bed awake, is another useful way to keep bed and wakefulness separate. The bedroom should represent a pleasant and calming place in which the child or young person feels comfortable when awake and relaxed when going to sleep.

Sleep-promoting behaviours

Getting up at the same time each day: ensuring that children wake at approximately the same time each morning, whether weekend or weekday, is an important means of regulating sleep–wake patterns and avoiding excessive night-to-night variability in sleep timings. Adolescents experience a natural delay in their circadian rhythms during this developmental period and many may start going to bed much later than they previously did as children (Roenneberg et al., 2007). This natural delay coupled with the need to rise early in the morning for school often means that many teenagers experience insufficient sleep throughout the week and so will sleep in later on the weekends. As such, sleeping in on weekends should be allowed if needed but should be limited to no later than approximately 10:00 am. Where this delay is more extreme and leading to problems with daytime functioning (particularly during the week), it may be a sign of a delayed sleep–wake phase disorder and warrants specialist assessment and treatment.

Bright mornings and dim evenings: light plays a central role in the daily synchronization of our circadian rhythms with our external environment. It is, in the main, morning light's effect on the body clock that maintains the rhythm and predictability of the timing of sleep–wake phases from day to day. Making sure children get regular morning exposure to sunlight is important in helping to maintain circadian rhythmicity, suppressing melatonin secretion, and increasing alertness. By contrast, avoiding evening light exposure and maintaining a dim light environment before bed encourages secretion of melatonin and reduces alertness.

Maintain a consistent bedtime and bedtime routine: consistent bedtime routines are associated with both better sleep and better daytime behaviour (Mindell et al., 2015; Mindell & Williamson, 2018). Regular bedtime routines offer a strong behavioural cue for sleep and give the child an opportunity to drop out of the active daytime state and into a more relaxed state that is conducive to sleep. Bedtime routines should typically consist of three or four calm activities that take place in the same order and at around the same time each night. Typical elements of a bedtime routine might include having a bath or shower, brushing teeth, reading a story, or being read a story by a parent, and a brief goodnight kiss or cuddle. For adolescents and older children, this might include a period of independent reading or listening to music. Bedtime routines should avoid any activities which are likely to result in stimulation (e.g. texting friends, videos, smartphone use, video gaming) that will impede sleep onset. As children develop, the timings of the bedtime routine may start to delay in line with their sleep need and circadian preference. In younger children, watching for signs of being ready for sleep (e.g. yawning, rubbing eyes, slowing down) is important, and bedtimes that are age inappropriate may contribute to difficulty settling (LeBourgeois et al., 2013). In adolescence, this can often become an explicit sticking point for families and negotiation of a quiet period before bed and a later bedtime may be more helpful than enforcing an earlier one.

Keep to an age-appropriate nap schedule: young children require naps to supplement night-time sleep. However, most children have begun to discontinue their daytime napping by around the age of 3 years. Resumption of daytime napping for children who have already discontinued their naps is likely to make sleep more difficult at night (also see 'Other common sleep problems').

Avoid caffeine and stimulants: caffeine, and other stimulants, are readily found in many commonly consumed energy drinks and soft drinks. When ingested, caffeine has the ability to temporarily alleviate, or obscure, sleepiness through its effects on several neurotransmitters involved in sleep. This disruption can be relatively long-lasting due to its elimination half-life of between 3 and 7 hours in adults. Use of caffeine to alleviate daytime sleepiness is not an effective means of dealing with that problem and should be discouraged in children regardless of whether or not they experience disturbed sleep.

Cognitive behavioural approaches

Where insomnia presents in adults, cognitive behavioural therapy for insomnia (CBT-I) is indicated as the recommended first-line treatment (National Institute for Health and Care Excellence, 2022). Although there is a paucity of high-quality clinical trials looking at CBT-I in children and young people, meta-analytic reviews suggest that CBT-I is also an effective treatment for school-age children and adolescents with insomnia (Åslund, Arnberg, Kanstrup, & Lekander, 2018; Blake et al., 2017). In infants and younger children, behavioural approaches (e.g. extinction-based approaches, see following section) are effective treatments for sleep disturbance (Mindell et al., 2006) and are also recommended at a guideline level (Morgenthaler et al., 2006).

Graduated extinction

The term '*extinction*' here refers to the discontinuation of reinforcement for a given behaviour (e.g. insisting on parental presence at bedtime) resulting in the termination of the behaviour. Unmodified extinction, also known as the 'cry it out' method, involves the parent or caregiver ignoring any undesired behaviours (e.g. calling out, crying) from bedtime until the following morning. The exceptions are when there is concern about safety or when the child is unwell. Although effective (Mindell et al., 2006) extinction-based approaches are often challenging for parents. This can be problematic as when parents are unable to follow them (e.g. when unable to tolerate the sounds of their child crying), intervening to facilitate the child's sleep onset becomes a strong reinforcer of the undesired behaviour, via an intermittent behavioural reinforcement schedule. As such, these approaches often benefit from modification and support to encourage adherence (Etherton, Blunden, & Hauck, 2016). Graduated extinction involves the parent putting their child to sleep and then checking in on them after a given period of time, briefly comforting them (without picking them up), and then leaving the room. Timing of checks can be kept the same (e.g. every 5 minutes), as needed (e.g. whenever the parent feels the need to check), or can increase in length over time (e.g. 5, 10, 15 minutes). The key element in this process is that the child learns to fall asleep without parental presence, hence *brief* checks. Night wakings that follow should reduce as the child learns to fall asleep independently; however, parental presence to resettle the child at night is acceptable.

Preparing for bed and the importance of relaxation

A common issue, particularly in older children and adolescents, is excessive pre-sleep worry. This is often focused on events of the day or those of tomorrow (e.g. social interactions at school, academic pressure), or indeed worry about sleep itself and the consequences of not sleeping well. Just as in adults, this being 'on edge' leads to difficulty 'switching off' and falling asleep. The 'fight-or-flight response' is an acute response to stress that, as an evolutionary adaptation, keeps us safe by allowing us to detect and respond appropriately to threat. A crucial part of this process is the maintenance of alertness and temporary suspension of our ability to fall asleep. In other words, even if primed for sleep, the body keeps itself alert and awake so that it can deal with any potential danger. While helpful for managing imminent external threat, the same process can keep us from falling asleep whenever we encounter frustration, irritation, or worry. Often the difficulty in falling asleep *itself* becomes a threat and perpetuates the state of arousal, often via 'sleep effort', the *active trying* to make sleep happen. Additionally, the fact that worry regularly takes place in bed, often while trying to sleep, leads to a disruption of a healthy association between being in bed and being asleep, and may develop into an association between being in bed and worry itself. An important part of being *ready* for sleep, therefore, is being in a relaxed state. Facilitation of a relaxed pre-sleep state can be done via the use of a range of cognitive and relaxation techniques. However, ensuring an appropriate, consistent, and regularly timed bedtime routine, no matter what age the child or young person, is generally a foundation. Winding down before bed should ideally be done in relatively dim light; this is important because evening secretion of the hormone melatonin is inhibited by light exposure and light has an alerting effect on our physiology. When considering the use of a relaxation technique prior to sleep, it is important to emphasize that this is done to induce a relaxed physiological state, rather than to induce sleep. The nuance here is important, because trying to relax in order to fall asleep is likely to lead to performance anxiety which will defeat the purpose of the exercise. There is no clear consensus on which relaxation strategies should be employed for people struggling to sleep, and it is likely that a wide range will be effective so long as they are acceptable to the individual and they are straightforward enough to follow. To this end, although not specifically relaxation techniques, mindfulness-based approaches to grounding and centring one in the present moment may also be helpful, and are best reinforced by practice during the day as well as at night.

Progressive muscle relaxation

Probably the most commonly used and best evidenced relaxation technique for people with insomnia is known as progressive muscle relaxation. Here, the person sits or lies down in a quiet place and allows the body to become comfortable and relaxed. To begin with, they can take several slow, deep breaths, breathing in through the nose and out through the mouth. Next, they should clench their right hand into a fist and hold it this way for approximately 10 seconds, focusing on the feeling of tension. After this, they can release the tension in their hand and focus on the relaxing sensation of the dissipation of tension. The sequence is then repeated with other parts of the body, typically including the other hand, the feet, legs, and thighs. In younger children, this can be facilitated by a parent to begin with and continued by the child once they feel confident in the technique.

Putting the day to rest and preparing for tomorrow

For some children, concerns about events of the day and being sufficiently prepared for the next day may interfere with winding down before bed. In instances of the former, these topics should be talked through and dealt with well in advance of the bedtime routine, so that any cognitive arousal has time to dissipate prior to winding down for bed. For older children and adolescents, this might take the form of a technique known as 'putting the day to rest'. Here, the individual takes around 15–20 minutes in the early evening and sits somewhere quiet and where they are not going to be disturbed with a pen and a notebook. They are encouraged to think through the events of the day and to note down some of the main points, including things about which they feel good and things which have troubled them. Next, they are encouraged to write down a brief 'to do' list with any outstanding jobs or tasks that require their attention, and to include steps that they can take to tie up these loose ends the following day. Thinking about the next day, they are encouraged to consider the things that they are looking forward to and anything that is causing them any worry. They can then add steps to deal with these on their 'to do' list. Next, they can be encouraged to leave the list somewhere safe and to set an alarm or reminder (e.g. on their phone) for a particular time the next day when they can come back to these tasks and concerns. When it comes to being in bed, they can remind themselves that they have already made a plan to deal with their list. Any new thoughts that come up during this time can be written on a piece of paper by their bedside and dealt with in a similar manner. In cases where children are concerned about being ready the next day, it may help to prepare school things, clothing, or other necessities before beginning the bedtime routine so that they can rest assured that they are sufficiently prepared. For younger children, a simplified approach might take the form of drawing a picture of their day and explaining it to their parent. Additionally, they might explore the various elements of the picture with their caregiver and together think carefully about what they might be worried about or looking forward to the next day.

The bed–sleep association and avoiding worrying in bed

Good sleepers exhibit a strong paired association between being in bed and sleep. For them, bed *means* sleep and there is little ambiguity about what happens once they get into bed at night. For people who struggle with sleep, this strong association becomes disrupted, leaving ambiguity about whether or not sleep will happen. People often spend time in bed *not sleeping*, instead spending their time worrying, trying to get to sleep (i.e. sleep effort), or even doing activating things simply to pass the time or entertain themselves (e.g. scrolling through social media on a smartphone). This has the effect of not only disrupting the bed–sleep association but also building up unhelpful associations between being in bed and doing things like worrying, trying to get to sleep, and so on.

Thinking about this with children and their parents can be done by way of an analogy. If we're asked by a friend to 'grab a tennis racket and to head down to the courts', our expectations are that we're off to play tennis, despite the fact that playing the game hasn't explicitly been mentioned. As long as we play tennis when we get to the tennis courts, we shall have no reason not to expect to play tennis whenever our friend next invites us to bring our racket and head down to the tennis courts. However, if when we arrive we don't actually play tennis and instead do other things, over just a few trips to the courts our clear expectations of playing tennis will have been eroded and we become less and less certain of whether or not we'll actually play. Furthermore, we might start associating going to the tennis courts with something other than tennis entirely. Getting the strong association back is not as hard as it might seem. All we need to do is to limit what we do on the tennis courts to just playing tennis. Whenever we find ourselves doing something else, we simply walk off the court until we're ready to play again. This way, the association is rebuilt and our expectation of playing tennis whenever we head to the courts will be re-established. In just the same way, keeping non-sleep activities out of bed is a helpful way to protect a strong bed–sleep association. Encouraging a child who spends time tossing and turning or worrying in bed to get out of bed whenever they notice them-selves worrying is a good start. It might be that they create a comfortable and specific place in their room to which they can retreat until they feel sleepy-tired, either by doing something enjoyable but non-stimulating (e.g. reading) or by doing an active relaxation exercise. This place is one in which they can 'give up' trying to make sleep happen and instead focus on relaxation. When they feel relaxed and sleepy once more, then they can return to bed and give sleep another chance.

Other common sleep problems

Several other sleep problems are commonly seen in children and young people and may benefit from low intensity intervention. These problems include nightmares, sleepwalking and sleep terrors, and delayed sleep–wake phase problems.

Nightmares

Nightmares, which occur during rapid eye movement (REM) sleep, are developmentally normal and do not in themselves constitute a sleep disorder. However, where they are commonly occurring and impacting sleep continuity and/or daytime function, they warrant intervention. Although several cognitive behavioural approaches have been shown to reduce nightmare symptoms, imagery rehearsal therapy has the most robust evidence base (Gieselmann et al., 2019). Imagery rehearsal therapy has been shown to be effective in both school-aged children (Simard & Nielsen, 2009) and adolescents (Krakow et al., 2001).

Sleepwalking and sleep terrors

Occurring in the transition to and from slow-wave (i.e. non-REM) sleep, and therefore typically during the first third of the night, sleepwalking and sleep terrors are manifestations of incomplete arousals from deep sleep. There is often a strong family history of these parasomnias, experiences of which are often made worse by insufficient sleep and daytime/pre-sleep autonomic arousal. As such, intervention to improve sleep onset and continuity difficulties may result in reduction of frequency and severity of episodes. In the case of sleepwalking, emphasis should be placed on ensuring the safety of the child (e.g. stairgates, locked windows and doors, keys hidden) and guiding them back to their bed with minimal interaction. Similarly, parents should be cautioned against actively intervening (e.g. rousing or talking to the child) with sleep terrors, as this may result in a complete awakening and further sleep disturbance. It is important to reassure parents that although distressing to watch, children do not have any recollection of their sleep terror and it is not indicative of the development of any psychopathology.

Delayed sleep–wake phase problems

A tendency towards a delay of the circadian rhythm in adolescence is developmentally normal, and often results in naturally later bedtimes. However, for many young people this developmental phenomenon results in a reduced opportunity to achieve sufficient sleep before being required to wake for school the following day. Additionally, when unable to sleep, young people may resort to using technology to pass the time, or else become worried (e.g. about how their difficulty falling asleep will affect function the following day), both of which may worsen outcomes. It is important to help the young person and their parents to understand that *consistent* difficulties falling asleep earlier at this age are often the result of a change to the biological timing of the body clock. This can help reduce any tension between the young person and parents. It is also prudent to encourage the young person to get into bed only when they are sleepy-tired (see 'The bed–sleep association and avoiding worrying in bed') and to remove any alerting stimuli (e.g. video games, smartphones) that may be negatively impacting sleep onset further. Where there is a moderate delay and where possible, encouraging parents to allow as much time for the young person to sleep in in the morning (e.g. by preparing for school the night before) may be helpful in reducing sleep debt associated with waking too early. Additionally, if the natural rise time of the young person (e.g. determined by allowing free-sleep during school holiday periods and using a sleep diary) is approximately 2 hours later than when they need to rise for school, exposure to morning sunlight (e.g. sitting next to a bright window for 30 minutes at breakfast) may be helpful in advancing the young person's bedtime. Bedtime can then be brought forward by 15 minutes every few days, along with exposure to sunlight on waking to continue to advance their sleep phase. Where there is a significant delay, or where this approach is ineffective, more specialist clinical support should be sought.

Further considerations

Unfortunately, despite the burden they place on children and their families, and their associations with other physical and mental health conditions, sleep problems often receive a disproportionately small degree of clinical attention. Sleep disorders are a varied group of conditions with diverse aetiologies and a wide range of clinical presentations. Additionally, there are some groups for whom problems with sleep are increasingly likely, such as those with neurodevelopmental disorders and intellectual disabilities. There are a range of symptoms that may be an indication of a disorder other than insomnia and warrant further specialist assessment. These symptoms include:

- Excessive daytime sleepiness (i.e. being unable to stay awake during the day; resumption of daytime napping when developmentally inappropriate).
- Respiratory pauses during sleep which may be associated with loud snoring, sounds of choking, or morning headaches.
- Difficulty falling asleep early and extreme difficulty waking in the morning.
- Falling asleep inappropriately early in the evening and waking extremely early in the morning.
- Frequent and disruptive nightmares with associated daytime impairment.
- Extreme sleepwalking or episodes of sleep terrors where there is a risk of harm to the child or young person.
- Episodes of stereotyped behaviours that take place at any point during the night and that may be indicative of nocturnal seizures.
- Sleep-disruptive muscular twitches or restlessness at night.

Chapter summary

Sleep problems in children and young people are common and varied. They are also often poorly understood and result in significant disruption to the lives of those affected, including to the lives of parents and family members. However, the majority of these problems can be treated using well-evidenced cognitive behavioural approaches. This is particularly important as the effective treatment of sleep problems not only improves sleep itself but also reduces the risk of other mental health problems and improves the ability of the child or young person and their family to function optimally during the day.

Conflicts of interest

Professor Espie is co-founder of and shareholder in Big Health Ltd, a company which specializes in the digital delivery of cognitive behavioural therapy for sleep improvement (Sleepio). Dr Gavriloff has been an employee of and continues to consult for Big Health Ltd. Dr Waite declares no conflicts of interest.

Recommended reading

- For further reading on behavioural treatment of childhood sleep problems, parents can be directed to *Sleeping Through the Night: How Infants, Toddlers and Their Parents Can Get a Good Night's Sleep* (Mindell, 2005) for babies and toddlers, and *Take Charge of Your Child's Sleep: The*

All-in-One Resource for Solving Sleep Problems in Kids and Teens (Owens & Mindell, 2005), for older children and adolescents.

- A comprehensive primer for clinicians on the assessment and treatment of paediatric sleep disorders is *A Clinical Guide to Pediatric Sleep: Diagnosis and Management of Sleep Problems* (Mindell & Owens, 2015).

References

Allen, S. L., Howlett, M. D., Coulombe, J. A., & Corkum, P. V. (2016). ABCs of SLEEPING: A review of the evidence behind pediatric sleep practice recommendations. *Sleep Medicine Reviews, 29*, 1–14.

Åslund, L., Arnberg, F., Kanstrup, M., & Lekander, M. (2018). Cognitive and behavioral interventions to improve sleep in school-age children and adolescents: A systematic review and meta-analysis. *Journal of Clinical Sleep Medicine, 14*(11), 1937–1947.

Beebe D. W. (2011). Cognitive, behavioral, and functional consequences of inadequate sleep in children and adolescents. *Pediatric Clinics of North America, 58*(3), 649–665.

Blake, M. J., Sheeber, L. B., Youssef, G. J., Raniti, M. B., & Allen, N. B. (2017). Systematic review and meta-analysis of adolescent cognitive-behavioral sleep interventions. *Clinical Child and Family Psychology Review, 20*(3), 227–249.

Blank, M., Zhang, J., Lamers, F., Taylor, A. D., Hickie, I. B., & Merikangas, K. R. (2015). Health correlates of insomnia symptoms and comorbid mental disorders in a nationally representative sample of US adolescents. *Sleep, 38*(2), 197–204.

Borbély, A. A. (1982). A two process model of sleep regulation. *Human Neurobiology, 1*(3), 195–204.

Borbély, A. A., Daan, S., Wirz-Justice, A., & Deboer, T. (2016). The two-process model of sleep regulation: A reappraisal. *Journal of Sleep Research, 25*(2), 131–143.

Cook, F., Conway, L. J., Giallo, R., Gartland, D., Sciberras, E., & Brown, S. (2020). Infant sleep and child mental health: A longitudinal investigation. *Archives of Disease in Childhood, 105*(7), 655–660.

Coons, S., & Guilleminault, C. (1984). Development of consolidated sleep and wakeful periods in relation to the day/night cycle in infancy. *Developmental Medicine & Child Neurology, 26*(2), 169–176.

Diekelmann, S., & Born, J. (2010). The memory function of sleep. *Nature Reviews. Neuroscience, 11*(2), 114–126.

Ednick, M., Cohen, A. P., McPhail, G. L., Beebe, D., Simakajornboon, N., & Amin, R. S. (2009). A review of the effects of sleep during the first year of life on cognitive, psychomotor, and temperament development. *Sleep, 32*(11), 1449–1458.

Espie, C. A., Broomfield, N. M., MacMahon, K. M., Macphee, L. M., & Taylor, L. M. (2006). The attention-intention-effort pathway in the development of psychophysiologic insomnia: A theoretical review. *Sleep Medicine Reviews, 10*(4), 215–245.

Etherton, H., Blunden, S., & Hauck, Y. (2016). Discussion of extinction-based behavioral sleep interventions for young children and reasons why parents may find them difficult. *Journal of Clinical Sleep Medicine, 12*(11), 1535–1543.

Gieselmann, A., Ait Aoudia, M., Carr, M., Germain, A., Gorzka, R., Holzinger, B., … Pietrowsky, R. (2019). Aetiology and treatment of nightmare disorder: State of the art and future perspectives. *Journal of Sleep Research, 28*(4), e12820. https://doi.org/10.1111/jsr.12820

Goldstein, T. R., Bridge, J. A., & Brent, D. A. (2008). Sleep disturbance preceding completed suicide in adolescents. *Journal of Consulting and Clinical Psychology, 76*(1), 84–91.

Hale, L., & Guan, S. (2015). Screen time and sleep among school-aged children and adolescents: A systematic literature review. *Sleep Medicine Reviews, 21*, 50–58.

Harvey, A. G. (2002). A cognitive model of insomnia. *Behaviour Research and Therapy, 40*(8), 869–893.

Hauri, P. (1977). *The sleep disorders: Current concepts*. Kalamazoo, MI: Scope Publications, Upjohn.

Henderson, J. M., France, K. G., Owens, J. L., & Blampied, N. M. (2010). Sleeping through the night: The consolidation of self-regulated sleep across the first year of life. *Pediatrics, 126*(5), e1081–e1087.

Hirshkowitz, M., Whiton, K., Albert, S. M., Alessi, C., Bruni, O., DonCarlos, L., . . ., & Adams Hillard, P. J. (2015). National Sleep Foundation's sleep time duration recommendations: Methodology and results summary. *Sleep Health, 1*(1), 40–43.

Honaker, S. M., & Meltzer, L. J. (2014). Bedtime problems and night wakings in young children: An update of the evidence. *Paediatric Respiratory Reviews, 15*(4), 333–339.

Krakow, B., Sandoval, D., Schrader, R., Keuhne, B., McBride, L., Yau, C. L., & Tandberg, D. (2001). Treatment of chronic nightmares in adjudicated adolescent girls in a residential facility. The Journal of adolescent health: official publication of the Society for Adolescent Medicine, 29(2), 94–100. https://doi.org/10.1016/s1054-139x(00)00195-6

LeBourgeois, M. K., Wright, K. P., Jr., LeBourgeois, H. B., & Jenni, O. G. (2013). Dissonance between parent-selected bedtimes and young children's circadian physiology influences nighttime settling difficulties. *Mind, Brain, and Education, 7*(4), 234–242.

Lodemore, M., Petersen, S. A., & Wailoo, M. P. (1991). Development of night time temperature rhythms over the first six months of life. *Archives of Disease in Childhood, 66*(4), 521–524.

Meltzer, L. J. (2010). Clinical management of behavioral insomnia of childhood: Treatment of bedtime problems and night wakings in young children. *Behavioral Sleep Medicine, 8*(3), 172–189.

Miller, M. A. (2015). The role of sleep and sleep disorders in the development, diagnosis, and management of neurocognitive disorders. *Frontiers in Neurology, 6*, 224.

Mindell, J. A. (2005). *Sleeping through the night: How infants, toddlers and their parents can get a good night's sleep* (2nd ed.). New York: William Morrow.

Mindell, J. A., Kuhn, B., Lewin, D. S., Meltzer, L. J., Sadeh, A., & American Academy of Sleep Medicine. (2006). Behavioral treatment of bedtime problems and night wakings in infants and young children. *Sleep, 29*(10), 1263–1276.

Mindell, J. A., Leichman, E. S., Composto, J., Lee, C., Bhullar, B., & Walters, R. M. (2016). Development of infant and toddler sleep patterns: Real-world data from a mobile application. *Journal of Sleep Research, 25*(5), 508–516.

Mindell, J. A., Leichman, E. S., Lee, C., Williamson, A. A., & Walters, R. M. (2017). Implementation of a nightly bedtime routine: How quickly do things improve? *Infant Behavior & Development, 49*, 220–227.

Mindell, J. A., Li, A. M., Sadeh, A., Kwon, R., & Goh, D. Y. (2015). Bedtime routines for young children: A dose-dependent association with sleep outcomes. *Sleep, 38*(5), 717–722.

Mindell, J. A., & Owens, J. A. (2015). *A clinical guide to pediatric sleep: Diagnosis and management of sleep problems* (3rd ed.). Philadelphia, PA: Wolters Kluwer.

Mindell, J. A., & Williamson, A. A. (2018). Benefits of a bedtime routine in young children: Sleep, development, and beyond. *Sleep Medicine Reviews, 40*, 93–108.

Morgenthaler, T. I., Owens, J., Alessi, C., Boehlecke, B., Brown, T. M., Coleman, J., Jr, . . ., & American Academy of Sleep Medicine (2006). Practice parameters for behavioral treatment of bedtime problems and night wakings in infants and young children. *Sleep, 29*(10), 1277–1281.

National Institute for Health and Care Excellence. (2020). *Insomnia: Clinical knowledge summary.* London: National Institute for Health and Care Excellence.

Owens, J. (2008). Classification and epidemiology of childhood sleep disorders. *Primary Care, 35*(3), 533–546, vii.

Owens, J., Adolescent Sleep Working Group, & Committee on Adolescence. (2014). Insufficient sleep in adolescents and young adults: An update on causes and consequences. *Pediatrics, 134*(3), e921–e932.

Owens, J. A., & Mindell, J. A. (2005). *Take charge of your child's sleep: The all-in-one resource for solving sleep problems in kids and teens.* Boston, MA: Da Capo.

Owens, J. A., Spirito, A., & McGuinn, M. (2000). The Children's Sleep Habits Questionnaire (CSHQ): Psychometric properties of a survey instrument for school-aged children. *Sleep, 23*(8), 1043–1051.

Palmer, C. A., & Alfano, C. A. (2017). Sleep and emotion regulation: An organizing, integrative review. *Sleep Medicine Reviews, 31*, 6–16.

Paruthi, S., Brooks, L. J., D'Ambrosio, C., Hall, W. A., Kotagal, S., Lloyd, R. M., . . ., & Wise, M. S. (2016). Recommended amount of sleep for pediatric populations: A consensus statement of the American Academy of Sleep Medicine. *Journal of Clinical Sleep Medicine, 12*(6), 785–786.

Rivkees, S. A. (2003). Developing circadian rhythmicity in infants. *Pediatrics, 112*(2), 373–381.

Roenneberg, T., Kuehnle, T., Juda, M., Kantermann, T., Allebrandt, K., Gordijn, M., & Merrow, M. (2007). Epidemiology of the human circadian clock. *Sleep Medicine Reviews, 11*(6), 429–438.

Sadeh, A. (2004). A brief screening questionnaire for infant sleep problems: Validation and findings for an internet sample. *Pediatrics, 113*(6), e570–e577.

Sadeh, A., Gruber, R., & Raviv, A. (2002). Sleep, neurobehavioral functioning, and behavior problems in school-age children. *Child Development, 73*(2), 405–417.

Sadeh, A., Tikotzky, L., & Kahn, M. (2014). Sleep in infancy and childhood: Implications for emotional and behavioral difficulties in adolescence and beyond. *Current Opinion in Psychiatry, 27*(6), 453–459.

Simard, V., & Nielsen, T. (2009). Adaptation of imagery rehearsal therapy for nightmares in children: A brief report. *Psychotherapy: Theory, Research, Practice, Training, 46*(4), 492–497.

Spielman, A. J., Caruso, L. S., & Glovinsky, P. B. (1987). A behavioral perspective on insomnia treatment. *Psychiatric Clinics of North America, 10*(4), 541–553.

Staton, S., Rankin, P. S., Harding, M., Smith, S. S., Westwood, E., LeBourgeois, M. K., & Thorpe, K. J. (2020). Many naps, one nap, none: A systematic review and meta-analysis of napping patterns in children 0–12 years. *Sleep Medicine Reviews, 50*, 101247.

Stickgold, R. (2005). Sleep-dependent memory consolidation. *Nature, 437*(7063), 1272–1278.

Van Cauter, E., Spiegel, K., Tasali, E., & Leproult, R. (2008). Metabolic consequences of sleep and sleep loss. *Sleep Medicine, 9*(Suppl 1), S23–S28.

Williamson, A. A., Mindell, J. A., Hiscock, H., & Quach, J. (2020). Longitudinal sleep problem trajectories are associated with multiple impairments in child well-being. *Journal of Child Psychology and Psychiatry, 61*(10), 1092–1103.

Xie, L., Kang, H., Xu, Q., Chen, M. J., Liao, Y., Thiyagarajan, M., . . ., & Nedergaard, M. (2013). Sleep drives metabolite clearance from the adult brain. *Science (New York, N.Y.), 342*(6156), 373–377.

14

Low intensity interventions for obsessive–compulsive disorder in children and adolescents

Georgina Krebs and Angela Lewis

Learning objectives

- Understand why low intensity interventions are important for obsessive–compulsive disorder in youth.
- Have an awareness of the evidence-based low intensity interventions available for children and young people with obsessive–compulsive disorder.
- Understand the challenges of implementing low intensity interventions in young people with obsessive–compulsive disorder.

Obsessive–compulsive disorder in children and adolescents

Obsessive–compulsive disorder (OCD) is characterized by persistent and unwanted intrusive thoughts, images and urges (obsessions), and repetitive behaviours or mental acts (compulsions) (American Psychiatric Association, 2013). OCD can encompass a wide range of obsessional worries and compulsive behaviours in children and adolescents (hereafter referred to as young people) (Box 14.1). Levels of insight can differ, with some young people readily acknowledging their obsessions and compulsions to be excessive and irrational, while others are convinced that their fears and behaviours are valid (American Psychiatric Association, 2013).

OCD usually emerges during childhood or adolescence (Dell'Osso et al., 2016) and has an estimated prevalence of approximately 2% in young people (Heyman et al., 2003; Zohar, 1999). The disorder causes marked impairment in family, academic, and social functioning (Lack et al., 2009; Piacentini, Bergman, Keller, & McCracken, 2003). Furthermore, OCD in youth is associated with increased risk of other psychiatric disorders in adulthood (Micali et al., 2010; Wewetzer et al., 2001). Without treatment, symptoms may wax and wane but often follow a chronic course (Mancebo et al., 2014; Wewetzer et al., 2001).

Box 14.1 Common obsessions and compulsions in young people with OCD

Obsessions	Compulsions
• Fear of dirt, germs, or certain illnesses.	• Excessive or ritualized washing or cleaning.
• Concerns with bodily waste or secretions (e.g. urine, faeces, semen).	• Excessive checking (e.g. taps, doors).
• Fear might harm self or others.	• Repeating routine activities (e.g. walking in and out of a room).
• Fear harm will come to self or others.	• Counting rituals.
• Fear of being responsible for an accident (e.g. a flood).	• Ordering and arranging items.
• Unwanted sexual thoughts or images (e.g. sexual acts with family member or children).	• Savings items that should be thrown away (e.g. wrappers and packaging).
• Fear of losing things.	• Reassurance seeking.
• Excessive concern about lucky/unlucky numbers or colours.	• Mental rituals.
• Fear of offending God or other religious entities.	• Rituals involving tapping or touching.
	• Performing behaviours until it feels 'just right'.

Note: these examples are adapted from the symptom checklist of the Children's Yale–Brown Obsessive Compulsive Scale (Scahill et al., 1997).

Why are low intensity treatments needed?

Over the last two decades, substantial evidence has accrued for the efficacy of cognitive behavioural therapy (CBT) for OCD in young people (Öst, Riise, Wergeland, Hansen, & Kvale, 2016; Watson & Rees, 2008) and it is a recommended first-line treatment (Avasthi, Sharma, & Grover, 2019; Geller & March, 2012; National Institute for Health and Clinical Excellence, 2005). However, in reality the majority of OCD sufferers fail to access CBT (Kohn, Saxenall, Levavill, & Saracenoll, 2004) or do so only after long delays (Garcia-Soriano, Rufer, Delsignore, & Weidt, 2014; Stengler et al., 2013). OCD is associated with greater delays in accessing treatment than many other psychiatric disorders (Kohn et al., 2004). This is concerning, particularly given that greater illness duration is predictive of poorer outcomes (Albert et al., 2019; Micali et al., 2010).

Obstacles to accessing CBT include individual, family, and cultural factors such as stigma, geographical isolation, inconvenience, and financial costs (Baer & Minichiello, 2008; Barton & Heyman, 2013; Goodwin, Koenen, Hellman, Guardino, & Struening, 2002; Marques et al., 2010), as well as service-related factors such as limited therapist capacity and lack of training/expertise (Keleher, Jassi, & Krebs, 2020; Nair et al., 2015). Low intensity (LI) treatments (i.e. those that involve less specialist therapist time; see Chapter 1) have the potential to reduce many of these barriers, thereby improving access.

What LI treatments are available for youth with OCD, and what is their evidence base?

Bibliotherapy

Several CBT self-help books have been written for young people with OCD (Derisley, Heyman, Robinson, & Turner, 2008; March & Benton, 2006; Wood & Fletcher, 2019). Their content mirrors that of therapist-delivered CBT protocols, emphasizing exposure and response prevention (ERP) (Table 14.1). Although the books are popular and widely used, there has been little research testing their efficacy. Several randomized controlled trials (RCTs) have demonstrated bibliotherapy to be efficacious for the treatment of OCD in *adulthood*, even in the absence of therapist support (Hauschildt, Schröder, & Moritz, 2016; Tolin et al., 2007; Vogel et al., 2014). However, it is essential to consider whether *young people* can meaningfully engage with and benefit from self-help books. Only one study has directly addressed this question (Robinson, Turner, Heyman, & Farquharson, 2013). In a small case series (n = 8), 11- to 16-year-olds with OCD were given *Breaking Free from OCD* (Derisley et al., 2008). Participants received brief weekly telephone calls from a therapist to monitor adherence and assess symptoms. The majority of participants reported that the book was easy to read and helpful for tackling their symptoms. Furthermore, significant OCD symptom reduction was observed for the group, although the degree of improvement was modest (19% symptom reduction) and was not evident across all outcome measures. The authors suggested that a greater level of therapist guidance may improve adherence and outcomes, as has been shown among adults (Pearcy, Anderson, Egan, & Rees, 2016).

Of note, self-help materials have also been evaluated as an adjunct to face-to-face CBT in youth with OCD. In an RCT, Bolton et al. (2011) compared brief CBT (on average five sessions) plus self-help with full CBT (12 sessions) and a waiting list control condition. The brief CBT plus self-help group showed equivalent outcomes to the full CBT group, and both had superior outcomes to the waiting list control group. These results suggest that self-help could be a useful supplement to CBT, and may provide an effective way of increasing treatment capacity in under-resourced services.

Table 14.1 Cognitive behaviour therapy self-help books available for young people with OCD

Title	Target age	Content		Information for parents
		Format	Main techniques	
Talking Back to OCD: The Program That Helps Kids and Teens Say 'No Way'—and Parents Say 'Way to Go' [a]	Children and adolescents	12 chapters divided into 2 sections: (A) 'Up Close but Not So Personal: A New Look at OCD for Parents (and Kids)' (B) 'Eight Steps for Getting Rid of Obsessions and Compulsions' Worksheets are included throughout	• Externalizing OCD • Constructing a symptom list ('Mapping OCD') • Rating anxiety using a 'fear thermometer' • ERP • Reward systems • Relapse prevention	Each chapter ends with 'Instructions for parents', providing guidance for parents on how to support their child through treatment and advice on withdrawing from rituals
Breaking Free from OCD: A CBT Guide for Young People and their Families [b]	11- to 16-year-olds	15 chapters, divided into 3 sections: (A) 'Understanding your OCD' (B) 'How to Recover from Your OCD' (C) 'OCD and the Bigger Picture' Worksheets are included throughout	• Psychoeducation, including understanding and rating anxiety • Formulation ('OCD trap') • Developing a hierarchy ('OCD ladder') • ERP • Using helpful thoughts • Responsibility pie charts • Relapse prevention	Each chapter ends with 'Advice for parents or carers', providing general tips on how to support their child as well as specific advice on withdrawing from rituals and dealing with reassurance-seeking
Stand Up to OCD! A CBT Self-Help Guide and Workbook for Teens [c]	12- to 17-year-olds	11 chapters divided into 2 sections: (A) 'Learning about OCD' (B) Workbook The first part of the book illustrates CBT techniques by following 3 young people through treatment. The second part includes worksheets	• Externalizing OCD • Psychoeducation, including anxiety habituation • Formulation ('compulsion cycle') • Behavioural experiments • Developing a hierarchy • ERP	No specific sections for parents

[a] March, J., & Benton, C. (2006). *Talking Back to OCD: The program that helps kids and teens say 'no way'—and parents say 'way to go'*. New York: The Guildford Press.

[b] Derisley, J., Heyman, I., Robinson, S., & Turner, C. (2008). *Breaking free from OCD: A CBT guide for young people and their families*. London: Jessica Kingsley Publishers.

[c] Wood, K., & Fletcher, D. (2019). *Stand up to OCD! A CBT self-help guide and workbook for teens*. London: Jessica Kingsley Publishers.

Internet CBT

Recent efforts have focused on developing internet-based CBT interventions for young people with OCD. Two such programmes have been developed (see Table 14.2 for details). *OCD? Not Me!* is aimed at 12- to 18-year-olds (Rees, Anderson, & Finlay-Jones,

Table 14.2 Internet cognitive behaviour therapy programmes available for young people with OCD

Title	Target age	Content		
		Format	Main techniques	Information for parents
OCD? Not me[a]	12- to 18-year-olds	• 8 stages/ modules, designed to be completed at the rate of 1 per week • Self-guided (i.e. no therapist input) • Interactive elements (i.e. programme responds to user input)	• Centred around metaphor of 'climbing OCD Mountain' • Psychoeducation, including anxiety habituation • Cognitive behaviour formulation of OCD ('OCD cycle') • Constructing an exposure hierarchy • ERP ('OCD Mountain challenges') • Consolidating gains	8 separate modules for parents, including strategies aimed at reducing levels of family distress and accommodation of OCD symptoms
Barninternetprojektet OCD (BIP OCD)[b]	Original version for 12- to 17-year-olds Junior version for 7- to 11-year-olds	• 12 sessions • Therapist-assisted • Interactive elements (i.e. programme responds to user input)	• Psychoeducation, including anxiety habituation • Rating anxiety • Cognitive behaviour formulation of OCD ('OCD cycle') • Constructing an exposure hierarchy (a 'goal ladder') • ERP • Cognitive strategies • Helpful thoughts • Relapse prevention	12 parallel sessions for parents, including strategies for reducing accommodation of OCD symptoms, parental coping, and supporting ERP tasks

[a] Lenhard, F., Andersson, E., Mataix-Cols, D., Rück, C., Vigerland, S., Högström, J., . . ., & Serlachius, E. (2017). Therapist-guided, internet-delivered cognitive-behavioral therapy for adolescents with obsessive-compulsive disorder: a randomized controlled trial. *Journal of the American Academy of Child & Adolescent Psychiatry*, 56(1), 10–19.

[b] Rees, C. S., Anderson, R. A., & Finlay-Jones, A. (2015). OCD? Not Me! Protocol for the development and evaluation of a web-based self-guided treatment for youth with obsessive-compulsive disorder. *BMJ Open*, 5(4), e007486.

Note: the original version of the adolescent OCD BIP programme included five sessions for parents.

Box 14.2 A case example of therapist-guided internet CBT

Caitlin was a 16-year-old girl with a recent diagnosis of moderately severe OCD. She lived in a village with her two siblings and father. She enjoyed school and generally achieved high grades, although recently her attendance had begun to decline. According to her father, Caitlin's behaviour had become challenging, particularly at times when he tried to resist accommodating her OCD.

Caitlin's OCD was characterized by obsessions relating to harm coming to her family and friends. Her compulsions included excessively checking that loved ones were safe by phoning or texting them, tapping surfaces in multiples of three, and repeating words and phrases in her head. She would also frequently seek reassurance from her father.

After being diagnosed with OCD, Caitlin was offered therapist-assisted internet CBT as an alternative to face-to-face CBT. Caitlin liked the idea of being able to schedule her treatment around school and other activities. Online treatment was also well received by her father, who had been worried about trying to arrange clinic appointments around work and childcare commitments.

Caitlin was told the name of the therapist who would be supporting her treatment, and the family were given log-in details for the 12-session programme. Caitlin and her father were able to log-in separately and could therefore work through their respective chapters at their own speed. Caitlin's father found the sessions on parental involvement in rituals particularly helpful, and realized that by accommodating Caitlin's compulsions he was inadvertently fuelling the problem. Caitlin was also enthusiastic about the programme and practised ERP tasks daily, diligently recording her anxiety ratings and quickly moving up her exposure hierarchy.

After 7 weeks, Caitlin's father contacted the therapist and raised concerns that Caitlin was distracting herself during ERP tasks. He was surprised by how low her recent anxiety ratings had been during ERP tasks and subsequently noticed that she had started to scroll through social media or listen to music during tasks. The therapist explained that distraction during ERP is a form of avoidance, and suggested Caitlin and her father review the psychoeducation material together to remind themselves of how avoidance fuels OCD. The therapist also advised Caitlin to break down some of her more challenging exposure tasks into more manageable steps. Caitlin decided to repeat some of her earlier tasks, this time working hard to resist distraction.

By the end of treatment, Caitlin's symptoms had decreased to the subclinical range, where they remained at 3-month follow-up. Her school attendance improved, and her father described the home environment as calmer. Caitlin said she valued having had the opportunity to take ownership of her treatment. Her father reflected that being able to maintain dialogue with the therapist had been important.

2015). The programme is fully *self-guided*, meaning that no therapist support is provided. In an uncontrolled trial, 132 young people engaged with the treatment and overall displayed a significant reduction in OCD symptoms (50% reduction on average; Rees & Anderson, 2016). Although further evaluation is required in the context of an RCT, the results are encouraging and suggest that online self-guided CBT could be an effective way of radically increasing access to CBT among adolescents with OCD.

The second internet CBT programme for young people with OCD is BIP (*Barninternetprojektet* in Swedish; see Box 14.2 for a case example). The original version was developed for adolescents (Lenhard et al., 2014) but has been modified for children (Aspvall et al., 2018). BIP OCD is *therapist guided*, meaning that an allocated therapist provides encouragement, feedback, and advice throughout treatment, primarily by sending messages through the BIP platform. Open trials have shown both the child and adolescent version to be associated with significant OCD symptom reduction and high levels of acceptability (Aspvall et al., 2018; Lenhard et al., 2014). The adolescent version has been further evaluated in an RCT, and shown to be efficacious relative to a waiting list control (Lenhard et al., 2017). In this trial, patients who received BIP OCD experienced a 40% reduction in their OCD symptoms on average, with less than 20 minutes of therapist input per patient per week. The adolescent programme has also been translated into English and evaluated in several other settings and countries, with promising results (Aspvall et al., 2020).

Although both self-guided and therapist-assisted internet CBT programmes show promise as LI treatments for OCD in young people, they are not yet widely available. At the time of writing, OCD? Not me! is only available to health professionals within Australia, and BIP OCD is being used solely in research contexts, although the intention is to eventually make it available for use in clinical settings.

Group CBT

Group CBT involves a single therapist supporting several young people simultaneously, making it a cost-effective format of delivery. There is preliminary evidence that group CBT may be as effective as individually delivered CBT (Barrett, Healy-Farrell, & March, 2004) and sertraline (Asbahr et al., 2005) in reducing OCD symptoms (Barrett et al., 2004) in young people. However, in these studies group CBT has been delivered by specialist therapists and involved 12–14 sessions. Further research is needed to determine the effectiveness of briefer group CBT programmes delivered by LI therapists.

Challenges to LI interventions and how to manage them

While there are multiple benefits to LICBT for OCD, there remain some challenges which should be considered.

Family accommodation of OCD

Parents commonly get drawn into facilitating their child's compulsions and avoidant behaviours and such 'accommodation' has been shown to be associated with poorer treatment outcomes (Monzani et al., 2020). Thus, it is often important to involve family members in treatment in order to directly tackle family accommodation. Including families in LI interventions may be difficult. It is important to be explicit at the outset that LI OCD treatment requires active involvement and commitment from parents as well as the young person. During treatment, therapists should ensure that parents understand that accommodating compulsions has the unwanted consequence of perpetuating OCD, and they should be encouraged to gradually withdraw from rituals with their child's agreement.

Insight

Some young people, particularly children, lack insight into the excessive and/or irrational nature of their obsessions and compulsions (Lewin et al., 2010). Those with poor insight may struggle to maintain adherence to a LI programme, which relies on some commitment to challenging established patterns of behaviour. Insight may improve with psychoeducation, as it can enable a young person to recognize their difficulties as being OCD. If insight continues to be limited a greater emphasis on parental involvement in treatment and use of parenting strategies (e.g. graded withdrawal from rituals, use of reward systems) is typically required.

Risk

When assessing OCD, there is a need to consider risk on multiple levels. This includes idiosyncratic risk that can arise as an unwanted consequence of compulsive behaviours and avoidance, such as restricted food intake due to contamination fears (Lewis, Stokes, Heyman, Turner, & Krebs, 2020; Veale, Freeston, Krebs, Heyman, & Salkovskis, 2009). Risk should be carefully assessed prior to starting LI treatment and monitored throughout. Where risk concerns are present, the suitability of a LI intervention should be considered with caution and only implemented with a parallel risk management in place (see Chapter X for further discussion on assessment and suitability for LI interventions).

Recommended measures

- Clinician administered: the Children's Yale–Brown Obsessive Compulsive Scale (Scahill, Riddle, McSwiggin-Hardin, & Ort, 1997).

- Parent and self-report: the Children's Obsessive Compulsive Inventory—Revised (Uher, Heyman, Turner, & Shafran, 2008).

Recommended reading

Lenhard, F., Andersson, E., Mataix-Cols, D., Rück, C., Vigerland, S., Högström, J., . . ., & Serlachius, E. (2017). Therapist-guided, internet-delivered cognitive-behavioral therapy for adolescents with obsessive-compulsive disorder: A randomized controlled trial. *Journal of the American Academy of Child & Adolescent Psychiatry, 56*(1), 10–19.

References

Albert, U., Barbaro, F., Bramante, S., Rosso, G., De Ronchi, D., & Maina, G. (2019). Duration of untreated illness and response to SRI treatment in obsessive-compulsive disorder. *European Psychiatry, 58*, 19–26.

American Psychiatric Association. (2013). *Diagnostic and statistical manual of mental disorders: DSM 5*. Arlington, VA: American Psychiatric Association.

Asbahr, F. R., Castillo, A. R., Ito, L. M., Latorre, M. R., Moreira, M. N., & Lotufo-Neto, F. (2005). Group cognitive-behavioral therapy versus sertraline for the treatment of children and adolescents with obsessive-compulsive disorder. *Journal of the American Academy of Child & Adolescent Psychiatry, 44*(11), 1128–1136.

Aspvall, K., Andrén, P., Lenhard, F., Andersson, E., Mataix-Cols, D., & Serlachius, E. (2018). Internet-delivered cognitive behavioural therapy for young children with obsessive–compulsive disorder: Development and initial evaluation of the BIP OCD Junior programme. *BJPsych Open, 4*(3), 106–112.

Aspvall, K., Lenhard, F., Melin, K., Krebs, G., Norlin, L., Nässtrom, K., . . ., & Serlachius, E. (2020). Implementation of internet-delivered cognitive behaviour therapy for pediatric obsessive-compulsive disorder: Lessons from clinics in Sweden, United Kingdom and Australia. *Internet Interventions, 20*, 100308.

Avasthi, A., Sharma, A., & Grover, S. (2019). Clinical practice guidelines for the management of obsessive-compulsive disorder in children and adolescents. *Indian Journal of Psychiatry, 61*(Suppl 2), 306–316.

Baer, L., & Minichiello, W. E. (2008). Reasons for inadequate utilization of cognitive-behavioral therapy for obsessive-compulsive disorder. *Journal of Clinical Psychiatry, 69*(4), 676.

Barrett, P., Healy-Farrell, L., & March, J. S. (2004). Cognitive-behavioral family treatment of childhood obsessive-compulsive disorder: A controlled trial. *Journal of the American Academy of Child & Adolescent Psychiatry, 43*(1), 46–62.

Barton, R., & Heyman, I. (2013). Obsessive–compulsive disorder in children and adolescents. *Paediatrics and Child Health, 23*(1), 18–23.

Bolton, D., Williams, T., Perrin, S., Atkinson, L., Gallop, C., Waite, P., & Salkovskis, P. (2011). Randomized controlled trial of full and brief cognitive-behaviour therapy and wait-list for paediatric obsessive-compulsive disorder. *Journal of Child Psychology and Psychiatry, 52*(12), 1269–1278.

Dell'Osso, B., Benatti, B., Hollander, E., Fineberg, N., Stein, D. J., Lochner, C., . . ., & Altamura, A. C. (2016). Childhood, adolescent and adult age at onset and related clinical correlates in obsessive-compulsive disorder: A report from the International College of Obsessive–Compulsive Spectrum Disorders (ICOCS). *International Journal of Psychiatry in Clinical Practice, 20*(4), 210–217.

Derisley, J., Heyman, I., Robinson, S., & Turner, C. (2008). *Breaking free from OCD: A CBT guide for young people and their families*. London: Jessica Kingsley Publishers.

Garcia-Soriano, G., Rufer, M., Delsignore, A., & Weidt, S. (2014). Factors associated with non-treatment or delayed treatment seeking in OCD sufferers: A review of the literature. *Psychiatry Research, 220*(1–2), 1–10.

Geller, D. A., & March, J. S. (2012). Practice parameter for the assessment and treatment of children and adolescents with obsessive-compulsive disorder. *Journal of the American Academy of Child & Adolescent Psychiatry*, *51*(1), 98–113.

Goodwin, R., Koenen, K. C., Hellman, F., Guardino, M., & Struening, E. (2002). Helpseeking and access to mental health treatment for obsessive-compulsive disorder. *Acta Psychiatrica Scandinavica*, *106*(2), 143–149.

Hauschildt, M., Schröder, J., & Moritz, S. (2016). Randomized-controlled trial on a novel (meta-) cognitive self-help approach for obsessive-compulsive disorder ('myMCT'). *Journal of Obsessive-Compulsive and Related Disorders*, *10*, 26–34.

Heyman, I., Fombonne, E., Simmons, H., Ford, T., Meltzer, H., & Goodman, R. (2003). Prevalence of obsessive-compulsive disorder in the British nationwide survey of child mental health. *International Review of Psychiatry*, *15*(1–2), 178–184.

Keleher, J., Jassi, A., & Krebs, G. (2020). Clinician-reported barriers to using exposure with response prevention in the treatment of paediatric obsessive-compulsive disorder. *Journal of Obsessive-Compulsive and Related Disorders*, *24*, 100498.

Kohn, R., Saxenall, S., Levavill, I., & Saracenoll, B. (2004). The treatment gap in mental health care. *Bulletin of the World Health Organisation*, *82*(11), 858–866.

Lack, C. W., Storch, E. A., Keeley, M. L., Geffken, G. R., Ricketts, E. D., Murphy, T. K., & Goodman, W. K. (2009). Quality of life in children and adolescents with obsessive-compulsive disorder: Base rates, parent–child agreement, and clinical correlates. *Social Psychiatry and Psychiatric Epidemiology*, *44*(11), 935–942.

Lenhard, F., Andersson, E., Mataix-Cols, D., Rück, C., Vigerland, S., Högström, J., . . ., & Serlachius, E. (2017). Therapist-guided, internet-delivered cognitive-behavioral therapy for adolescents with obsessive-compulsive disorder: A randomized controlled trial. *Journal of the American Academy of Child & Adolescent Psychiatry*, *56*(1), 10–19.e12.

Lenhard, F., Vigerland, S., Andersson, E., Ruck, C., Mataix-Cols, D., Thulin, U., . . ., & Serlachius, E. (2014). Internet-delivered cognitive behavior therapy for adolescents with obsessive-compulsive disorder: An open trial. *PLoS One*, *9*(6), e100773.

Lewin, A. B., Bergman, R. L., Peris, T. S., Chang, S., McCracken, J. T., & Piacentini, J. (2010). Correlates of insight among youth with obsessive-compulsive disorder. *Journal of Child Psychology and Psychiatry*, *51*(5), 603–611.

Lewis, A., Stokes, C., Heyman, I., Turner, C., & Krebs, G. (2020). Conceptualizing and managing risk in pediatric OCD: Case examples. *Bulletin of the Menninger Clinic*, *84*(1), 3–20.

Mancebo, M. C., Boisseau, C. L., Garnaat, S. L., Eisen, J. L., Greenberg, B. D., Sibrava, N. J., . . ., & Rasmussen, S. A. (2014). Long-term course of pediatric obsessive–compulsive disorder: 3 years of prospective follow-up. *Comprehensive Psychiatry*, *55*(7), 1498–1504.

March, J., & Benton, C. (2006). *Talking back to OCD: The program that helps kids and teens say 'no way'—and parents say 'way to go'*. New York: Guildford Press.

Marques, L., LeBlanc, N. J., Weingarden, H. M., Timpano, K. R., Jenike, M., & Wilhelm, S. (2010). Barriers to treatment and service utilization in an internet sample of individuals with obsessive-compulsive symptoms. *Depression and Anxiety*, *27*(5), 470–475.

Micali, N., Heyman, I., Perez, M., Hilton, K., Nakatani, E., Turner, C., & Mataix-Cols, D. (2010). Long-term outcomes of obsessive–compulsive disorder: Follow-up of 142 children and adolescents. *British Journal of Psychiatry*, *197*(2), 128–134.

Monzani, B., Vidal-Ribas, P., Turner, C., Krebs, G., Stokes, C., Heyman, I., . . ., & Stringaris, A. (2020). The role of paternal accommodation of paediatric OCD symptoms: Patterns and implications for treatment outcomes. *Journal of Abnormal Child Psychology*, *48*(10), 1313–1323.

Nair, A., Wong, Y. L., Barrow, F., Heyman, I., Clark, B., & Krebs, G. (2015). Has the first-line management of paediatric OCD improved following the introduction of NICE guidelines? *Archives of Disease in Childhood*, *100*(4), 416–417.

National Institute for Health and Care Excellence. (2005). *Obsessive-compulsive disorder: Core interventions in the treatment of obsessive-compulsive disorder and body dysmorphic disorder*. London: National Institute for Health and Care Excellence.

Öst, L.-G., Riise, E. N., Wergeland, G. J., Hansen, B., & Kvale, G. (2016). Cognitive behavioral and pharmacological treatments of OCD in children: A systematic review and meta-analysis. *Journal of Anxiety Disorders*, *43*, 58–69.

Pearcy, C. P., Anderson, R. A., Egan, S. J., & Rees, C. S. (2016). A systematic review and meta-analysis of self-help therapeutic interventions for obsessive–compulsive disorder: Is therapeutic contact key to overall improvement? *Journal of Behavior Therapy and Experimental Psychiatry, 51*, 74–83.

Piacentini, J., Bergman, R. L., Keller, M., & McCracken, J. (2003). Functional impairment in children and adolescents with obsessive-compulsive disorder. *Journal of Child and Adolescent Psychopharmacology, 13*(2, Suppl 1), 61–69.

Rees, C. S., & Anderson, R. A. (2016). Online obsessive-compulsive disorder treatment: Preliminary results of the 'OCD? Not Me!' self-guided internet-based cognitive behavioral therapy program for young people. *JMIR Mental Health, 3*(3), e29.

Rees, C. S., Anderson, R. A., & Finlay-Jones, A. (2015). OCD? Not Me! Protocol for the development and evaluation of a web-based self-guided treatment for youth with obsessive-compulsive disorder. *BMJ Open, 5*(4), e007486.

Robinson, S., Turner, C., Heyman, I., & Farquharson, L. (2013). The feasibility and acceptability of a cognitive-behavioural self-help intervention for adolescents with obsessive-compulsive disorder. *Behavioural and Cognitive Psychotherapy, 41*(1), 117–122.

Scahill, L., Riddle, M. A., McSwiggin-Hardin, M., & Ort, S. I. (1997). Children's Yale–Brown Obsessive Compulsive Scale: Reliability and validity. *Journal of the American Academy of Child & Adolescent Psychiatry, 36*(6), 844–852.

Stengler, K., Olbrich, S., Heider, D., Dietrich, S., Riedel-Heller, S., & Jahn, I. (2013). Mental health treatment seeking among patients with OCD: Impact of age of onset. *Social Psychiatry and Psychiatric Epidemiology, 48*(5), 813–819.

Tolin, D. F., Hannan, S., Maltby, N., Diefenbach, G. J., Worhunsky, P., & Brady, R. E. (2007). A randomized controlled trial of self-directed versus therapist-directed cognitive-behavioral therapy for obsessive-compulsive disorder patients with prior medication trials. *Behavior Therapy, 38*(2), 179–191.

Uher, R., Heyman, I., Turner, C. M., & Shafran, R. (2008). Self-, parent-report and interview measures of obsessive-compulsive disorder in children and adolescents. *Journal of Anxiety Disorders, 22*(6), 979–990.

Veale, D., Freeston, M., Krebs, G., Heyman, I., & Salkovskis, P. (2009). Risk assessment and management in obsessive–compulsive disorder. *Advances in Psychiatric Treatment, 15*(5), 332–343.

Vogel, P. A., Solem, S., Hagen, K., Moen, E. M., Launes, G., Håland, Å. T., . . ., & Himle, J. A. (2014). A pilot randomized controlled trial of videoconference-assisted treatment for obsessive-compulsive disorder. *Behaviour Research and Therapy, 63*, 162–168.

Watson, H. J., & Rees, C. S. (2008). Meta-analysis of randomized, controlled treatment trials for pediatric obsessive-compulsive disorder. *Journal of Child Psychology and Psychiatry, 49*(5), 489–498.

Wewetzer, C., Jans, T., Müller, B., Neudörfl, A., Bücherl, U., Remschmidt, H., . . ., & Herpertz-Dahlmann, B. (2001). Long-term outcome and prognosis of obsessive–compulsive disorder with onset in childhood or adolescence. *European Child & Adolescent Psychiatry, 10*(1), 37–46.

Wood, K., & Fletcher, D. (2019). *Stand up to OCD! A CBT self-help guide and workbook for teens.* London: Jessica Kingsley Publishers.

Zohar, A. H. (1999). The epidemiology of obsessive-compulsive disorder in children and adolescents. *Child and Adolescent Psychiatric Clinics of North America, 8*(3), 445–460.

15

Low intensity interventions for autistic children and young people

Erin J. Libsack, Morgan L. McNair, Joseph Giacomantonio, Peter Felsman, and Matthew D. Lerner

Learning objectives

- Increase knowledge of evidence-based treatments for core and co-occurring symptoms in autism spectrum disorder.
- Elucidate ongoing research in autism spectrum disorder interventions as well as future directions.
- Summarize clinical implications of various intervention modalities, such as technological implementations and alternative providers.
- Discuss autism spectrum disorder-specific implementation and optimization challenges and potential solutions, for example, the distillation and matching model approach.

Description of the disorder and diagnostic criteria

Autism spectrum disorder (ASD) is a lifelong neurodevelopmental disorder estimated to affect 1 in 54 children (Maenner et al., 2020). ASD is characterized by persistent impairments in social communication and interaction and restricted, repetitive patterns of behaviour, interests, or activities (American Psychiatric Association, 2013).

Introduction: rationale and evidence-base for low intensity interventions for autistic youth

In addition to the core deficits associated with ASD, autistic youth are more likely to experience common mental disorders than their non-autistic peers (Rosen, Mazefsky, Vasa, & Lerner, 2018). Approximately 70% of autistic youth experience at least one co-occurring psychiatric disorder, while 40% experience two or more (Hossain et al., 2020; Rosen et al., 2018). In addition to increasing the psychological and emotional burden experienced by autistic youth, the presence of co-occurring psychiatric disorders also increases the monetary costs and time commitment associated with accessing mental healthcare services (see Chapter 5). These costs emphasize the heightened need for cost-effective and easily accessible low intensity (LI) interventions for autistic youth.

Despite being a relatively new field within ASD research, LI interventions have been developed and applied to a variety of treatment targets including sleep problems (Loring, Johnston, Gray, et al., 2016; Loring, Johnston, Shui, et al., 2018), oral language (Ingersoll & Wainer, 2013; Popovic, Starr, & Koegel, 2020), social skills (Apple, Billingsley, Schwartz, & Carr, 2005; Charlop-Christy, Le, & Freeman, 2000; Corbett et al., 2014; Flynn & Healy, 2012; Kasari, Rotheram-Fuller, Locke, & Gulsrud, 2012; Marro et al., 2019), adaptive skills (e.g. functional communication, daily living skills; Campbell, Morgan, Barnett, & Spreat, 2015; Charlop-Christy et al., 2000; Shrestha, Anderson, & Moore, 2013, 2013), symptomatology associated with co-occurring psychiatric conditions like anxiety (Hepburn, Blakeley-Smith, Wolff, & Reaven, 2016; Storch et al., 2020) and attention deficit hyperactivity disorder (ADHD; Yerys et al., 2019; Vahabzadeh, Keshav, Salisbury, & Sahin, 2018), and executive functioning skills (e.g. attention, working memory, cognitive flexibility; de Vries, Prins, Schmand, & Geurts, 2015; Simmons, Paul, & Shic, 2016). Although interest in LI interventions for autistic youth has increased recently, most published research remains limited to small sample sizes and pilot methodology. Evidence-based research collected from large-scale randomized controlled trials, inclusion of active control groups, and replication studies are largely still lacking (Hollis et al., 2017; Lounds Taylor et al., 2012). Here we offer a window into the growing field of LI intervention research within the extant ASD literature.

LI interventions for autistic youth: modalities of treatment delivery

Treatment duration of LI interventions for autistic youth ranges from single-session interventions to courses of one or two weekly sessions administered over 2–24 weeks. Standard and long-term ASD interventions are often longer than comparable treatments for other populations, usually ranging from 12 to 16+ weeks in length and sometimes including several intervention hours/week (Perihan et al., 2020). Because ASD youth often need more time for repeated or targeted practice (Clarke, Hill, & Charman, 2016), even LI interventions may be delivered over longer periods of time to maximize uptake. Such LI interventions reduce burden on, or eliminate the need for, highly trained clinicians to deliver treatments, thus reducing the cost of treatment provision, promoting community dissemination of evidence-based treatments, and increasing treatment accessibility for a wide range of patients. LI interventions used with autistic youth have demonstrated promising feasibility, acceptability, and significant therapeutic effects across many target behaviours and delivery modalities.

Technology

Interventions for autistic youth with co-occurring conditions have employed various technological modalities. Telehealth, whether implemented by a clinician via video conferencing (Hepburn et al., 2016) or by a real-time, clinician-coached parent (Wacker et al., 2013), has been found to be feasible and effective. For example, the telehealth adaptation of the Facing Your Fears programme for anxiety in autistic youth/adolescents (ages 7–19 years) demonstrated small to medium effects sizes and was found acceptable by both parents and their children (Hepburn et al., 2016).

Video modelling and video self-monitoring involve identifying target behaviours and creating videos where either someone (parent, therapist, etc.) performs the behaviours in steps (i.e. video modelling) or the child is videotaped performing the target task in steps (i.e. video self-monitoring). The child is instructed to watch the video before the target behaviour needs to be performed and then tries to complete the task steps (independently or with prompts) until mastery (Bellini & Akullian, 2007). These intervention methods have been successfully used to teach social skills (Apple et al., 2005; Charlop-Christy et al., 2000; Flynn & Healy, 2012) as well as adaptive skills (Campbell et al., 2015; Charlop-Christy et al., 2000; Shrestha et al., 2013) to small samples of autistic children of varying ages and developmental levels.

Some interventions for autistic children and adolescents have utilized virtual reality environments to target core ASD symptoms (e.g. social communication difficulties) and co-occurring psychological disorders like specific phobia (Maskey et al., 2019) and ADHD (Vahabzadeh et al., 2018). Despite establishing good feasibility and acceptability metrics, virtual reality interventions have demonstrated inconsistent findings across participants (Maskey et al., 2019) and may be subject to expectancy effects (Vahabzadeh et al., 2018).

Computer-based interventions and electronic applications have been developed to target various challenges common in ASD such as face processing (Tanaka et al., 2010), affect recognition (Thomeer et al., 2015), executive functioning skills (de Vries et al., 2015), and flexible relational responding (Murphy, Lyons, Kelly, Barnes-Holmes, & Barnes-Holmes, 2019). While all treatments resulted in improvements of their target behaviours in school-aged children, only the affect recognition computer-based intervention demonstrated large effect sizes. Further, the executive functioning intervention had high attrition rates and did not show differential effects from controls (de Vries et al., 2015), while the computerized program for relational responding decreased response time but did not significantly increase response accuracy nor intelligence scores (Murphy et al., 2019). Some tablet and/or iPad™ applications have also been developed to provide LI interventions to autistic children, including a personal digital assistant (PDA) programme created to aid independent

transitioning between activities for autistic adolescents with no intellectual disability (Palmen, Didden, & Verhoeven, 2012) and applications targeting social communication in young children under 6 years (Fletcher-Watson et al., 2016) as well
as cognitive control in autistic young adolescents with co-occurring ADHD (Yerys
et al., 2019). While all applications were found acceptable by users, only the PDA
and cognitive control programmes demonstrated significant improvements in target
behaviours.

Ecological momentary assessment (EMA; Stone & Shiffman, 1994) uses notification prompts on smartphones or other portable digital devices to collect real-time
data on behaviours, moods, and experiences in natural environments. Although
few studies have evaluated the feasibility of utilizing EMA with autistic youth (Khor,
Gray, Reid, & Melvin, 2014) or adults (Gerber, Girard, Scott, & Lerner, 2019), EMA
technology provides ecologically valid, rich information on both objective and subjective behavioural patterns and shows promise as a potential LI therapeutic tool for
autistic individuals. For example, in a recent study (Alda, 2018; Gerber et al., 2019),
EMA was used to administer an intervention aimed at increasing attention to facial
emotions during real-world social interactions. Every day for 1 week, participants in
all conditions received an approximately 5-minute training session on how to identify and log all *in vivo* social interaction, and were instructed to do so (they also received random-interval reminder prompts 12 times per day throughout the week).
In the 'active' condition, participants were also instructed to log the emotion of the
person with whom they were interacting, with the goal of increasing attention to facial emotions. This study demonstrates the utility of EMA for both tracking social
behaviour (a key outcome) and delivering the LI intervention of prompted *in vivo*
social-emotional attention. Thus, EMA provides a promising avenue for maintaining
engagement in treatment and promoting independent progress towards treatment
goals outside of a therapy session, while simultaneously providing clinicians with
accurate, real-time data about treatment progress.

Alternative treatment providers and settings

Many LI interventions for autistic youth utilize parents and caregivers as alternative service providers to further increase treatment accessibility and to encourage
generalization of skills beyond clinical settings. Furthermore, evidence suggests
that increasing parents' involvement in their child's treatment and/or coordinating
care across treatment settings (e.g. home and school) may reduce parental stress
and change parental perceptions of their child's problem behaviours. For example,
shifting parental attribution of motive for their child's emotional outbursts from
wilful opposition to difficulty appropriately expressing and regulating emotions
due to core social communication skills deficits may increase parental motivation
and agency in supporting their child's therapeutic progress, potentially augmenting
the effectiveness of interventions for autistic youth (D'Elia et al., 2014; Mesibov &

Shea, 2010; Panerai et al., 2009). Parent- and caregiver-mediated LI interventions for autistic youth have been shown to significantly reduce impairment and internalizing symptoms in autistic youth with co-occurring anxiety but without intellectual disability (ages 6–17 years; Storch et al., 2020), increase toddlers' joint attention (ages 22–36 months; Kasari, Gulsrud, Paparella, Hellemann, & Berry, 2015), and improve use of spontaneous language in young children with language delays (ages 44–80 months; Ingersoll & Wainer, 2013), demonstrating small to large effect sizes. Additionally, brief (two to six sessions) parent-mediated interventions have demonstrated small effect sizes for decreasing parental stress and increasing parental coping, improving child joint attention, verbal and motor imitation, social engagement, and adaptive skills in children (ages 2–6 years; Manohar, Kandasamy, Chandrasekaran, & Rajkumar, 2019), improving sleep hygiene and reducing daytime problem behaviours in autistic youth/adolescents with insomnia (Loring et al., 2016, 2018; Papadopoulos et al., 2022), and have shown preliminary evidence of increasing the frequency of young children's social initiations (ages 3–4 years; Popovic et al., 2020).

Contextually mediated LI intervention approaches aim to leverage the *physical setting* to reduce barriers to treatment by delivering interventions outside of traditional clinical settings and, instead, within the places where children may already (choose to) be. Implementing interventions within naturalistic, non-therapeutic, and/or recreational environments reduces barriers to access and increase opportunities for engagement by bringing interventions into pre-established venues where autistic youths already learn and play, while also encouraging generalization of skills to new settings. Classroom peers, teachers, and theatre directors have all been used as vehicles for delivery of evidence-based LI interventions for autistic youth in such non-clinical settings. Findings from several teacher-implemented LI interventions for autistic youth show significant improvements in joint attention in preschool-aged children (Lawton & Kasari, 2012) as well as large to very large effect sizes for educational outcomes (Ruble, McGrew, Toland, Dalrymple, & Jung, 2013) and improvements in active social engagement, adaptive communication, social skills, executive functioning, and problem behaviours (Morgan et al., 2018) in elementary school children. Peer-mediated interventions provide indirect social skills training (as opposed to direct, didactic instruction) and demonstrate moderate effect sizes for increasing social connections and social skills in elementary school settings (Kasari et al., 2012), while theatre-based social skills programmes for autistic youth/adolescents (ages 8–17) have demonstrated medium to large effect sizes for improvements across social skills domains (Corbett et al., 2016, 2019; Lerner, Mikami, & Levine, 2011; Lerner & Levine, 2007).

Brief interventions and truncated adaptations

Brief interventions and truncated adaptations of more time-intensive treatment protocols have been utilized in mechanism-focused research aimed at isolating the 'active ingredients' of specific interventions. For example, a scalable, single-session, computer-guided growth mindset intervention shown to reduce anxiety and depression symptoms and increase perceived behavioural control in non-autistic adolescents (Schleider & Weisz, 2018) has recently been adapted for use with autistic youth/adolescents and is currently being tested in this population (Gerber, Giacomantonio, Uriarte, Schleider, & Lerner, 2020). In terms of brief interventions, Zhou and colleagues have adapted a brief (two-session) romantic relationship workshop (Davila et al., 2017; Zhou & Davila, 2019) for improving social communication, romantic competence, healthy relationship functioning, and well-being for autistic young adults. Truncated versions of theatre-based social skills programmes have also demonstrated acceptability and treatment outcomes for adolescents comparable to their full-length treatment counterparts (Corbett et al., 2014; Marro et al., 2019). Lastly, therapist-implemented LI interventions adapted for outpatient settings have been shown to be feasible, acceptable, and demonstrate effectiveness for increasing social engagement, language, and play skills in young children (Ingersoll, Wainer, Berger, & Walton, 2017), while LI adaptations of social skills groups show moderate effect sizes for improving adaptive functioning and core ASD symptoms in children ages 7–17 years when used as an adjunct to standard models of care (Jonsson et al., 2019; Olsson et al., 2017).

Challenges

Duration of treatment represents one challenge of implementing LI interventions with autistic youth. While duration of LI interventions are significantly truncated compared to the time-intensive structure of typical interventions for autistic individuals, 6.5–12.5 treatment hours per week may still be considered intensive by some practitioners (Eldevik, Eikeseth, Jahr, & Smith, 2006; Peters-Scheffer Didden, Mulders, & Korzilius, 2010). Second, some co-occurring conditions may present differently in the context of ASD (e.g. anxiety; White, Oswald, Ollendick, & Scahill, 2009); thus, measures developed for and used in non-ASD clinical populations may not adequately capture treatment response/symptom change in autistic individuals. Third, some autistic youth may need supplementary materials like social stories, visual schedules, and checklists to fully engage with and comprehend treatment content, and these components should be considered during the design of LI interventions for autistic youth. Lastly, to date, LI interventions for autistic individuals have focused primarily on children who have parents and teachers to support implementation, while older adolescents transitioning out of highly structured home and educational environments and into adulthood have received significantly less attention (Lounds Taylor et al., 2012).

Potential solutions

The distillation and matching model (DMM) provides one promising framework for addressing these challenges. The DMM involves (1) distilling: breaking down or filtering treatment programmes or manuals into units of techniques; and (2) matching: summarizing client, setting, or other contextual factors relevant for selecting empirically supported techniques (Chorpita, Daleiden, & Weisz, 2005). Evidence shows that using such a framework to guide *modular* treatment for child mental health problems (where techniques are deployed flexibly, based on a child's presenting problems) outperforms standard, manualized treatment approaches (where therapeutic techniques are delivered in a pre-set order) for youth with anxiety, depression, and conduct disorder (Weisz et al., 2012). For example, research has shown that autistic individuals have difficulties with social problem-solving (Channon, Charman, Heap, Crawford, & Rios, 2001; Russo-Ponsaran et al., 2015), and these challenges have traditionally been treated en masse. However, using the DMM approach, social problem-solving can be broken down into discrete steps (e.g. problem identification, goal selection, solution selection), and then the specific element most pertinent for a given individual can be targeted, thus allowing for a more nuanced approach to intervention and skills learning. The DMM approach for ASD would allow clinicians to develop context-appropriate interventions based on techniques (whether developed in autistic or non-autistic populations; e.g. practising emotion recognition, exposure) and designed to maximize cost-effectiveness (e.g. truncating interventions with needlessly long durations; using peer or self-guided treatment provision where possible). Taking a DMM approach to treating autistic youth requires standardizing more treatment outcome measures for use in autistic populations but will ultimately result in more cost-effective treatments.

What is the future?

Going forward, we expect to see more testing of truncated versions of existing interventions (e.g. Corbett et al., 2014) and more adapting of LI interventions from other populations (e.g. Quach, Hiscock, Ukoumunne, & Wake, 2011; Schleider & Weisz, 2018) to autistic youth (Gerber et al., 2020; Papadopoulos et al., 2022). Additionally, we expect more research on non-behavioural LI interventions (e.g. repetitive transcranial magnetic stimulation; Wang et al., 2016), and on interventions that combine delivery modalities (e.g. both peer-mediated and child-assisted interventions; Kasari et al., 2012). There is also ample opportunity to evaluate the cost-effectiveness of existing programmes that have yet to be empirically tested (e.g. additional variants on LI summer camp interventions; Kasthurirathne, Alana, & Ansaldo, 2018) as well as potential benefits of capitalizing on established dissemination. Finally, LI interventions can be a useful tool for increasing access to evidence-based practices for diverse populations of autistic youth, and research into LI interventions would benefit from prioritizing the involvement and expertise of researchers of diverse backgrounds (e.g. autistic researchers; black, indigenous, and people of colour; Jones, & Mandell, 2020).

Chapter summary

There is growing interest in the developing field of LI interventions for autistic individuals. However, empirical research on LI interventions in the context of ASD remains limited. The need for large-scale randomized controlled trials and further intervention adaptations for young autistic people provides a springboard for future research.

Recommended measures

- Brief Observation of Social Communication Change (BOSCC; Kim, Grzazdinski, Martinez, & Lord, 2019).

Recommended reading

Self-help resources

Gaus, V. L. (2011). *Living well on the spectrum: How to use your strengths to meet the challenges of Asperger syndrome/high-functioning autism*. New York: Guilford Press.

Harpur, J., Lawlor, M., & Fitzgerald, M. (2004). *Succeeding in college with Asperger's syndrome: A student guide*. London: Jessica Kingsley Publishers.

Holliday Willey, L. (2003). *Asperger syndrome in adolescence: Living with the ups, the downs, and things in between*. London: Jessica Kingsley Publishers.

Sainsbury, C. (2009). *Martian in the playground: Understanding the schoolchild with Asperger's syndrome* (2nd ed.). Thousand Oaks, CA: SAGE Publications Ltd.

References

Alda, A. (2018). *If I understood you, would I have this look on my face?: My adventures in the art and science of relating and communicating*. New York: Penguin Random House LLC.

American Psychiatric Association. (2013). *Diagnostic and statistical manual of mental disorders* (5th ed.). Arlington, VA: American Psychiatric Association.

Apple, A. L., Billingsley, F., Schwartz, I. S., & Carr, E. G. (2005). Effects of video modeling alone and with self-management on compliment-giving behaviors of children with high-functioning ASD. *Journal of Positive Behavior Interventions, 7*(1), 33–46.

Bellini, S., & Akullian, J. (2007). A meta-analysis of video modeling and video self-modeling interventions for children and adolescents with autism spectrum disorders. *Exceptional Children, 73*(3), 264–287.

Campbell, J. E., Morgan, M., Barnett, V., & Spreat, S. (2015). Handheld devices and video modeling to enhance the learning of self-help skills in adolescents with autism spectrum disorder. *OTJR: Occupation, Participation and Health, 35*(2), 95–100.

Channon, S., Charman, T., Heap, J., Crawford, S., & Rios, P. (2001). Real-life-type problem-solving in Asperger's syndrome. *Journal of Autism and Developmental Disorders, 31*(5), 461–469.

Charlop-Christy, M. H., Le, L., & Freeman, K. A. (2000). A comparison of video modeling with in vivo modeling for teaching children with autism. *Journal of Autism and Developmental Disorders, 30*(6), 537–552.

Chorpita, B. F., Daleiden, E. L., & Weisz, J. R. (2005). Identifying and selecting the common elements of evidence based interventions: A distillation and matching model. *Mental Health Services Research, 7*(1), 5–20.

Clarke, C., Hill, V., & Charman, T. (2016). School based cognitive behavioural therapy targeting anxiety in children with autistic spectrum disorder: A quasi-experimental randomised controlled trail incorporating a mixed methods approach. *Journal of Autism and Developmental Disorders, 47*(12), 3883–3895.

Corbett, B. A., Ioannou, S., Key, A. P., Coke, C., Muscatello, R., Vandekar, S., & Muse, I. (2019). Treatment effects in social cognition and behavior following a theater-based intervention for youth with autism. *Developmental Neuropsychology, 44*(7), 481–494.

Corbett, B. A., Key, A. P., Qualls, L., Fecteau, S., Newsom, C., Coke, C., & Yoder, P. (2016). Improvement in social competence using a randomized trial of a theatre intervention for children with autism spectrum disorder. *Journal of Autism and Developmental Disorders, 46*, 658–672.

Corbett, B. A., Swain, D. M., Coke, C., Simon, D., Newsom, C., Houchins-Juarez, N., . . ., & Song, Y. (2014). Improvement in social deficits in autism spectrum disorders using a theatre-based, peer-mediated intervention. *Autism Research, 7*(1), 4–16.

de Vries, M., Prins, P. J., Schmand, B. A., & Geurts, H. M. (2015). Working memory and cognitive flexibility-training for children with an autism spectrum disorder: A randomized controlled trial. *Journal of Child Psychology and Psychiatry, 56*(5), 566–576.

D'Elia, L., Valeri, G., Sonnino, F., Fontana, I., Mammone, A., & Vicari, S. (2014). A longitudinal study of the TEACCH program in different settings: The potential benefits of low intensity intervention in preschool children with autism spectrum disorder. *Journal of Autism and Developmental Disorders, 44*(3), 615–626.

Davila, J., Mattanah, J., Bhatia, V., Latack, J. A., Feinstein, B. A., Eaton, N. R., . . ., & Zhou, J. (2017). Romantic competence, healthy relationship functioning, and well-being in emerging adults. *Personal Relationships, 24*(1), 162–184.

Eldevik, S., Eikeseth, S., Jahr, E., & Smith, T. (2006). Effects of low-intensity behavioral treatment for children with autism and mental retardation. *Journal of Autism and Developmental Disorders, 36*(2), 211–224.

English, O., Wellings, C., Banerjea, P., & Ougrin, D. (2019). Specialized therapeutic assessment-based recovery-focused treatment for young people with self-harm: Pilot study. *Frontiers in Psychiatry, 10*, 895.

Fletcher-Watson, S., Petrou, A., Scott-Barrett, J., Dicks, P., Graham, C., O'Hare, A., . . ., & McConachie, H. (2016). A trial of an iPadTM intervention targeting social communication skills in children with autism. *Autism, 20*, 771–782.

Flynn, L., & Healy, O. (2012). A review of treatments for deficits in social skills and self-help skills in autism spectrum disorder. *Research in Autism Spectrum Disorders, 6*(1), 431–441.

Gerber, A. H., Girard, J. M., Scott, S. B., & Lerner, M. D. (2019). Alexithymia—not autism—is associated with frequency of social interactions in adults. *Behaviour Research and Therapy, 123*, 103477.

Gerber, A. H., Giacomantonio, J., Uriarte, V. N., Schleider, J., & Lerner, M. D. (2020). Single-Session Growth-Mindset Intervention Improves Perceived Control and Depression in Youth with ASD: A Pilot RCT. Poster at the *Autism Spectrum/Developmental Disorders Special Interest Group Exposition at the Annual Convention of the Association for Behavioral and Cognitive Therapies*, Philadelphia, PA, November 19–22.

Hepburn, S. L., Blakeley-Smith, A., Wolff, B., & Reaven, J. A. (2016). Telehealth delivery of cognitive-behavioral intervention to youth with autism spectrum disorder and anxiety: A pilot study. *Autism, 20*(2), 207–218.

Hollis, C., Falconer, C. J., Martin, J. L., Whittington, C., Stockton, S., Glazebrook, C., & Davies, E. B. (2017). Annual research review: Digital health interventions for children and young people with mental health problems—a systematic and meta-review. *Journal of Child Psychology and Psychiatry, 58*(4), 474–503.

Hollocks, M. J., Lerh, J. W., Magiati, I., Meiser-Stedman, R., & Brugha, T. S. (2019). Anxiety and depression in adults with autism spectrum disorder: A systematic review and meta-analysis. *Psychological Medicine*, *49*(4), 559–572.

Hossain, M. M., Khan, N., Sultana, A., Ma, P., McKyer, E. L. J., Ahmed, H. U., & Purohit, N. (2020). Prevalence of comorbid psychiatric disorders among people with autism spectrum disorder: An umbrella review of systematic reviews and meta-analyses. *Psychiatry Research*, *287*, 112922.

Ingersoll, B., & Wainer, A. (2013). Initial efficacy of Project ImPACT: A parent-mediated social communication intervention for young children with ASD. *Journal of Autism and Developmental Disorders*, *43*(12), 2943–2952.

Ingersoll, B. R., Wainer, A. L., Berger, N. I., & Walton, K. M. (2017). Efficacy of low intensity, therapist-implemented Project ImPACT for increasing social communication skills in young children with ASD. *Developmental Neurorehabilitation*, *20*(8), 502–510.

Jones, D. R., & Mandell, D. S. (2020). To address racial disparities in autism research, we must think globally, act locally. *Autism*, *24*(7), 1587–1589.

Jonsson, U., Olsson, N. C., Coco, C., Görling, A., Flygare, O., Råde, A., . . ., & Bölte, S. (2019). Long-term social skills group training for children and adolescents with autism spectrum disorder: A randomized controlled trial. *European Child and Adolescent Psychiatry*, *28*(2), 189–201.

Kasari, C., Rotheram-Fuller, E., Locke, J., & Gulsrud, A. (2012). Making the connection: Randomized controlled trial of social skills at school for children with autism spectrum disorders. *Journal of Child Psychology and Psychiatry*, *53*(4), 431–439.

Kasari, C., Gulsrud, A., Paparella, T., Hellemann, G., & Berry, K. (2015). Randomized comparative efficacy study of parent-mediated interventions for toddlers with autism. *Journal of Consulting and Clinical Psychology*, *83*(3), 554–563.

Kasthurirathne, R., Alana, L., & Ansaldo, J. (2018). Improvising social skills for teens with ASD: Through improv, teens can tap into their inner comedian while building social-communication skills. See how an Indiana University camp does it. *The American Speech-Language-Hearing Association Leader*, *23*(5), 38–41.

Kenny, L., Hattersley, C., Molins, B., Buckley, C., Povey, C., & Pellicano, E. (2016). Which terms should be used to describe autism? Perspectives from the UK autism community. *Autism*, *20*(4), 442–462.

Khor, A. S., Gray, K. M., Reid, S. C., & Melvin, G. A. (2014). Feasibility and validity of ecological momentary assessment in adolescents with high-functioning autism and Asperger's disorder. *Journal of Adolescence*, *37*(1), 37–46.

Kim, S. H., Grzadzinski, R., Martinez, K., & Lord, C. (2019). Measuring treatment response in children with autism spectrum disorder: Applications of the Brief Observation of Social Communication Change to the Autism Diagnostic Observation Schedule. *Autism*, *23*(5), 1176–1185.

Lawton, K., & Kasari, C. (2012). Teacher-implemented joint attention intervention: Pilot randomized controlled study for preschoolers with autism. *Journal of Consulting and Clinical Psychology*, *80*(4), 687–693.

Lerner, M., & Levine, K. (2007). The Spotlight Program: An integrative approach to teaching social pragmatics using dramatic principles and techniques. *Journal of Developmental Processes*, *2*, 91–102.

Lerner, M., Mikami, A. Y., & Levine, K. (2011). Socio-dramatic affective-relational intervention for adolescents with Asperger syndrome & high functioning autism: Pilot study. *Autism*, *15*, 21–42.

Levy, S. E., Giarelli, E., Lee, L. C., Schieve, L. A., Kirby, R. S., Cunniff, C., . . ., & Rice, C. E. (2010). Autism spectrum disorder and co-occurring developmental, psychiatric, and medical conditions among children in multiple populations of the United States. *Journal of Developmental and Behavioral Pediatrics*, *31*(4), 267–275.

Leyfer, O.T., Folstein, S.E., Bacalman, S., Davis, N.O., Dinh, E., Morgan, J., . . ., & Lainhart, J.E. (2006). Comorbid psychiatric disorders in children with autism: Interview development and rates of disorders. *Journal of Autism and Developmental Disorders*, *36*(7), 849–861.

Loring, W. A., Johnston, R., Gray, L., Goldman, S., & Malow, B. (2016). A brief behavioral intervention for insomnia in adolescents with autism spectrum disorders. *Clinical Practice in Pediatric Psychology*, *4*(2), 112–124.

Loring, W. A., Johnston, R. L., Shui, A. M., & Malow, B. A. (2018). Impact of a brief behavioral intervention for insomnia on daytime behaviors in adolescents with autism spectrum disorders. *Journal of Contemporary Psychotherapy*, *48*(3), 165–177.

Lounds Taylor, J., Dove, D., Veenstra-VanderWeele, J., Sathe, N. A., McPheeters, M. L., Jerome, R. N., & Warren, Z. (2012). *Interventions for adolescents and young adults with autism spectrum disorders.* Comparative Effectiveness Review No. 65. Rockville, MD: Agency for Healthcare Research and Quality.

Maenner, M. J., Shaw, K. A., Baio, J., Washington, A., Patrick, M., DiRienzo, M., . . ., & Lopez, M. (2020). Prevalence of autism spectrum disorder among children aged 8 years—Autism and Developmental Disabilities Monitoring Network, 11 Sites, United States, 2016. *Morbidity and Mortality Weekly Report. Surveillance Summaries, 69*(4), 1–12.

Marro, B. M., Kang, E., Hauschild, K. M., Normansell, K. M., Abu-Ramadan, T. M., & Lerner, M. D. (2019). Social performance-based interventions promote gains in social knowledge in the absence of explicit training for youth with autism spectrum disorder. *Bulletin of the Menninger Clinic, 83*(3), 301–325.

Manohar, H., Kandasamy, P., Chandrasekaran, V., & Rajkumar, R. P. (2019). Brief parent-mediated intervention for children with autism spectrum disorder: A feasibility study from South India. *Journal of Autism and Developmental Disorders, 49*(8), 3146–3158.

Maskey, M., Rodgers, J., Grahame, V., Glod, M., Honey, E., Kinnear, J., . . ., & Parr, J. R. (2019). A randomised controlled feasibility trial of immersive virtual reality treatment with cognitive behaviour therapy for specific phobias in young people with autism spectrum disorder. *Journal of Autism and Developmental Disorders, 49*(5), 1912–1927.

Mazza, M., Mariano, M., Peretti, S., Masedu, F., Pino, M. C., & Valenti, M. (2017). The role of theory of mind on social information processing in children with autism spectrum disorders: A mediation analysis. *Journal of Autism and Developmental Disorders, 47*(5), 1369–1379.

Mesibov, G. B., & Shea, V. (2010). The TEACCH program in the era of evidence-based practice. *Journal of Autism and Developmental Disorders, 40*(5), 570–579.

Morgan, L., Hooker, J. L., Sparapani, N., Reinhardt, V. P., Schatschneider, C., & Wetherby, A. M. (2018). Cluster randomized trial of the classroom SCERTS intervention for elementary students with autism spectrum disorder. *Journal of Consulting and Clinical Psychology, 86*(7), 631–644.

Murphy, C., Lyons, K., Kelly, M., Barnes-Holmes, Y., & Barnes-Holmes, D. (2019). Using the Teacher IRAP (T-IRAP) interactive computerized programme to teach complex flexible relational responding with children with diagnosed autism spectrum disorder. *Behavior Analysis in Practice, 12*(1), 52–65.

Murphy, C. M., Ellie Wilson, C., Robertson, D. M., Ecker, C., Daly, E. M., Hammond, N., . . ., & McAlonan, G. M. (2016). Autism spectrum disorder in adults: Diagnosis, management, and health services development. *Neuropsychiatric Disease and Treatment, 12*, 1669–1686.

Olsson, N. C., Flygare, O., Coco, C., Görling, A., Råde, A., Chen, Q., . . ., & Tammimies, K. (2017). Social skills training for children and adolescents with autism spectrum disorder: A randomized controlled trial. *Journal of the American Academy of Child and Adolescent Psychiatry, 56*(7), 585–592.

Palmen, A., Didden, R., & Verhoeven, L. (2012). A personal digital assistant for improving independent transitioning in adolescents with high-functioning autism spectrum disorder. *Developmental Neurorehabilitation, 15*(6), 401–413.

Panerai, S., Zingale, M., Trubia, G., Finocchiaro, M., Zuccarello, R., Ferri, R., & Elia, M. (2009). Special education versus inclusive education: The role of the TEACCH program. *Journal of Autism and Developmental Disorders, 39*(6), 874–882.

Papadopoulos, N., Sciberras, E., Hiscock, H., Williams, K., McGillivray, J., Mihalopoulos, C., . . ., & Rinehart, N. (2022). Sleeping Sound Autism Spectrum Disorder (ASD): A randomised controlled trial of a brief behavioural sleep intervention in primary school-aged autistic children. *Journal of Child Psychology and Psychiatry*.

Perihan, C., Burke, M., Bowman-Perrott, L., Bicer, A., Gallup, J., Thompson, J., & Sallese, M. (2020). Effects of cognitive behavioral therapy for reducing anxiety in children with high functioning ASD: A systematic review and meta-analysis. *Journal of Autism and Developmental Disorders, 50*(6), 1958–1972.

Peters-Scheffer, N., Didden, R., Mulders, M., & Korzilius, H. (2010). Low intensity behavioral treatment supplementing preschool services for young children with autism spectrum disorders and severe to mild intellectual disability. *Research in Developmental Disabilities, 31*(6), 1678–1684.

Popovic, S. C., Starr, E. M., & Koegel, L. K. (2020). Teaching initiated question asking to children with autism spectrum disorder through a short-term parent-mediated program. *Journal of Autism and Developmental Disorders, 50*(10), 3728–3738.

Quach, J., Hiscock, H., Ukoumunne, O. C., & Wake, M. (2011). A brief sleep intervention improves outcomes in the school entry year: a randomized controlled trial. *Pediatrics, 128*(4), 692–701.

Robison, J. E. (2019). Talking about autism—thoughts for researchers. *Autism Research, 12*(7), 1004–1006.

Rosen, T. E., Mazefsky, C. A., Vasa, R. A., & Lerner, M. D. (2018). Co-occurring psychiatric conditions in autism spectrum disorder. *International Review of Psychiatry, 30*(1), 40–61.

Ruble, L. A., McGrew, J. H., Toland, M. D., Dalrymple, N. J., & Jung, L. A. (2013). A randomized controlled trial of COMPASS web-based and face-to-face teacher coaching in autism. *Journal of Consulting and Clinical Psychology, 81*(3), 566–572.

Russo-Ponsaran, N. M., McKown, C., Johnson, J. K., Allen, A. W., Evans-Smith, B., & Fogg, L. (2015). Social-emotional correlates of early stage social information processing skills in children with and without autism spectrum disorder. *Autism Research, 8*(5), 486–496.

Schleider, J., & Weisz, J. (2018). A single-session growth mindset intervention for adolescent anxiety and depression: 9-month outcomes of a randomized trial. *Journal of Child Psychology and Psychiatry, 59*(2), 160–170.

Shrestha, A., Anderson, A., & Moore, D. W. (2013). Using point-of-view video modeling and forward chaining to teach a functional self-help skill to a child with autism. *Journal of Behavioral Education, 22*(2), 157–167.

Simmons, E. S., Paul, R., & Shic, F. (2016). Brief report: A mobile application to treat prosodic deficits in autism spectrum disorder and other communication impairments: A pilot study. *Journal of Autism and Developmental Disorders, 46*(1), 320–327.

Sinclair, J. (2013). Why I dislike 'person first' language. *Autonomy, the Critical Journal of Interdisciplinary Autism Studies, 1*(2), 2–3.

Stone, A. A., & Shiffman, S. (1994). Ecological momentary assessment (EMA) in behavioral medicine. *Annals of Behavioral Medicine, 16*(3), 199–202.

Storch, E. A., Schneider, S. C., De Nadai, A. S., Selles, R. R., McBride, N. M., Grebe, S. C., . . ., & Lewin, A. B. (2019). A pilot study of family-based exposure-focused treatment for youth with autism spectrum disorder and anxiety. *Child Psychiatry and Human Development, 51*(2), 209–219.

Tanaka, J. W., Wolf, J. M., Klaiman, C., Koenig, K., Cockburn, J., Herlihy, L., . . ., & Schultz, R. T. (2010). Using computerized games to teach face recognition skills to children with autism spectrum disorder: The Let's Face It! program. *Journal of Child Psychology and Psychiatry, 51*(8), 944–952.

Thomeer, M. L., Smith, R. A., Lopata, C., Volker, M. A., Lipinski, A. M., Rodgers, J. D., . . ., & Lee, G. K. (2015). Randomized controlled trial of mind reading and in vivo rehearsal for high-functioning children with ASD. *Journal of Autism and Developmental Disorders, 45*, 2115–2127.

Vahabzadeh, A., Keshav, N. U., Salisbury, J. P., & Sahin, N. T. (2018). Improvement of attention-deficit/hyperactivity disorder symptoms in school-aged children, adolescents, and young adults with autism via a digital smartglasses-based socioemotional coaching aid: Short-term, uncontrolled pilot study. *Journal of Medical Internet Research Mental Health, 5*(2), e25.

Vivanti, G. (2020). Ask the editor: What is the most appropriate way to talk about individuals with a diagnosis of autism? *Journal of Autism and Developmental Disorders, 50*(2), 691–693.

Wacker, D. P., Lee, J. F., Dalmau, Y. C. P., Kopelman, T. G., Lindgren, S. D., Kuhle, J., . . ., & Waldron, D. B. (2013). Conducting functional communication training via telehealth to reduce the problem behavior of young children with autism. *Journal of Developmental and Physical Disabilities, 25*(1), 35–48.

Wang, Y., Hensley, M. K., Tasman, A., Sears, L., Casanova, M. F., & Sokhadze, E. M. (2016). Heart rate variability and skin conductance during repetitive TMS course in children with autism. *Applied Psychophysiology and Biofeedback, 41*(1), 47–60.

Weisz, J. R., Chorpita, B. F., Palinkas, L. A., Schoenwald, S. K., Miranda, J., Bearman, S. K., . . ., & Gray, J. (2012). Testing standard and modular designs for psychotherapy treating depression, anxiety, and conduct problems in youth: A randomized effectiveness trial. *Archives of General Psychiatry, 69*(3), 274–282.

White, S.W., Oswald, D., Ollendick, T., & Scahill, L. (2009). Anxiety in children and adolescents with autism spectrum disorders. *Clinical Psychology Review*, *29*(3), 216–229.

Yerys, B. E., Bertollo, J. R., Kenworthy, L., Dawson, G., Marco, E. J., Schultz, R. T., & Sikich, L. (2019). Brief report: Pilot study of a novel interactive digital treatment to improve cognitive control in children with autism spectrum disorder and co-occurring ADHD symptoms. *Journal of Autism and Developmental Disorders*, *49*(4), 1727–1737.

Zhou, J., & Davila, J. (2019). Romantic competence behavior during problem solving among emerging adult dating couples: Development of an observational coding system. *Personal Relationships*, *26*(3), 448–465.

16

Low intensity interventions for children with Tourette syndrome and tic disorders

Charlotte Sanderson, Charlotte L. Hall, and Tara Murphy

Learning objectives

- To understand how tic disorders and Tourette syndrome present in children and young people.
- To consider how co-occurring mental health problems commonly present alongside tic disorders and impact treatment.
- To explore how evidence-based low intensity interventions may be used to support children and young people with tics and other presenting difficulties.

What are tic disorders and Tourette syndrome?

Around 20% of children will experience some form of tic (i.e. involuntary, repetitive movement or vocalization). In many cases, these 'transient', simple tics will not require clinical evaluation or intervention and may remit within months of onset. However, around 1% of the population experience more persistent, complex, or severe motor and/or vocal tics (Scharf, Miller, Mathews, & Ben-Shlomo, 2012) that can significantly impact quality of life and daily functioning. Tourette syndrome represents the more severe form of tic disorders and is diagnosed where both vocal and motor tics are present for more than 1 year. Typically, tics begin at around 6–7 years of age and peak at 8–12 years before declining, though for a minority they persist through late adolescence and into adulthood (Leckman et al., 1989).

Tic disorders rarely present on their own. It is estimated that around 85% of individuals have at least one other co-occurring psychiatric condition, with comorbid attention deficit hyperactivity disorder (54%), obsessive–compulsive disorders (50%), and anxiety (36%) being most common (Hirschtritt et al., 2015). Co-occurring conditions may have implications for behavioural treatments (Sanderson et al., 2020), and can be associated with greater functional impairment and distress than tics themselves (Bernard et al., 2009).

Behavioural interventions in tic disorders

This chapter provides a brief overview of the three core behavioural treatments for tics: comprehensive behavioural intervention for tics (CBIT), which includes habit reversal training (HRT), and exposure and response prevention (ERP). Access to therapies is more limited compared with medication (Cuenca et al., 2015) which has resulted in a growing interest in adaptations to treatment. Preliminary evidence has highlighted the potential for existing effective behavioural tic treatments to be delivered in briefer formats, and via alternative modalities (e.g. online/group interventions) that may help to widen access and referral pathways. We explore how these may be modified for low intensity (LI) delivery, drawing upon available evidence. We consider how co-occurring conditions may be addressed within/alongside brief tic-focused interventions, presenting a case study of a young person with tics and social anxiety. Readers less familiar with tic disorders are encouraged to consult the 'Recommended reading' list at the end of the chapter.

Comprehensive behavioural intervention for tics

The largest clinical trials, and arguably the strongest evidence, to date for behavioural treatments for tics in both youth and adults has been for CBIT (McGuire, et al., 2014)—a multicomponent manualized intervention that combines HRT with relaxation skills and functional analysis to promote a positive, supportive environment (Verdellen, van der Griendt, Kriens, Oostrum, & Chang, 2011; Woods et al., 2008). In HRT, the individual first learns to recognize the urge to tic (a sensory phenomenon termed the 'premonitory urge', similar to the need to sneeze or itch) through self-monitoring and awareness building. Starting with the most bothersome tic(s), they are then taught to apply physically incompatible movements or sounds (i.e. a 'competing response') to 'block' the tic. Treatments incorporating HRT have shown tic reductions of 30–100% (Andrén et al., 2022), with medium to large effect sizes relative to control interventions (McGuire et al., 2014).

Exposure and response prevention

Also centred around developing tic awareness and control, in ERP the patient learns to build tolerance to the premonitory urge by *withholding* all tics. Through exposure exercises, they practise withholding vocal/motor tics when the urge is very strong and for increased lengths of time. While less researched, ERP protocols have shown at least equivalent treatment effects to HRT in terms of tic reduction (Andrén et al., 2019; van de Griendt, van Dijk, Verdellen, & Verbraak, 2018). Some clinicians particularly advocate ERP where there are multiple impairing tics, or where other presenting factors (such as obsessive–compulsive symptoms) may also indicate an ERP-based intervention (Sanderson et al., 2020).

LI and digital adaptations

In their 'original' format, CBIT/HRT and ERP protocols were developed for individual, face-to-face delivery (Piacentini et al., 2010; Verdellen et al., 2004) over ten sessions. However, recent studies have highlighted that abbreviated or less resource-intensive treatments may be feasible and effective, and that embracing diverse treatment modalities may be key to implementing LI interventions. In a pilot randomized controlled trial (RCT) in Sweden, Andren et al. (2019) found that an adapted online self-help ERP protocol with therapist and parent support led to significant reductions in tic severity, with less than 30 minutes of therapist input per week. While an equivalent HRT group did not show significant tic reduction in this small trial, improvements in tic-related impairment and quality of life were still noted. In Israel, a pilot study using an internet-based guided self-help comprehensive behavioral intervention for tics (ICBIT) for young people aged between 7 and 18 years showed good feasibility. Reductions in tic severity and improved youth global impairment and functioning were maintained at 6 months post treatment (Rachamim et al., 2022). Recently published, the Online Remote Behavioural Intervention for Tics (ORBIT) trial (Hall et al., 2019; Hollis et al., 2021) is the first large-scale RCT examining the cost-effectiveness and long-term efficacy of an online, therapist-guided behavioural therapy (ERP) relative to supported psychoeducation for tics which supported delivery of treatment with this modality. Previously, various online resources have been available to children and parents, such as 'TicHelper.com' based on an existing CBIT protocol (Conelea & Wellen, 2017) but these await programme-specific, published research outcomes.

Further investigating the potential of digital technologies and parental input, Singer, McDermott, Ferenc, Specht, and Mahone (2020) developed an instructional HRT-based DVD guide for parent delivery, and compared outcomes with a face-to-face, therapist-led protocol. While tic reductions were equivalent in both groups, high dropout (approximately 70%) was noted among those completing the DVD-based treatment. Face-to-face assessments and/or telephone contact in the earlier stages of digital treatment courses may help to engage families and promote stronger adherence, over a pure self-help approach.

Other studies have focused on briefer treatment courses or group delivery to potentially widen access and/or improve service efficiencies. Of particular note is a feasibility study that sought to address limited treatment provision among younger children (younger than 9 years) with chronic tics, using a brief six-session intervention. The CBIT-JR study (Bennett et al., 2019) integrated HRT strategies in a game-format with parental guidance to reduce attention to/accommodation of tics, showing significant tic reduction at up to 1 year.

Group interventions, which offer the opportunity to treat multiple patients (both in adults and children) simultaneously, have also shown promising outcomes in terms of tic reduction and user acceptability (Dabrowski, et al., 2018; Nissen, Kaergaard, Laursen, Parner, & Thomsen, 2018). Beyond potential cost savings for services, additional benefits of the group format may also be meeting other young people with tics, building self-efficacy, and practice in explaining tics to peers. While not strictly 'LI', there has been recent interest in brief 'intensive' interventions, delivered either in individual or group format (Heijerman-Holtgrefe et al., 2020). Being able to access as few as 1–2 days of focused face-to-face treatment, followed by remote telephone follow-up support, may be valuable to families who would struggle to attend extended weekly face-to-face sessions.

Challenges and solutions for LI interventions in tic disorders

Dose–response effects and therapeutic contact

Although dose–response relationships are poorly understood, meta-analytic data suggest that trials with more therapy sessions may produce greater effect sizes (McGuire et al., 2014). However, it is unclear whether this is linked to actual therapist contact, or longer treatment/follow-up duration. In an extended case series, Ricketts et al. (2016) found that adherence and treatment responsiveness to a six-session adapted CBIT protocol designed for delivery by multidisciplinary team staff members (e.g. nurse practitioners) was generally lower than achieved in the original CBIT trial (Piacentini et al., 2010). Beyond possible dose–response effects, this may reflect specific challenges in translating behavioural therapies to primary care settings. Feedback from practitioners highlighted clinician time burden, space limitations, and challenges in training/supporting non-mental health professionals to deliver psychological interventions as key considerations for multidisciplinary teams. Future trials should therefore carefully assess the role of therapeutic contact hours and treatment duration, as well as who delivers treatments, on treatment efficacy. In multifaceted therapies such as CBIT, it is also important to examine which treatment components are the key mediators of change and for whom.

Addressing co-occurring conditions

The majority of young people presenting for behavioural therapy for tic disorders will have additional mental health or neurodevelopmental needs. An in-depth examination of the implications of co-occurring conditions is beyond the scope of this chapter and the available research at present; however, it is important to consider some complexities that additional needs may present.

Consideration should, however, be given to ordering of treatment based on which presenting problem causes most impairment. Co-occurring conditions should generally not be considered a contraindication for behavioural therapy for tics. If tics are the most impairing difficulty to the individual but attention deficit hyperactivity disorder and anxiety symptoms impact treatment efficacy, then it may be important to address these symptoms prior to treating tics (McGuire et al., 2014; Sukhudolsky et al., 2017). Some additional symptoms may also interfere with the treatment process, or exacerbate tics. For example, where disruptive behaviours are present, parental attention to tics (both positive and negative) may be reinforcing of tic behaviours and limit therapeutic gains from HRT/ERP. A brief parent-focused behavioural intervention (e.g. McGuire et al., 2015) is worth considering in such cases, and may boost parental efficacy and confidence in supporting a child through subsequent behavioural therapy for tics. It is also not uncommon for parents and/or young people to attribute wider-ranging difficulties and impairment to tics, and also seek total 'cure' from behavioural therapy. Therefore, comprehensive psychoeducation that sets realistic expectations for therapy and considers the 'whole child' including other underlying difficulties (and strengths) is a crucial way to start treatment (Nussey, Pistrang, & Murphy, 2013). Involving family, carers, and teachers in this work can be valuable.

As motor and vocal tics can be challenging to manage in public situations, social anxiety and worries about others' perceptions can exacerbate distress and maintain difficulties. The following case study outlines how cognitive work, functional analysis, and family engagement can complement a brief tic-focused intervention to address these common complexities.

Case study

Yvonne is a 16-year-old girl living in a rural area of the UK with her parents. She was diagnosed with Tourette syndrome aged 7 years, and later with high functioning autism at age 11. She developed complex vocal and motor tics around the age of 13 that caused distress. Her father regularly commented on the tics and her teachers asked her why she did the movements. She avoided school and social activities, even online activities, that she had previously enjoyed.

Yvonne was seen at a local child and adolescent mental health service. Assessment revealed that Yvonne's education, home life, and activities of daily living were impacted by social anxiety secondary to tics in addition to pain from a complex head and shoulder tic and a simple torso tic which involved jerking her lower back. The Yale Global Tic Severity Scale (YGTSS; Leckman, 1989) was completed, indicating moderate severity and impairment from tics in the preceding week (YGTSS = 64, including impairment score = 30). A care plan was formulated locally to manage the social anxiety, and a referral was made to a national specialist clinic for young people with complex Tourette syndrome for tic-focused intervention. At the specialist clinic, Yvonne and her family were offered an online group-based intervention. The intervention comprised of four online appointments conducted via video conference. The first appointment was for 2 hours and focused on psychoeducation about tics. Information covered the natural history of tics, their understood causes and prognosis, and how treatment would not cure tics but could help Yvonne to manage symptoms. One week later, Yvonne engaged with a group-based online course of ERP for a further three sessions which lasted for 3–7 hours per session and were offered to young people and parents who joined at different times. Yvonne was one of nine young person attendees and break-out rooms were used during the intervention in which young people worked together. In the first day of the ERP programme, Yvonne learnt about the premonitory urge, response prevention (controlling tics for as long as possible without provoking the urge), and habituation (a reduction in the urge over time when she blocked the tic). A functional analysis helped to understand where the tics were most bothersome and frequent which gave Yvonne insight into where to apply the ERP technique and to change element of her environment so that the tics were not so interferring at these times, such as after school. She also developed exposure strategies to make the urge very strong while withholding tics for prolonged periods. A couple of days later, on the second day of the programme, she practised using the exposure technique, modelling and describing it to other people in the group. She practised often between sessions using techniques such as seeing a video of herself ticcing and looking at her stomach to make the urge to tic very strong. She resisted ticcing when the urge was strong and allowed the sensation to subside. By the third session, she could control the tics for long periods even when the urge was strong.

Yvonne then attended four individual sessions of cognitive behavioural therapy for social anxiety which helped her to identify situations that she had avoided and develop cognitive skills to re-integrate back into these situations. She learnt to speak assertively to friends about tics, using role play and decision-making, which were delivered by the local child and adolescent mental health service.

Three months after completing treatment, Yvonne achieved a YGTSS score of 12, with impairment of 0. She reported feeling more confident in her ability to manage her tics and life in general. Yvonne was particularly pleased that she had attended 3 weeks at school with full attendance.

What is the future?

Limited access to evidence-based therapies remains a key challenge in service provision for tic disorders. Recent research has highlighted digital technologies as a promising means of improving provision. Large-scale RCTs, such as the ORBIT Trial (Hollis et al., 2021), will be important in establishing the efficacy and cost-effectiveness of these interventions, as well as acceptability to users. To support ERP/HRT practice 'on the go', future research should consider how app-based technologies can also be integrated such as the BT Coach tic App or TicTimer Web (Black et al., 2020).

Tic disorders are increasingly recognized as part of a broader spectrum, and rarely present on their own. Clinicians working with young people with neurodevelopmental difficulties such as autism should be mindful of the impact of tic disorders and of the evidence-based treatments available. Here we have discussed promising evidence that brief interventions may be feasible as stand-alone therapies or as part of modular treatments for children and young people. However, high-quality research (including RCTs) into the efficacy of truly LI interventions is needed, exploring in finer detail dose–response effects, 'active' treatment content, and suitability for different populations and settings.

Chapter summary

- Tic disorders are common and often occur alongside other mental health/neurodevelopmental difficulties.
- Behavioural therapies are recommended as first-line interventions for tic disorders, but access to these is limited.
- LI adaptations using briefer protocols and/or alternative modes of delivery such as online, therapist-guided self-help have potential to widen access.

Recommended Tourette syndrome-specific measures

- Yale Global Tic Severity Scale (YGTSS; Leckman, 1989).
- Child and Adolescent Gilles de la Tourette Syndrome-Quality of Life Scale (C&A GTS-QOL; Su et al., 2017).

Recommended reading

- European/North American practice guidelines for the treatment of tic disorders (Pringsheim et al., 2019; Andrén et al., 2021).

References

Andrén, P., Aspvall, K., de la Cruz, L. F., Wiktor, P., Romano, S., Andersson, E., . . ., & Mataix-Cols, D. (2019). Therapist-guided and parent-guided internet-delivered behaviour therapy for paediatric Tourette's disorder: A pilot randomised controlled trial with long-term follow-up. *BMJ Open, 9*(2), e024685.

Andrén, P., Jakubovski, E., Murphy, T. L., Woitecki, K., Tarnok, Z., Zimmerman-Brenner, S., . . ., & Verdellen C. (2022). European clinical guidelines for Tourette syndrome and other tic disorders-version 2.0. Part II: Psychological interventions. *European Journal of Child Adolescent Psychiatry*, *31*(3), 403–423. doi:10.1007/s00787-021-01845-z. Epub 2021 Jul 27. PMID: 34313861; PMCID: PMC8314030.ver.

Bearman, S. K., & Weisz, J. R. (2015). Comprehensive treatments for youth comorbidity—evidence-guided approaches to a complicated problem. *Child and Adolescent Mental Health*, *20*(3), 131–141.

Bennett, S. M., Capriotti, M., Bauer, C., Chang, S., Keller, A. E., Walkup, J., . . ., & Piacentini, J. (2019). Development and open trial of a psychosocial intervention for young children with chronic tics: The CBIT-JR Study. *Behavior Therapy*, *51*(4), 659–669.

Bernard, B. A., Stebbins, G. T., Siegel, S., Schultz, T. M., Hays, C., Morrissey, M. J., . . ., & Goetz, C. G. (2009). Determinants of quality of life in children with Gilles de la Tourette syndrome. *Movement Disorders*, *24*(7), 1070–1073.

Black, J. K., Koller, J. M., & Black, K. J. (2020). TicTimer Web: Software for measuring tic suppression remotely. *F1000Res.* 9, 1264. doi:10.12688/f1000research.26347.2. PMID: 33824720; PMCID: PMC7993402.

Conelea, C. A., & Wellen, B. C. M. (2017). Tic treatment goes tech: A review of TicHelper.com. *Cognitive and Behavioral Practice*, *24*(3), 374–381.

Cuenca, J., Glazebrook, C., Kendall, T., Hedderly, T., Heyman, I., Jackson, G., . . ., & Hollis, C. (2015). Perceptions of treatment for tics among young people with Tourette syndrome and their parents: A mixed methods study. *BMC Psychiatry* 15, 46.

Dabrowski, J., King, J., Edwards, K., Yates, R., Heyman, I., Zimmerman-Brenner, S., & Murphy, T. (2018). The long-term effects of group-based psychological interventions for children with Tourette syndrome: A randomized controlled trial. *Behavior Therapy*, *49*(3), 331–343.

Hall, C. L., Davies, E. B., Andren, P., Murphy, T., Bennett, S. D., Brown, B. J., . . ., & Hollis, C. (2019). Investigating a therapist-guided, parent-assisted remote digital behavioural intervention for tics in children and adolescents—'Online Remote Behavioural Intervention for Tics' (ORBIT) Trial: Protocol of an internal pilot study and single-blind randomised controlled trial. *BMJ Open*, *9*(1), e027583.

Heijerman-Holtgrefe, A. P., Verdellen, C. W. J., van de Griendt, J. M. T. M., Beljaars, L. P. L., Kan, K. J., Cath, D., . . ., & Utens, E. M. W. J. (2020). Tackle your tics: Pilot findings of a brief, intensive group-based exposure therapy program for children with tic disorders. *European Journal of Child Adolescent Psychiatry*, *30*(3), 461–473.

Hirschtritt, M. E., Lee, P. C., Pauls, D. L., Dion, Y., Grados, M. A., Illmann, C., . . ., & Mathews, C. A. (2015). Lifetime prevalence, age of risk, and genetic relationships of comorbid psychiatric disorders in Tourette syndrome. *JAMA Psychiatry*, *72*(4), 325–333.

Hollis, C., Hall, C. L., Jones, R., Marston, L., Novere, M. L., Hunter, R., . . ., & Murray E. (2021). Therapist-supported online remote behavioural intervention for tics in children and adolescents in England (ORBIT): A multicentre, parallel group, single-blind, randomised controlled trial. *Lancet Psychiatry*, *8*(10), 871–882. doi:10.1016/S2215-0366(21)00235-2. Epub 2021 Sep 1. Erratum in: *Lancet Psychiatry*. 2022 Jan;9(1):e1. Erratum in: *Lancet Psychiatry*. 2021 Dec 3; PMID: 34480868; PMCID: PMC8460453.

Leckman, J. F., Riddle, M. A., Hardin, M. T., Ort, S. I., Swartz, K. L., Stevenson, J., Cohen, D. J. (1989). The Yale Global Tic Severity Scale: Initial testing of a clinician-rated scale of tic severity. *Journal of the American Academy of Child and Adolescent Psychiatry*, *28*(4), 566–573.

McGuire, J. F., Piacentini, J., Brennan, E. A., Lewin, A. B., Murphy, T. K., Small, B. J., & Storch, E. A. (2014). A meta-analysis of behavior therapy for Tourette syndrome. *Journal of Psychiatric Research*, *50*, 106–112.

McGuire, J. F., Ricketts, E. J., Piacentini, J., Murphy, T. K., Storch, E. A., & Lewin, A. B. (2015). Behavior therapy for tic disorders: An evidenced-based review and new directions for treatment research. *Current Developmental Disorders Reports*, *2*(4), 309–317.

Nissen, J. B., Kaergaard, M., Laursen, L., Parner, E., & Thomsen, P. H. (2018). Combined habit reversal training and exposure response prevention in a group setting compared to individual training: A randomized controlled clinical trial. *European Child & Adolescent Psychiatry*, *28*(1), 57–68.

Nussey, C., Pistrang, N., & Murphy, T. (2013). How does psychoeducation help? A review of the effects of providing information about Tourette syndrome and attention-deficit/hyperactivity disorder. *Child: Care, Health and Development, 39*(5), 617–627.

Piacentini, J., Woods, D. W., Scahill, L., Wilhelm, S., Peterson, A. L., Chang, S., . . ., & Walkup, J. T. (2010). Behavior therapy for children with Tourette disorder: A randomized controlled trial. *JAMA, 303*(19), 1929–1937.

Pringsheim, T., Okun, M. S., Müller-Vahl, K., Martino, D., Jankovic, J., Cavanna, A. E., . . ., & Piacentini, J. (2019). Practice guideline recommendations summary: Treatment of tics in people with Tourette syndrome and chronic tic disorders. *Neurology, 92*(19), 896–906.

Rachamim, L., Zimmerman-Brenner, S., Rachamim, O. Mualem, H., Zingboim, N., & Rotstein, M. (2022). Internet-based guided self-help comprehensive behavioral intervention for tics (ICBIT) for youth with tic disorders: A feasibility and effectiveness study with 6 month-follow-up. *European Child & Adolescent Psychiatry, 31*(2), 275–287.

Ricketts, E. J., Goetz, A. R., Capriotti, M. R., Bauer, C. C., Brei, N. G., Himle, M. B., . . ., & Woods, D. W. (2016). A randomized waitlist-controlled pilot trial of voice over internet protocol-delivered behavior therapy for youth with chronic tic disorders. *Journal of Telemedicine & Telecare, 22*(3), 153–162.

Sanderson, C. L., Verdellen, C., Debes, N., Tarnok, Z., Van de Griendt, J. M. T. M., . . ., & Murphy, T. (2022). *Co-occurring conditions in tic disorders and Tourette syndrome: A guideline for delivering and adapting behavioral therapies.* Manuscript submitted for publication.

Scharf, J. M., Miller, L. L., Mathews, C. A., & Ben-Shlomo, Y. (2012). Prevalence of Tourette syndrome and chronic tics in the population-based Avon longitudinal study of parents and children cohort. *Journal of the American Academy of Child and Adolescent Psychiatry, 51*(2), 192–201.e195.

Singer, H. S., McDermott, S., Ferenc, L., Specht, M., & Mahone, M. (2020). Efficacy of parent-delivered, home-based therapy for tics. *Paediatric Neurology, 106*, 17–23.

Su, M. T., McFarlane, F., Cavanna, A. E., Termine, C., Murray, I., Heidemeyer, L., . . ., & Murphy, T. (2017). The English Version of the Gilles de la Tourette Syndrome-Quality of Life Scale for Children and Adolescents (C&A-GTS-QOL). *Journal of Child Neurology, 32*(1), 76–83.

Sukhodolsky, D. G., Woods, D. W., Piacentini, J., Wilhelm, S., Peterson, A. L., Katsovich, L., . . ., & Scahill, L. (2017). Moderators and predictors of response to behavior therapy for tics in Tourette syndrome. *Neurology, 88*(11), 1029–1036.

van de Griendt, J. M. T. M., van Dijk, M. K., Verdellen, C. W., & Verbraak, M. J. P. M. (2018). The effect of shorter exposure versus prolonged exposure on treatment outcome in Tourette syndrome and chronic tic disorders—an open trial. *International Journal of Psychiatry in Clinical Practice, 22*(4), 262–267.

Verdellen, C. W., Keijsers, G. P., Cath, D. C., & Hoogduin, C. A. (2004). Exposure with response prevention versus habit reversal in Tourettes syndrome: a controlled study. *Behaviour Research and Therapy, 42*(5), 501–511.

Verdellen, C., van de Griendt, J., Hartmann, A., Murphy, T., & ESSTS Guidelines Group (2011). European clinical guidelines for Tourette syndrome and other tic disorders. Part III: Behavioural and psychosocial interventions. *European Journal of Child & Adolescent Psychiatry, 20*(4), 197–207.

Verdellen, C., van der Griendt, J., Kriens, S., Oostrum, I., & Chang, I. (2011). *Tics: Therapist manual & workbook for children.* Amsterdam: Boom Cure & Care.

Woods, D. W., Piacentini, J., Chang, S., Deckersbach, T., Ginsburg, G., Peterson, A., . . ., & Wilhelm, S. (2008). *Managing Tourette syndrome: A behavioral intervention for children and adults therapist guide.* Oxford: Oxford University Press.

17

Low intensity interventions for mental health problems in children with chronic physical illness

Matteo Catanzano and Sophie D. Bennett

Learning objectives

- To understand how common mental health problems may present in children and young people with a chronic physical illness.
- To understand how evidence-based low intensity interventions may be used in the context of medical complexity in children and young people.
- To consider the extent to which standard interventions may need adapting for this group.

Introduction

Chronic physical illnesses or long-term conditions are defined as those:

- Lasting for at least 3 months.
- Causing functional impairment.
- Necessitating medical care.
- Where cure is considered unlikely.

Common chronic physical illnesses in children include asthma, eczema, and diabetes. Some chronic physical illnesses, particularly neurological conditions, are associated with increased rates of intellectual and/or neurodevelopmental disabilities such as autism spectrum disorder. Rates of mental health disorders are elevated in children with a chronic physical illness compared to children who are otherwise healthy, but the most common mental health disorders in this group are the same as the most common in children without a chronic physical illness: anxiety disorders (Pinquart & Shen, 2011a), depressive disorders (Pinquart & Shen, 2011b), and disruptive behaviour disorders (Adams, Chien, & Wisk, 2019; Pinquart & Shen, 2011c). This chapter describes how low intensity (LI) and/or brief interventions may be used to treat these common mental health disorders in the context of chronic physical illness. Such interventions may have particular value in this population given children with chronic physical illness may already have multiple medical appointments resulting in missed school and work. While mental health professionals also work with psychological aspects of living with a chronic physical illness, such as adjustment and/or medication adherence, these interventions are beyond the scope of the present chapter. However, such problems may be associated with a common mental health problem; for example, poor medication adherence may be associated with depression, and such mental health problems may be treated using brief and/or LI interventions.

Identifying mental health difficulties in children with chronic physical illness

Mental health problems in the context of chronic physical illness are known to be under-recognized and under-treated (Welch, Shafran, Heyman, Coughtrey, & Bennett, 2018). There are many reasons for this, but they include diagnostic overshadowing, with the physical health condition being prioritized over mental health problems. Clinicians may assume that a mental health problem is understandable in the context of the illness, or an inherent part of the illness and therefore not able to be treated. A key first step in treatment of the mental health problems is therefore to identify them. Instruments used in routine child and adolescent mental health services, such as the Strengths and Difficulties Questionnaire (SDQ), have been shown to be effective in detecting the presence of an emotional or behavioural disorder in those with chronic physical illness (Glazebrook, Hollis, Heussler, Goodman, & Coates, 2003; Hysing, Elgen, Gillberg, Lie, & Lundervold, 2007). Various feasibility studies have shown that using a standardized online diagnostic assessment tool, the Development and Well-being Assessment (DAWBA) can be an acceptable and feasible way to diagnose common mental health disorders in young people with chronic physical illness (Bennett et al., 2019; Hysing et al., 2007). Providing a self-referral option, as well as actively asking young people/carers in paediatric clinic waiting rooms if they think they would benefit from support around emotions and/or behaviour, may also increase detection of mental health problems (Catanzano et al., 2021).

The evidence for brief and LI treatments for children with a chronic physical illness

Standard evidence-based interventions can be effective for treating mental health disorders in the context of chronic physical illness in children (Moore et al., 2019) and LI interventions are efficacious in treating adult mental health disorders in the context of chronic physical illness (Beatty & Lambert, 2013). A systematic review and meta-analysis investigated the evidence base for brief and LI interventions for mental health difficulties in children and young people who have a chronic physical illness (Catanzano et al., 2020). Twelve studies were found to meet the inclusion criteria. Evidence was therefore limited, although results suggested that LI and brief interventions are effective in this group. LI and brief treatments for anxiety demonstrated a large effect size.

Examples of using LI interventions

The extent to which interventions need to be adapted for the presence of chronic physical illness is a matter of debate and not clear from current evidence, as no trials directly compare standard evidence-based therapies with those adapted for chronic physical illness. While modifications to the structure may be required, such as having shorter sessions, adaptations to the content of interventions may not be needed. There is inherent personalization of any psychological intervention, for example, using examples from the client's own experience to illustrate a concept such as thought challenging. In the case of chronic physical illness, this may include challenging thoughts related to the illness. We do not consider such personalization to be 'adaptations' to the intervention, but instead good practice (see Chapter 9 on fidelity and flexibility).

In the absence of trials of formally adapted therapy, if children with a chronic physical illness meet diagnostic criteria for a mental health disorder, it is most parsimonious to use the guidance pertaining to the treatment of that disorder (see chapters in Section 2B). In cases in which there is additional comorbidity such as intellectual disability or autism spectrum disorder, standard evidence-based interventions may still be used, with minor modifications to account for the needs of the young person (see Chapters 9 and 15). The following case example considers how standard evidence-based treatments can be adhered to while maintaining sufficient flexibility to be suitable for the needs of a child with a chronic physical illness.

Telephone delivered guided self-help for separation anxiety and behavioural difficulties

Philippa is a 9-year old girl with a genetic condition associated with intellectual and physical disability and necessitating frequent paediatric hospital visits. She was screened for mental health problems using the parent-reported SDQ as part of a routine hospital appointment. The SDQ identified elevated emotional and behavioural difficulties. These were further discussed with Philippa's mother, Kate, who said that Phillipa often became very upset when she was asked to stop the activity that she was doing, sometimes becoming physically violent towards her mother and sister. She also became distressed when apart from Kate in the house, meaning that Kate was unable to spend even 5 minutes separated from Philippa at home. This was the first time that Kate had been asked about Philippa's emotions and behaviour.

Intervention description

Philippa was offered a six-session guided self-help intervention. This was implemented as part of a stepped care approach, in which this LI intervention was offered as a first-step treatment while patients awaited child and adolescent mental health services appointments for higher intensity treatments where necessary. The intervention comprised self-help handouts on different topics (see below), which were sent out via email each week, followed by weekly 30-minute telephone calls from a psychology graduate under supervision. The intervention content itself was not modified for the presence of a chronic physical illness.

Main components of intervention

- *Goal setting:* parents were invited to attend the paediatric hospital for an initial brief 45-minute face-to-face assessment, during which they were encouraged to identify up to three goals for treatment during the first session. These goals were then monitored and rated on a scale of 0–10 at each session (where 0 is no progress towards goals and 10 is the goal has been met).
- *Weekly measurement:* in addition to goals, parents completed weekly symptom measures. See Chapter 8 for further information on using outcome measures in LI therapy.
- *Written self-help materials:* the session content was the same as that used in standard evidence-based intervention, in this case for behavioural difficulties, based on principles of reinforcement and social learning theory. Worksheets covered special time, praise, active ignoring, effective instruction-giving, rewards, school progress monitoring, and planning for the future.
- *Ten weekly telephone calls:* weekly support calls with a therapist were arranged in advance. Calls lasted up to 30 minutes. As a guided self-help intervention, the purpose of these phone calls was to briefly discuss the new worksheets for the week, and to discuss the implementation of the previous week's strategy as well as solve any problems that had occurred during the week. If appropriate, parents could repeat the week's strategy rather than introduce a new one, until the strategy was implemented reliably.

The intervention for Philippa was focused on a behavioural parenting approach for behavioural difficulties. Treatment for anxiety may have also been an option given the SDQ scores and presenting separation anxiety; however, a behavioural intervention delivered via parents was considered preferable due to the additional behavioural difficulties, as behavioural interventions may target both. It was therefore important to provide Philippa's parent with psychoeducation around the relationship between physical health problems and mental health to ensure that she did not feel blamed. This was paired with clear information separating the cause from the intervention. In some cases, we have used the analogy of aspirin which works to treat a headache, regardless of the cause.

Kate set the following goals for treatment:

1. For Philippa to be able to be alone in a room in the house without Kate for 5 minutes.
2. For Philippa to respond calmly when asked to turn off her tablet.

Kate attended all telephone sessions, although had to reschedule some due to Phillipa's ill health. Work towards goal 1 needed liaison with the medical team, as Philippa could not be safely left alone for extended periods. In addition, Kate felt very guilty ignoring some of Philippa's calls as she was worried that Phillipa may have been genuinely ill and needed her help. With discussion from the medical team, we were able to discuss how long and in what circumstances Phillipa could be left alone. Kate realized that she was able to tell the difference between a distressed call versus Phillipa calling for her attention, and with support from the therapist, was able to ignore the calls for attention and praise Philippa's independent play. She had learnt that ignoring was in Phillipa's best interest and she was not being unkind by doing so. The goals set at the beginning of therapy were fully met by the end of the 6-week guided self-help intervention. In her own words, 'it doesn't have to take a long time, it can be six phone calls, it doesn't have to be intense, it's something that's simple, that as long as you do it, it can have a huge impact on the family's life'.

Challenges in implementing LI interventions in the context of chronic physical illness

The major challenges in implementing LI interventions in these groups are the same as those faced when delivering higher intensity interventions: the question of how much to modify the intervention, real limitations on health, and concerns around safety and delivery when there are several external factors including other medical appointments. There are also issues of measurement; it is not clear whether standardized measures are able to pick up on the changes in this complex group.

Potential solutions

Regarding modifications, while evidence for adapting content for the context of chronic physical illness is equivocal, some changes to the format/delivery of interventions have been identified as potentially helpful both in the literature (Bennett et al., 2015; Morey & Loades, 2021) and from clinical experience. The most obvious is the need for increased flexibility around appointments, both as cancellations/non-attendances from illness are more likely in this group, but also as families and young people may already be very time poor due to existing medical appointments and unplanned emergency admissions.

Evidence-supported treatment can be personalized in the same way as those for children without a chronic physical illness. For example, using more behavioural than cognitive strategies for treating anxiety in a young person with a mild intellectual disability. As chronic physical illnesses vary, specific strategies may need to be personalized to the individual. For example, it might be that a young person with an inflammatory joint condition previously enjoyed running and had become low in mood after a flare-up had made it impossible for them to continue. In such a case, the LI therapist would need to consider alternative forms of exercise (e.g. swimming) with the young person when doing behavioural activation. From experience, we have found that it is best to liaise with the medical team and bring these issues of personalization to supervision. Nursing staff or other health professionals are often able to tell you what would or would not be a safe and appropriate activity given the diagnosis and level of severity. Using goal-based outcomes in addition to standardized measures is key in ensuring that the intervention meets the needs of the family.

What is the future?

There are still several gaps in the literature. Trials of brief parenting interventions for disruptive behaviour and brief interventions for depression are lacking but have been shown to be effective in young people without a long-term physical health condition and/or in a high intensity format in children with a long-term physical health condition. Larger, high-quality trials targeting elevated anxiety symptoms need to replicate the preliminary findings in the review (Catanzano et al., 2020) and include longer-term follow-ups. As a number of LI evidence-based treatments for anxiety for children without a long-term physical health condition already exist, these could be tested in future trials. Trials evaluating stepped care approaches for young people with a long-term physical health condition need to be conducted to establish who benefits from LI treatment who may need to be 'stepped up' and how services can best be organized to meet rising demands.

Chapter summary

In summary, LI interventions appear to be feasible and acceptable in children with chronic physical illnesses and show preliminary effectiveness. Although the research is not conclusive, it appears that LI interventions can be used without a need for major adaptation but instead ensuring personalization through goal-based outcomes and flexibility in delivery.

Recommended measures

We recommend using quality of life measures such as the Pediatric Quality of Life Inventory (Varni, Seid, & Kurtin, 2001) and goal-based outcomes in addition to the standardized outcomes measures used for mental health disorders in children who do not have a chronic physical illness.

Recommended reading

Bennett, S. D., Coughtrey, A. E., Heyman, I., Greally, S., Clarkson, H., Bhattacharyya, T., . . ., & Shafran, R. (2018). Guided self-help for mental health disorders in children and young people with chronic neurological conditions: A qualitative evaluation. *European Journal of Paediatric Neurology, 22*(4), 620–631.

Bennett, S. D., Heyman, I., Varadkar, S., Coughtrey, A. E., & Shafran, R. (2017). Simple or complex? A case study of physical and mental health co-morbidity. *The Cognitive Behaviour Therapist, 10*, e18.

Catanzano, M., Bennett, S. D., Kerry, E., Liang, H., Heyman, I., Coughtrey, A. E., ... & Shafran, R. (2021). Evaluation of a mental health drop-in centre offering brief transdiagnostic psychological assessment and treatment for children and adolescents with long-term physical conditions and their families: a single-arm, open, non-randomised trial. *Evidence-based mental health, 24*(1), 25–32.

Catanzano, M., Bennett, S. D., Sanderson, C., Patel, M., Manzotti, G., Kerry, E., . . ., & Shafran, R. (2020). Brief psychological interventions for psychiatric disorders in young people with long term physical health conditions: A systematic review and meta-analysis. *Journal of Psychosomatic Research, 136*, 110187.

Moore, D. A., Nunns, M., Shaw, L., Rogers, M., Walker, E., Ford, T., . . ., & Thompson Coon, J. (2019). Interventions to improve the mental health of children and young people with long-term physical conditions: linked evidence syntheses. *Health Technology Assessment, 23*(22), 1–164.

Thabrew, H., Stasiak, K., Hetrick, S. E., Donkin, L., Huss, J. H., Highlander, A., . . ., & Merry, S. N. (2018). Psychological therapies for anxiety and depression in children and adolescents with long-term physical conditions. *Cochrane Database of Systematic Reviews, 12*(12), CD012488.

Thabrew, H., Stasiak, K., Hetrick, S. E., Wong, S., Huss, J. H., & Merry, S. N. (2018). eHealth interventions for anxiety and depression in children and adolescents with long-term physical conditions. *Cochrane Database of Systematic Reviews, 8*(8) CD012489.

References

Adams, J. S., Chien, A. T., & Wisk, L. E. (2019). Mental illness among youth with chronic physical conditions. *Pediatrics, 144*(1), e20181819.

Beatty, L., & Lambert, S. (2013). A systematic review of internet-based self-help therapeutic interventions to improve distress and disease-control among adults with chronic health conditions. *Clinical Psychology Review, 33*(4), 609–622.

Bennett, S., Shafran, R., Coughtrey, A., Walker, S., & Heyman, I. (2015). Psychological interventions for mental health disorders in children with chronic physical illness: A systematic review. *Archives of Disease in Childhood, 100*(4), 308–316.

Bennett, S. D., Heyman, I., Coughtrey, A. E., Buszewicz, M., Byford, S., Dore, C.J., . . ., & Shafran, R. (2019). Assessing feasibility of routine identification tools for mental health disorder in neurology clinics. *Archives of Disease in Childhood, 104*(12), 1161–1166.

Catanzano, M., Bennett, S. D., Kerry, E., Liang, H., Heyman, I., Coughtrey, A. E., ... & Shafran, R. (2021). Evaluation of a mental health drop-in centre offering brief transdiagnostic psychological assessment and treatment for children and adolescents with long-term physical conditions and their families: a single-arm, open, non-randomised trial. Evidence-based mental health, 24(1), 25–32.

Catanzano, M., Bennett, S. D., Sanderson, C., Patel, M., Manzotti, G., Kerry, E., . . ., & Shafran, R. (2020). Brief psychological interventions for psychiatric disorders in young people with long term physical health conditions: A systematic review and meta-analysis. *Journal of Psychosomatic Research, 136,* 110187.

Glazebrook, C., Hollis, C., Heussler, H., Goodman, R., & Coates, L. (2003). Detecting emotional and behavioural problems in paediatric clinics. *Child Care, Health and Development, 29*(2), 141–149.

Hysing, M., Elgen, I., Gillberg, C., Lie, S., & Lundervold, A.J. (2007). Chronic physical illness and mental health in children. Results from a large-scale population study. *Journal of Child Psychology and Psychiatry, and Allied Disciplines, 48*(8), 785–792.

Moore, D. A., Nunns, M., Shaw, L., Rogers, M., Walker, E., Ford, T., . . ., & Thompson Coon, J. (2019). Interventions to improve the mental health of children and young people with long-term physical conditions: linked evidence syntheses. *Health Technology Assessment, 23*(22), 1–164.

Morey, A., & Loades, M. E. (2021). How has cognitive behaviour therapy been adapted for adolescents with comorbid depression and chronic illness? A scoping review. *Child and Adolescent Mental Health, 26*(3), 252–264.

Pinquart, M., & Shen, Y. (2011a). Anxiety in children and adolescents with chronic physical illnesses: A meta-analysis. *Acta Paediatrica, 100*(8), 1069–1076.

Pinquart, M., & Shen, Y. (2011b). Behavior problems in children and adolescents with chronic physical illness: A meta-analysis. *Journal of Pediatric Psychology, 36*(9), 1003–1016.

Pinquart, M., & Shen, Y. (2011c). Depressive symptoms in children and adolescents with chronic physical illness: An updated meta-analysis. *Journal of Pediatric Psychology, 36*(4), 375–384.

Varni, J. W., Seid, M., & Kurtin, P. S. (2001). PedsQL 4.0: Reliability and validity of the Pediatric Quality of Life Inventory version 4.0 generic core scales in healthy and patient populations. *Medical Care, 39*(8), 800–812.

Welch, A., Shafran, R., Heyman, I., Coughtrey, A., & Bennett, S. (2018). Usual care for mental health problems in children with epilepsy: A cohort study. *F1000Research, 7,* 1907.

18

A problem-solving self-help approach for family and friends of young people with first-episode psychosis

Terence V. McCann and Dan I. Lubman

Learning objectives

- To understand the experience of caring for young people with first-episode psychosis.
- To consider the evidence base for low intensity interventions for carers.
- To understand the usefulness of, and how to use, a problem-solving self-help approach for carers in supporting a young person with first-episode psychosis.

Introduction

The term 'psychosis' refers to a condition that affects the mind and where the person has some loss of contact with reality. Symptoms of psychosis can alter the person's thoughts, beliefs, emotions, senses, and behaviours. The term 'first-episode psychosis' (FEP; or 'early psychosis') relates to the first occasion a person experiences an episode of psychosis, and where the symptoms are severe, persist for over a week, and disrupt their daily activities.

Primary carers have a critical role to play in supporting a relative or friend with FEP. However, caregiving can be challenging, demanding, and is often protracted, and carers can be faced by fluctuating levels of physical, emotional, and financial hardship (Kuipers, Onwumere, & Beddington, 2010; McCann, Lubman, & Clark, 2011b). There are limited evidence-based support materials to assist carers in this situation. This chapter considers how a low intensity problem-solving intervention may be beneficial for carers of young people with FEP.

A primary (or informal) carer is the main person (aside from health, social, or voluntary care providers) responsible for assisting with activities of daily living, supporting, and advocating on behalf of the young person with FEP (McCann et al., 2011b).

Carers frequently experience a wide range of strong, often conflicting emotions as they struggle to comprehend what is happening to their loved one. Parents can experience helplessness, loss of control, and guilt, or blame themselves for their family member's condition, perceiving it as a sign of poor parenting (Nystrom & Svensson, 2004). Others criticize themselves for not seeking help earlier, misinterpreting psychotic symptoms as typical adolescent behaviour (Reed, 2008). Different emotions can develop as, in some young people, the long-lasting nature of psychotic illness emerges. As a consequence, parents can grieve for the loss of the child they once knew, realizing their hopes, dreams, and aspirations for the young person are unlikely to be accomplished (Jungbauer, Stelling, Dietrich, & Angermeyer, 2004). Carers can experience stigma and social exclusion, because the carer and the young person may be perceived as equally at fault (Angermeyer, Schulze, & Dietrich, 2003).

Despite these difficulties, there are some beneficial outcomes for carers. For some, the turmoil brought about by FEP culminates in a period of personal growth and strengthening of family relationships. Some report their relationship improves and deepens, bringing the carer and the young person closer into a deeper and more fulfilling relationship (Jungbauer et al., 2004; Kartalova-O'Doherty & Tedstone Doherty, 2008).

Evidence base for interventions for family and friends in a FEP context

Family interventions are acceptable and effective for young people with FEP and relatives but are costly and resource intensive, restricting their reach and penetration. A systematic review and meta-analysis of family interventions (Claxton, Onwumere, & Fornells-Ambrojo (2017), found they were effective in reducing relapse in people with schizophrenia-spectrum conditions as well as psychological distress among carers. While they were also effective in reducing psychotic symptoms at follow-up, improvements were not sustained at the end of treatment. Carers receiving family interventions were more likely to change from high to low expressed emotion (a measure of the quality of social interaction between an individual with mental disorder and a carer; Bebbington & Kuipers, 1994), and were less likely to criticize or engage in conflict communication. However, they had no impact on a carer's emotional overinvolvement.

Family interventions are an integral part of the treatment programme for FEP Chien, Thompson, Lubman, & McCann, 2016; Miklowitz et al., 2014). Family interventions can be subdivided into 'high' and 'low' intensity; however, there are no standard definitions of these terms, and there is a continuum between the two.

- High intensity interventions are characterized by moderate to high levels of face-to-face health professional involvement, typically requiring specific training. They may be conducted on a one-to-one or group basis, are usually underpinned by a specific theoretical approach, and may be directive or non-directive. The duration can be variable, and the overall costs of interventions are high. Examples include one-to-one or group therapy.

- Low intensity interventions are characterized by low or no level of health professional involvement and time. Where they are involved in the delivery, health professionals typically require minimal training and interventions are often delivered remotely. In most cases, the interventions are underpinned by a theoretical approach. Recipients often determine the pace and frequency of intervention, and the duration can be variable, with the overall cost usually substantially less than high intensity interventions. Examples include peer-led psychoeducational groups, guided or non-facilitated self-help bibliotherapy (therapy in book-form), and computer-delivered therapy.

A problem-solving-based self-help manual

Initially, we conducted a qualitative study of 20 first-time primary carers to understand their experience of caring for young adults with FEP. Findings highlighted caregiving was a burdensome, unpredictable, and roller-coaster experience. Carers often felt responsible for the young person's illness; however, eventually most came to terms with the changes in the young person. The relationship between carer and young person frequently became closer and deeper, and it was important for both to maintain hope for the future (McCann et al., 2011b). Carers experienced stigma, which they responded to in one of two ways: by being open in disclosing the young person's illness to others or, alternatively, by being secretive (McCann, Lubman, & Clark, 2011c). Carers reported contrasting experiences with general practitioners, and experienced service-focused and carer-focused barriers in accessing FEP services (McCann, Lubman, & Clark, 2011a).

Based on the findings of the qualitative study, a review of literature, and contributions from experts in the field, we developed a self-help manual entitled *Reaching Out: Supporting a Family Member or Friend with First-Episode Psychosis*, the first guided self-help programme to focus on carers of young people with FEP. The manual was evaluated in a randomized controlled trial of 124 carers. Results showed carers who completed the manual had a better experience of caring when supporting their relative than the control group. These effects were maintained throughout the 3-month duration of the study and were evident 10 weeks later. By the end of the study, carers using the manual also experienced a greater reduction in unhelpful attitudes about having to give extra support to the young person with FEP. The level of psychological distress diminished at a greater rate in those receiving the manual compared to the control group, but this difference was not maintained at follow-up.

There was partial support for the beneficial effect of the manual on expressed emotion. The influence on *critical comments* made by carers towards the young person approached significance, with the intervention group reporting fewer of these comments than the control group. There was no significant difference between the groups for carer *emotional overinvolvement*.

On completion of the study, a random sample of 24 carers who received the manual were interviewed to evaluate its usefulness. Findings highlighted its helpfulness in promoting their own well-being and enhancing their understanding of, and equipping them to support, young people with FEP. It was deemed comprehensive, well written, easy-to-read, understandable, and informative (McCann & Lubman, 2014). There was also strong support to retain the book-form format, with small modifications, as it was accessible, suitable to use in a broad range of settings, could be re-read, and reduced travel to specialist services for family interventions.

What does the intervention look like?

The self-help manual was based on Nezu, Maguth Nezu, and D'Zurilla's (2007)[1] approach to problem-solving. The approach is premised on equipping individuals with problem-solving skills and attitudes to enable them to adjust and adapt to challenging situations in their day-to-day lives (Bell & D'Zurilla, 2009).

There are five major dimensions or steps in dealing with real-life problems (D'Zurilla & Nezru, 2007, p. 11). Two dimensions focus on 'problem orientation', while three dimensions focus on people's 'problem-solving styles'.

Problem orientation dimensions

Problem orientation is a metacognitive process that principally has a motivational role in the way an individual thinks about social problem-solving, and has two dimensions (Bell & D'Zurilla, 2009).

1. *Positive problem orientation* (helpful) is aligned with 'successful problem-solving', where the individual has a propensity to (a) perceive a problem as a challenge and can result in beneficial outcomes, (b) view it as solvable rather than insolvable, (c) believe in one's capacity to solve the problem, (d) recognize problem-solving takes time and perseverance, and (e) commit oneself to addressing the problem with diligence rather than delaying or avoiding the problem.
2. *Negative problem orientation* (unhelpful) is an incorrect way of responding to a problem, where the person has a proclivity to (a) perceive a problem as a major risk to well-being, (b) doubt one's capacity to address it successfully, and (c) readily become exasperated and dismayed when faced with the problem.

[1] With the permission of Springer Publishing Company, New York.

Problem-solving styles

Problem-solving styles are the cognitive and behavioural approaches a person implements to understand problems and find solutions or methods of coping with them (Bell & D'Zurilla, 2009). There are three problem-solving styles.

1. *Rational problem-solving* (positive problem orientation) is a constructive, rational, and systematic way of addressing problems. A person displaying this style consciously and systematically draws on four major problem-solving skills: (a) identifies and defines the problem, (b) 'brainstorms or generates a range of potential solutions, (c) considers possible outcomes and consequences of each solution and selects the best or most suitable solution, and (d) implements then monitors and evaluates the outcome of the chosen solution.
2. *Impulsivity/carelessness style* (negative problem orientation) is an incorrect approach to problem-solving. An individual exhibiting this style is unsuccessful in addressing the problem, characterized by one or more of the following behaviours: impulsive, narrow-minded, rushed, careless, or unsystematic approach.
3. *Avoidance style* (negative problem orientation) is an incorrect approach to problem-solving. A person displaying this style procrastinates or delays, avoids addressing the problem, puts things off for as long as possible, and tries to shift responsibility to others for dealing with the problem.

Problem-solving self-assessment test

Before learning the problem-solving approach, it is important for carers to self-evaluate their current problem-solving strengths and limitations, attitudes and beliefs, and areas requiring the most practice. One way to do this is to use the 25-item (revised short version) self-assessment test. The test contains five scales assessing the five dimensions: two focusing on problem-solving orientation (e.g. 'Sometimes even difficult problems have a way of moving my life forward in positive ways') and three focusing on problem-solving styles (e.g. 'When making decisions, I think carefully about my many options') (Nezu et al., 2007, p. 14).

ADAPT problem-solving framework

Once carers have obtained a greater understanding of their problem-solving strengths and weaknesses, and what they need to concentrate on improving, the next step is to consider the ADAPT method of effective problem-solving (Nezu et al., 2007). The underlying premise of ADAPT is that an individual can adapt and

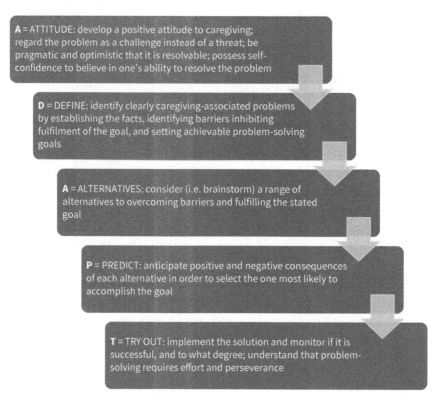

Figure 18.1 ADAPT method of problem-solving.

become better at problem-solving and coping with life's stresses. There are five sequential steps to effective problem-solving (Figure 18.1).

Effective communication

The following case study on effective communication is abstracted from McCann, Lubman, and Boardman's (2021) book *The Carer's Guide to Schizophrenia: A Concise Problem-solving Resource for Family and Friends.*[2] In addition to adopting a problem-solving approach, emphasis is placed on carers:

- Adopting an open and collaborative approach to problem-solving with the young person.
- Focusing on one problem at a time.
- Using positive language, building the young person's self-esteem and confidence, and giving encouragement.
- Communicating in a supportive, respectful, caring way that helps promote the young person's recovery and prevents relapse.

[2] With the permission of Jessica Kingsley Publishers, London.

The book chapter on effective communication contains five sections focusing on enhancing carer's communication skills: (1) effective communication skills, (2) communicating when the person is unwell, (3) communicating during a psychotic episode and other difficult periods, (4) communicating using helpful language, and (5) communication within the family (expressed emotion). This is then followed by a case study using the ADAPT framework.

One of the five sections is elaborated upon below.

Communicating when the young person is unwell

Conversation may be difficult when the young person is unwell during the acute phase of the disorder and at times throughout the recovery phase, but there are straightforward ways to improve this. A sample of some helpful tips that carers can use during these phases include:

- Face the young person and maintain appropriate eye contact.
- Always treat the person with respect.
- Avoid making promises you cannot keep.
- Be sensitive to what the person is telling you; try to see things from their perspective.
- Avoid arguing with the person, no matter how logical you think your argument is, and how illogical you think their responses are.
- Try to convey a message of hope by assuring the person that help is available and things can get better.

Problem-solving case study

Carers are then presented with a sample case study, using the ADAPT problem-solving framework.

Carrie is Jordan's mum and his primary carer. They both live together. Problem: for the past week, Jordan has not spoken to Carrie.

ADAPT problem-solving framework

Attitude
Adopt a positive, optimistic attitude.

Define
Define the problem. State the facts, identify obstacles, and specify a goal.
Jordan used to speak to Carrie every day about all sorts of things. For the past month, he has spoken less and less to her. Throughout the past week he has not said a word to her. Carrie does not want to have an argument with Jordan about the problem. Carrie's goal is to attempt to re-open communication and have a short conversation with Jordan within 1 week.

ADAPT problem-solving framework

Alternatives

Generate a list of different alternatives for overcoming the problem and achieving a goal.

1. Carrie could try to initiate conversations with Jordan about topics he likes.
2. Carrie could speak to him regularly and include him in conversations, even if he does not respond, just to let him know she is there. For example, saying 'Hello', asking him if he wants a drink, telling him what she will do today, remarking about what is in the newspaper, and just giving him a smile.
3. Carrie could do nothing and allow him to be silent in the hope that he will speak to her again when he feels ready to.

Predict

Predict the helpful and unhelpful consequences for each alternative. Choose the best one to achieve your goal that minimizes costs and maximizes benefits.

Alternatives	Helpful consequences	Unhelpful consequences
Alternative 1	Carrie demonstrates she wants to talk to Jordan Jordan might speak to Carrie again	Jordan still does not speak to Carrie. She does not know much about what he is interested in
Alternative 2	Carrie demonstrates she wants to talk to Jordan and wishes to include him in her conversations Jordan speaks to Carrie again	Jordan still does not speak to Carrie
Alternative 3	Jordan may initiate conversation by himself and speak regularly to Carrie	Jordan still does not speak to Carrie Jordan may feel ignored, which may only make matters worse

Try out

Try out the solution in 'real life'. See if it works, and evaluate it.

Carrie tried Alternative 2 for 1 week. Jordan sometimes showed interest when she spoke to him but he didn't respond, nor did he initiate conversation with her.

Problem solved? No. Jordan still does not speak to Carrie. Try Alternative 1 instead.

After reviewing the sample case study, carers are asked to think of a communication problem they are currently experiencing with the young person. They are then asked to briefly describe the situation and the problem and proceed to completing a blank ADAPT chart.

Chapter summary

Problem-solving bibliotherapy is an alternative, non-threatening, cost-effective, low intensity intervention for FEP, with potentially good reach and penetration, in comparison to other more complex and resource-intensive family interventions. It can be used by carers more or less independently of healthcare professionals; however, it seems to work best when integrated with other therapeutic approaches (Campbell & Smith, 2003). Bibliotherapy gives carers the chance to refamiliarize themselves with material at a later date. It increases access to support for carers whose caregiving and other commitments, and geographical, financial, and other constraints prevent them from accessing face-to-face family interventions.

Recommended reading

McCann, T. V., Lubman, D. I., & Boardman, G. (2021). *The carer's guide to schizophrenia: A concise problem-solving resource for family and friends.* London: Jessica Kingsley Publishers.

References

Angermeyer, M. C., Schulze, B., & Dietrich, S. (2003). Courtesy stigma. A focus group study of relatives of schizophrenia patients. *Social Psychiatry and Psychiatric Epidemiology, 38*(10), 593–602.

Bebbington, P., & Kuipers, L. (1994). The predictive utility of expressed emotion in schizophrenia: an aggregate analysis. *Psychological Medicine, 24*(3), 707–718.

Bell, A. C., & D'Zurilla, T. J. (2009). Problem-solving therapy for depression: A meta-analysis. *Clinical Psychology Review, 29*(4), 348–353.

Campbell, L. F., & Smith, T. P. (2003). Integrating self-help books into psychotherapy. *Journal of Clinical Psychology, 59*(2), 177–186.

Chien, W. T., Thompson, D. R., Lubman, D. I., & McCann, T. V. (2016). A randomized controlled trial of clinician-supported problem-solving bibliotherapy for family caregivers of people with first-episode psychosis. *Schizophrenia Bulletin, 42*(6), 1457–1466.

Claxton, M., Onwumere, J., & Fornells-Ambrojo, M. (2017). Do family interventions improve outcomes in early psychosis? A systematic review and meta-analysis. *Frontiers in Psychology, 8,* 371.

D'Zurilla, T. J., & Nezru, A. M. (2007). *Problem-solving therapy: A positive approach to clinical intervention* (3rd ed.). New York: Springer.

Jungbauer, J., Stelling, K., Dietrich, S., & Angermeyer, M. C. (2004). Schizophrenia: Problems of separation in families. *Journal of Advanced Nursing, 47*(6), 605–613.

Kartalova-O'Doherty, Y., & Tedstone Doherty, D. (2008). Coping strategies and styles of family carers of persons with enduring mental illness: A mixed methods analysis. *Scandinavian Journal of Caring Sciences, 22*(1), 19–28.

Kuipers, E., Onwumere, J., & Beddington, P. (2010). Cognitive model of caregiving in psychosis. *British Journal of Psychiatry, 196*(4), 259–265.

McCann, T. V., & Lubman, D. I. (2014). Qualitative process evaluation of a problem-solving guided self-help manual for family carers of young people with first-episode psychosis. *BMC Psychiatry, 14,* 168.

McCann, T. V., Lubman, D. I., & Boardman, G. (2021). *The carer's guide to schizophrenia: A concise problem-solving resource for family and friends.* London: Jessica Kingsley Publishers.

McCann, T. V., Lubman, D. I., & Clark, E. (2011a). First-time primary caregivers' experience accessing first-episode psychosis services. *Early Intervention in Psychiatry, 5*(2), 156–162.

McCann, T. V., Lubman, D. I., & Clark, E. (2011b). First-time primary caregivers' experience of caring for young adults with first-episode psychosis. *Schizophrenia Bulletin, 37*(2), 381–388.

McCann, T. V., Lubman, D. I., & Clark, E. (2011c). Responding to stigma: First-time caregivers of young people with first-episode psychosis. *Psychiatric Services, 62*(5), 548–550.

Miklowitz, D. J., O'Brien, M. P., Schlosser, D. A., Addington, J., Candan, K. A., Marshall, C., . . ., & Cannon, T. D. (2014). Family-focused treatment for adolescents and young adults at high risk for psychosis: results of a randomized trial. *Journal of the American Academy of Child and Adolescent Psychiatry, 53*(8), 848–858.

Nezu, A. M., Maguth Nezu, C., & D'Zurilla, T. J. (2007). *Solving life's problems: A 5-step guide to enhanced wellbeing.* New York: Springer Publishing Company.

Nystrom, M., & Svensson, H. (2004). Lived experiences of being a father of an adult child with schizophrenia. *Issues in Mental Health Nursing, 25*(4), 363–380.

Reed, S. (2008). First-episode psychosis: A literature review. *International Journal of Mental Health Nursing, 17*(2), 85–91.

SECTION 3

IMPLEMENTATION AND SERVICE ORGANIZATION

19

Supervision and case management in low intensity interventions

Vicki Curry and Lesley French

Learning objectives

- To define what is meant by supervision in the context of low intensity work with children and young people.
- To understand the value and purpose of supervision in this context, including models of and research into supervision.
- To provide suggestions for good practice in the implementation of supervision with the low intensity workforce, including potential challenges and solutions.

Introduction and context

Demand for qualified child mental health practitioners continues to outstrip supply. As described in Chapter 22, the rapid training and development of a new workforce, equipped to deliver low intensity (LI) interventions for children and young people (CYP) in a variety of community settings and schools, was developed to address this deficit in England. The supervision context, described in this chapter, lies within the implementation of this national programme.

Definitions of supervision

Clinical supervision is generally understood to be a formal process of support and learning for practitioners which enables the supervisee to develop competence and gradually assume responsibility for their own practice. This chapter considers the importance and clinical implementation of clinical supervision in LI interventions. It is important to mention that support for practitioners requires both case management and clinical supervision. Case management refers to the review of whole case-loads, undertaken regularly, and where all referrals are held in mind in relation to risk and progress, not just those 'brought' by the practitioners. Clinical supervision refers to the shared understanding of the presenting difficulties of the young person, the formulation and content of the intervention plan, and the use of outcome measures to assess progress and outcomes. For child well-being practitioners in England, case management supervision usually occurs in weekly one-to-one meetings with the manager or supervisor. Clinical supervision is recommended to occur weekly, either one-to-one or in a small group.

Both tasks are essential for good client outcomes and the clinical supervisor needs to be sighted on appropriate case numbers and the range of cases, particularly for newly qualified practitioners. Where the function of these two types of supervision is held by different colleagues, it is important in the delivery of LI interventions that the clinical supervisor is sighted on throughput of cases and efficient use of practitioner time linked to good outcomes for families and to the wider objective about improving access to services (see Reiser, Watkins, & Milne, 2014). Both supervision functions should be about optimizing good practice and developing practitioner skills in the delivery of evidence-based interventions to significant numbers of families.

There is an organizational expectation for most services providing mental health interventions that (1) supervision will occur and that (2) supervisees will present work in an open and collaborative way to allow for maximum learning and development. However, even in established and lengthy clinical trainings there is a lack of parallel accreditation of supervisors from professional bodies alongside training programmes (Roth & Pilling, 2008). For example, a study of newly qualified educational psychologists in the UK showed only a third receiving professional supervision and many practitioners reporting pressure to practise outside competencies because of a lack of access to supervision (Silva, Newman, Guiney, Valley-Gray, & Barrett, 2016). Supervision skills are often not taught on clinical psychology courses (Falendar, 2018). Furthermore, the literature on efficacy of treatment does not elicit the contribution or differential value that the presence of 'good' supervision might make to client outcomes (Roth & Pilling, 2008). This is true of the current training programmes in the UK for the LI workforce where clinical supervision is undertaken by on-site practitioners. Further investigation to differentiate the impact of supervision on client outcomes alongside the training programmes is required.

Principles of good supervision within CYP services include collaboration, respect, reflection, skills development, service user feedback, and use of routine outcome measures (ROMs) to capture client progress (Law, 2014).

Some models of supervision provide a multifaceted view of a focus on the client, intervention strategies, the supervisee's focus on their own process, and the organizational context of the work (Hawkins & Shohet, 2012). Diversity and power dynamics, whether visible or unstated, provide an important focus for all supervisors and require ongoing and active attention in the supervisory relationship (Burnham, Alvis Palma, & Whitehouse, 2008). In addition, in part driven by supervision capacity, there is an increasing requirement to provide supervision in groups, which requires skills in developing shared responsibility and alliance to enable each group member to be an active part of the supervision process (Proctor, 2008).

Case management supervision

Case management supervision provides an opportunity to review an entire case-load. Importantly, it is a space to assess and monitor risk in relation to CYP on the practitioner's case load. It also identifies issues such as CYP who may be being seen for longer than would be recommended when they should be 'stepped up' to full therapy; and CYP who may be being discharged too early by a practitioner keen to demonstrate that they are delivering service targets.

Case management supervision is fast-paced, meaning that the practitioner has to present a great deal of clinical information quickly, clearly, and accurately to their supervisor. By keeping to a strict format, it should be possible to discuss at least ten CYP in an hour's supervision session. This is only possible if the practitioner and supervisor work together efficiently and stick to a predetermined and highly struc-tured format. The practitioner must be organized and well prepared for the session with all the required information to hand in the correct format.

Some electronic client health record management systems automatically select cases for discussion according to set criteria so that no one gets missed in the system that is there to protect them. Some systems can be set to provide a weekly list of cli-ents who should be discussed in supervision. For this system to be effective, it is necessary to be meticulous in the submission of ROMs (see Chapter 8). Without this data, it would not be possible to run an automated system of alerts for supervision. In the absence of electronic system options, practitioners and supervisors should work together to develop a system, such as keeping a log of caseloads, including cer-tain information such as red/amber/green (RAG) ratings to monitor risk.

The decision to bring certain CYP to traditional clinical supervision is usually down to the practitioner to decide. However, in case management supervision, CYP are dis-cussed based on predetermined criteria at particular points in their care pathway, and, if possible, through an automated system as already mentioned (Box 19.1).

Case management supervision generally starts with an overview of the practitioner's caseload numbers which allows the supervisor to check whether the practitioner's caseload size is appropriate. Supervision then progresses to discussion of CYP in

---

Box 19.1 Criteria for taking cases to case management supervision

- All new clients.
- All clients discussed, at the very least, 4-weekly.
- Any clients with risk issues.
- All clients with high scores on outcome measures.
- All clients who have missed appointments or not been contacted recently by the practitioner.
- Any client for whom the practitioner would like additional support.

categories as per the Box 19.1. This type of supervision ensures that CYP are reviewed at the start of their care pathway and then at least once after that. For instance, a practitioner might say 'I have 36 young people on my caseload and I have ten to discuss today. I have three new cases, two for 4-weekly review, one for increased risk, two that have high scores and do not seem to be making any progress, and two that I would like to seek advice on please.' If there is an electronic system that automatically raises all the cases for supervision, the supervisor might add another case (e.g. 'I see DF has been seen for more than the usual number of sessions for behavioural activation and yet does not seem to be making much progress in his scores, let's add him to the list too please'; 'I see two cases there that missed their last appointments and it looks like you haven't been able to contact them, we need to talk about them too').

Purpose and value of clinical supervision

There is broad agreement about the key purposes of clinical supervision in the literature, namely an enhancement of the experience of the supervisee in the workplace; a focus on outcomes of the intervention for the family; attention to case management issues (numbers, range of cases, complexity); clinical governance or assurance for the organization; skills development for the supervisee; and a form of support for the supervisee in managing the emotional demands of working at times with distressed families (Richards, Chellingsworth, Hope, Turpin, & Whyte, 2010). One of the key challenges for the LI supervisor is clinical governance, that is, safeguarding the effective management of the high volume of cases seen by the LI supervisee.

While most organizations accept there is value to the supervision process in relation to quality assurance issues, there is also evidence that the presence of effective supervision is an important factor in mental health, well-being, and job satisfaction at work (Hammig, 2017). This is particularly salient given the current challenges in workforce retention across CYP services.

The importance of supervision has been recognized in the development of the CYP LI training programmes in England, where a 1-year course for supervisors, which teaches both the CYP LI interventions and also theory and practice in relation to case management and clinical skills supervision, has been developed to support the new workforce of LI practitioners.

It is also important to recognize that trainees and practitioners in the LI workforce may have less clinical and work experience than those with training in other interventions and by association require greater scaffolding about the expectations of supervision. For example, the ability to attend supervision with a succinct summary of the key aspects of the clinical presentation, including a description of the problem and treatment goals, hypotheses regarding the development/maintenance of the CYP's difficulties (e.g. using the five-areas model—see Chapter XX), and outcome measures, and reviewing an audio recording of a session and bringing the correct section of recording to review in supervision are skills in their own right, and need to be taught as other competencies.

Box 19.2 Helpful Aspects of Supervision Questionnaire (H.A.S.Q.)

Your Name (optional):

Date of supervision:

1. Please rate how helpful this supervision was overall:

Very unhelpful	Fairly unhelpful	Neither helpful nor unhelpful	Fairly helpful	Very helpful
1	2	3	4	5

2. Of the events which occurred in this supervision, which one do you feel was the most helpful for you personally? It might be something you said or did, or something the supervisor said or did. Can you say why it was helpful?

3. How helpful was this particular event? Rate this on the scale:

Very unhelpful	Fairly unhelpful	Neither helpful nor unhelpful	Fairly helpful	Very helpful
1	2	3	4	5

4. Did anything else of particular importance happen during this supervision? Include anything else which may have been helpful, or anything which might have been unhelpful.

© 2007, Derek Milne and Chris Dunkerley

During the supervisors' training courses, the process of supervision itself is actively evaluated by the supervisee using tools such as the Helpful Aspects of Supervision Questionnaire (HASQ) tool (Milne, Aylott, Fitzpatrick, & Ellis, 2008; Reiser, Cliffe, & Milne, 2018; Box 19.2) which provides immediate feedback to the supervisor. Training on use of the SAGE, a scale for rating competence in supervision (Milne, Reiser, Cliffe, & Raine, 2011), also assists supervisors in evaluating the development of competencies which are set out systematically and which form a basis for shared learning and improvement of the supervision process. Training on collaborative use of feedback for the supervisor builds on the knowledge that self-rated competence increases with experience but independently observed (assessed) competence does not (Tracey, Wampold, Lichtenberg, & Goodyear, 2014).

Theory and research that guides good practice in LI supervision

Ideas about what constitutes good supervision are informed by different parts of the literature but there is general international agreement on supervision competencies and helpful reviews are available (Falender & Shafranske, 2017; Gonsalvez, Hamid, Savage, & Livni, 2017; Johnston & Milne, 2012; Ladany, 2014; Milne, 2017;

Rønnestad, Orlinsky, Schröder, Skovholt, & Willutzki, 2019). We set out the key learning points from this research for effective supervision of the LI workforce in the following sections.

Implementing effective LI supervision

1. *Prioritize the supervisory alliance.* The nature of the supervisory relationship is crucial. A weak supervisory alliance has been linked with negative consequences, including reduced disclosure and greater anxiety from the supervisee and a more negative experience of supervision; whereas a more positive relationship has been shown to predict professional development, clinician competence and client outcomes (e.g. Falender, Shafranske, & Ofek, 2014; Palomo, Beinart, & Cooper, 2010). Supervisees like supervisors to be open and supportive, and to attend to personal and professional well-being. Creating a culture of reflection and allowing multiple perspectives is also a factor within the therapeutic alliance that has been associated with good practice in supervision.

2. *Attend to issues of culture and diversity.* A multisystemic approach to supervision is also crucial, ensuring consideration of issues such as gender, race, sexuality, disability, class, and religion. Falender and Shafranske (2017) outline the potential negative impact of having a 'Western lens on clinical supervision' (p. 89), highlighting how increasing diversity in the supervisory triad (clients, supervisees, and supervisors) interacts in complex ways with the power hierarchy inherent in both the supervisory and therapeutic relationships. The Social GGRRAAACCEEESSS model (Burnham et al., 2008; Burnham, 2012) provides a useful acronym to represent different aspects of belief, power, lifestyle, and culture that it is important to bear in mind and articulate in the supervision process.

3. *Be organized about supervision.* Factors such as ensuring consistency and protected time for supervision have also been found to be important (e.g. Milne et al., 2008); as well as the need for mutual agreement between supervisee and supervisor on the goals and task of supervision (Bordin, 1983). It is recommended that supervision contracts are collaboratively drawn up between the supervisor and supervisee, and this is a requirement of training courses, although these are still often not formally done in practice (Cookson, Sloan, Dafters, & Jahoda, 2014). See Box 19.3 for an example supervision contract.

4. *Consider supervisee cycles of learning.* One theory that is helpful to bear in mind in relation to the supervisory process is Vygotsky's (1986) zone of proximal development (ZPD). This educational theory emphasizes the social aspect of learning, and the importance of support provided to children by adults in the development of their knowledge and understanding. The ZPD is the distance between what a learner cannot do, and what they can do with help and guidance from 'a more knowledgeable other' (Box 19.4). In order to facilitate learning, the learner requires the presence of an individual with

Box 19.3 Sample Supervision Contract (BABCP)

This contract was drawn up on (date):

Between Supervisee:
(print names)
and Supervisor

A copy of this contract will be held by both the Supervisor and Supervisee. This contract will change as and when necessary and with prior consultation.

Frequency / Length

- Supervision sessions will be held weekly
- A minimum of one hour will be available for individual supervision
- If a supervision session is missed, the Supervisor takes responsibility to rearrange an alternative date as soon as possible.

Confidentiality

- Supervisee accepts that work issues may be discussed, when appropriate, with other managers.
- Supervisee accepts that any arising issues may be discussed with practice tutors on the CWP/EMHP/ RtT course (e.g.IT, number of cases, and progress).
- The Supervisee is entitled to have issues concerning the quality of his/her work to be overt and open to his/her involvement.
- Supervisee and Supervisor are to inform each other of anything that needs to be kept confidential.
- Supervisee accepts that their supervision records will move with them in the event of transfer of Supervisor.
- Supervisee accepts that following their departure, supervision records will be kept in line with the Service's clinical governance procedure.

Supervisee's Rights

- To uninterrupted time in a private venue.
- To be respected within a framework of social differences
- To Supervisor's attention, ideas and guidance.
- To receive feedback.
- To set part of the agenda.
- To ask questions.
- To expect Supervisor to carry out agreed action or provide an appropriate explanation, within an agreed time frame.
- To state when over/under worked including CWP/EMHP course demands.
- To have his/her development/training needs met.
- To challenge ideas and guidance in a constructive way.

Supervisee's Responsibilities

- To routinely bring videos to supervision.
- To be proactive.
- To have a predominantly problem-solving approach.
- To accept feedback positively.
- To update Supervisor and provide relevant information.
- To prepare for supervision, and to keep their copy of the supervision record in a secure location.
- To bring issues, concerns and problems.
- To maintain the agreement.
- To identify development / training needs and engage in agreed activities.
- To give feedback to supervisors (e.g. using the HASQ- Helpful Aspects of Supervision Questionnaire)

Supervisor's Rights

- To bring concerns/issues about Supervisee's work.
- To question Supervisee about his/her work and workload.
- To give Supervisee constructive feedback on his/her work performance.
- To negotiate around Supervisee's work/workload.
- To observe Supervisee's practice and to initiate supportive / corrective action as required.

Supervisor's Responsibilities

- To set a clear agenda for each session with the supervisee(s)
- To make sure supervision sessions happen as agreed and to keep a record of the meeting.
- To create a supervision file for each Supervisee containing their supervision records and other documents relating to their employment and development.
- To ensure that Supervisee is clear about his/her role and responsibilities.
- To ensure Supervisee is clear regarding their employment status e.g. induction, probation, temporary, permanent.
- To record the supervision session and to store securely (and in line with local clinical governance policy).
- To ensure that Supervisee is kept up-to-date with departmental/local authority policy and procedures.
- To monitor Supervisee's performance, including work and attendance.
- To set standards and assess the Supervisee against these.
- To know what Supervisee is doing and how it is being done.
- To deal with problems as they impact on the Supervisee's performance.
- To support Supervisee and the agreed personal development plan.

Feedback and Outcome Tools

- The supervisee to bring outcome data (ROMS) to discuss in supervision Supervisor and Supervisee to use POD to track client progress Recording Mechanisms
- The Supervisor and Supervisee to keep notes and actions from supervision in line with their service clinical governance guidance.

Conflict

- Every effort should be made to resolve any conflict within supervision.
- In exceptional circumstances, where this cannot be achieved, the Supervisee has recourse to the Supervisor's line manager.

Signed by: ....   Date: ....
(Supervisee)

Signed by: ....   Date: ....
(Supervisor)

more knowledge and expertise than themselves; some form of social interaction with this 'more knowledgeable other' that allows them to observe and practise their skills; and the provision of supportive activities to guide them through this process.

A key concept associated with Vygotsky's theory is that of 'scaffolding' (Wood, Bruner, & Ross, 1976), defined as a process 'that enables a child or

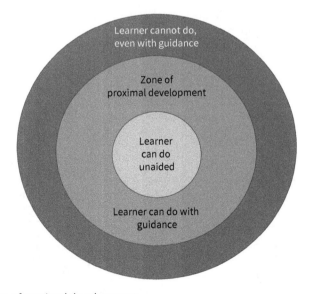

Figure 19.1 Zone of proximal development.

novice to solve a task or achieve a goal that would be beyond his unassisted efforts' (p. 90). This theory describes how a more competent individual can provide temporary support, matched to the needs of the learner, that enables them to achieve success in an activity they would not have been able to do alone; and then gradually remove this support. Through this process, the learner becomes able to carry out the activity unaided. Both the concepts of ZPD and scaffolding are clearly relevant to the nature of the CBT-informed interventions delivered by these LI practitioners, which incorporate the practitioner supporting CYP and parents/carers in developing new knowledge and skills that promote emotional well-being (Fuggle, Dunsmuir, & Curry, 2013). They can also clearly be applied to the process of supervision, in which a 'more knowledgeable other' (the supervisor) guides the supervisee in the development of their theoretical and practical understanding and skills in delivering these interventions.

Another educational theory, Kolb's (1984) experiential learning cycle, has been particularly influential in the field of supervision (Figure 19.2).

This cycle postulates four stages of learning: doing/having an experience; reviewing/reflecting on the experience; concluding/learning from the experience; and planning/trying out what you have learned. The cycle may be entered at any point, but the practitioner must then follow it sequentially for successful learning to take place and, critically, be reinforced by active strategies in supervision such as role play and rehearsal.

5. *Share supervisor knowledge.* Supervisees value the supervisor having expertise and knowledge (Gonsalvez et al., 2017). However, in line with the concepts of the ZDP and scaffolding outlined above, the way this is shared will vary as the supervisee develops, moving from information giving/educational scaffolding (*what* to do) to a more collaborative discussion of process issues (*how* to do it) (Johnston & Milne, 2012).

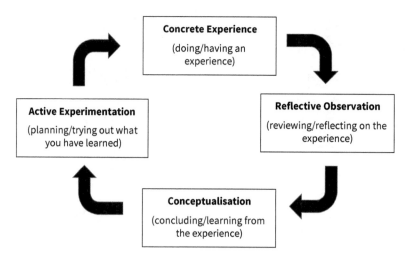

Figure 19.2 The experiential learning cycle (Kolb, 1984).

6. *Use ROMs.* There is some evidence regarding the benefits of outcome-informed supervision (e.g. Reese et al., 2009). This might include supporting supervisees with the complexity and nuances of using ROMs in LI interventions; encouraging the use of ROMs to guide decisions about who to prioritize for discussion in both case management and clinical supervision; monitoring the progress of CYP; and identifying themes in feedback from different clients to support the development of the supervisee's practice (Swift et al., 2015). Supervisors' confidence with and competence in ROMs sends an important signal to supervisees about evidence-based practice and mirrors the teaching in training programmes (see Law, 2014). Similarly, the supervisors routinely requesting feedback using simple session-by-session methods such as the HASQ (Box 19.2) both improves practice and models collaborative learning.

7. *Incorporate direct observation.* Historically, supervision has been a process conducted in privacy and viewed predominantly as a reflective space provided for the supervisee to reflect and learn from practice. However, the use of audio/video recordings, multimodal teaching such as live demonstration, and role play have been shown to have a highly positive impact on supervisees' learning (Beidas, Cross, & Dorsey, 2014; O'Donovan, Clough, & Petch, 2017; Weck, Kaufmann, & Witthöft, 2017). Studies have found practitioner self-assessment alone to be unreliable and it has been known for some time that supervisees can give a partial account of sessions, withholding aspects of the intervention which might be negatively viewed (Ladany, 2014; Yourman & Farber, 1996). In the UK, studies indicate there may be an established cultural shift towards the use of audio/video material in supervision (Townend, 2002, vs Reiser & Milne, 2016; Gonsalvez et al., 2017), and it is increasingly a course requirement in workforce development programmes; although this is not necessarily the case in other countries (Weck, Kaufmann, & Witthöft, 2017).

8. *Provide competence-focused feedback.* Giving feedback is another factor associated with supervisee learning; particularly feedback that relates to specific competencies (Weck, Kaufmann, & Hofling, 2017). There are some formal rating forms on different aspects of therapeutic practice which can help supervisors with this, although there are often problems with inter-rater reliability and there are relatively few developed for use with CYP. Given this, it may be that these are best used to guide formative rather than summative feedback in supervision, and to be part of a broader way of monitoring adherence to therapeutic models and supervisee performance. Where there is a need to use these for summative purposes, such as for assessment on training courses, it is crucial that this is just one of a range of ways of assessing competence, and that robust procedures for moderation of marking are in place (Ferguson, Harper, Platz, Sloan, & Smith, 2016; Loades & Armstrong, 2016; Roth, Myles-Hooton, & Branson, 2019).

9. *Consider the context of the child LI workforce.* Certain contextual elements of the child LI workforce will have an impact on the nature of supervision. Firstly, it is a relatively new workforce in England involving the training of hundreds of new practitioners. Those trained specifically in LI, such as in the CYP mental health

programme in England workforce, may be trained only in a small number of relatively manualized approaches. Secondly, consequently, there is a need for a greater focus on developing skills in specific therapeutic approaches than in more routine child and adolescent mental health services (CAMHS) supervision. Supervisors will need a good working knowledge of these models to be able to support the development of their practice, and screen out cases according to complexity or presenting difficulties that this workforce is not trained to treat (see Chapter 7 on assessment and Chapter 22 for an overview). Thirdly, LI practitioners with exclusively LI caseloads have a high number of short-term cases, so it is important to ensure adequate case management in addition to practice-focused supervision. Finally, a mixture of individual and group supervision is often recommended, allowing supervisees to benefit in learning from each other and supervisors to manage the number of practitioners they often have to support. Although group supervision can be very beneficial (Mastoras & Andrews, 2011), it requires additional skills of facilitation in the supervisor to manage group processes which are beyond the scope of this chapter. The Group Supervision Alliance Model (Proctor, 2008) provides useful support for supervisors in this area.

Implications of the literature and LI context on supervision practice

Set the right context for supervision

The supervisor and supervisee should work together to agree a supervision agreement (sometimes called a supervision 'contract', although it is not a legally enforceable document). This will include practical issues such as frequency and length of supervision, as well as goals and tasks of supervision. For those trained exclusively in LI approaches, there may be a need for a greater amount of supervision than might traditionally be provided to their more highly trained and experienced CAMHS colleagues, and it is important to incorporate both case management and clinical supervision. It is also crucial to hold a stance of 'cultural humility' (Falender & Shafranske, 2017) and to ensure discussion of multicultural and diversity issues.

Agree a structure for supervision sessions

An agenda should be collaboratively agreed at the start of the supervision session. The supervisee should be encouraged to prepare for supervision beforehand. This will include thinking about which cases they want to discuss, and bringing information to facilitate this discussion (e.g. a working formulation diagram, succinct additional background information, client ROMs, session recordings, and a supervision question). The supervisor should support the supervisee in prioritizing cases and topics for discussion, and this might usefully include using ROMs from the assessment or intervention session or looking at themes from client feedback, or issues that arose in relation to direct observation of the supervisee's practice.

Vary the content of supervision sessions

Supervision should ensure a balance of reflective discussion as well as active strategies to support supervisees in moving round the experiential learning cycle. The techniques and strategies employed will helpfully include:

- Demonstration by the supervisor.
- Role play.
- Review of risk and supervisee/client safety.
- Review of clinical methods and their guidelines.
- Review of appropriate choice of treatment materials.
- Reference to models and theories and their links to practice; use of video/audio/ direct observation.
- Reflection and Socratic discussion.
- Discussing client ROMs.
- Agreeing homework.

Incorporate direct observation and competency-based feedback

It is helpful for supervisors to provide supervisees with competency-based feedback, and also to encourage the supervisee to self-reflect. Good areas of focus include:

- What went well in the role play/video/audio clip?
- Are there any things they might do differently next time?
- Relate feedback to relevant competency frameworks, to help socialize them to the models and support their skill development.

Make use of group and individual supervision

In a group setting, supervisees can observe and reflect on their own practice and also on the practice of their colleagues, both of which facilitate learning. The provision of additional individual supervision is important, however, as this gives the supervisee space to discuss their own personal issues and development in a safe space. A helpful framework is provided in the stages of supervision set out by Inskipp and Proctor (2001) using group relations theory. Formative aspects (establishing the group), normative aspects (culture and purpose), and restorative aspects (learning and reflection) reflect the development of the supervisory group identity, maturity, and moving from supervisor led to supervisor facilitation.

Gather supervisee feedback

This might take the form of routine use of feedback rating forms, for example, the HASQ noted previously or at least asking for verbal feedback at the end of the session. Reviews of supervision should be regularly undertaken.

Keep a record of all supervision sessions

Examples of an individual supervision record and supervision log are provided in Boxes 19.4 and 19.5.

Box 19.4 Record of Supervision

Supervisor ....   **Supervisee** ....

Date ....   **Client Initials**.........................

Type (please circle) face to face/ telephone/Teams/Zoom

Methods used (please circle) case discussion, recording, role-play, direct observation

Supervision Questions

Summary of discussion

Actions

To bring back for next session

Box 19.5 Log of supervision given

LOG OF SUPERVISION GIVEN

Practice Diary and Supervision Log

Name of Supervisee(s):...

Date	Supervisee(s)	Individual or Group	Duration of contact	Content	Methods
		TOTAL HOURS			

LOG OF SUPERVISION RECEIVED

Practice Diary and Supervision Log

Name of Supervisee:...

Name of supervisor ....

Modality of supervisor ....

Date	Supervisee	Individual or Group	Duration of contact	Content	Methods
		TOTAL HOURS			

Challenges

There remain considerable challenges in implementing and sustaining adequate structures of supervisory support for LI practitioners, many of whom will be inexperienced at entry to training and to deliver a small number of manualized interventions. Supervisors need to understand these interventions and know how to screen in appropriate cases for a cohort of practitioners who are trained to see a high number of short-term cases. Service leads and commissioners need to be sighted on the need to employ enough supervisors to support these practitioners and to give these supervisors sufficient authority in the system to gate-keep referrals to prevent LI practitioners from being asked to provide interventions outside of their competencies. There is also some evidence that low intensity practitioners are very quickly moving on to other professional training programmes where career progression appears more established, rather than becoming senior practitioners or supervisors within the LI workforce in England. These factors further impact the lack of trained supervisors for this group and present a significant risk to sustaining and developing the workforce as a whole.

Potential solutions

At the time of writing, the process of beginning professional accreditation for LI practitioners has begun at a national level in England. In addition, senior low intensity roles are being introduced, e.g. the senior practitioner role. It is hoped that this will mitigate the risk of a perceived lack of status for these workers in the wider service and make them more in line with other professional training courses, where there is a structural link between progression-including into more senior and supervisory roles-and greater levels of renumeration. As noted above, a one-year postgraduate certificate course in supervision is available for supervisors new to the LI workforce. These courses have the remit of increasing the pool of staff trained in both LI interventions and also in supervision theory and practice, thus enabling them to deliver the right kind of evidence-based supervision to support the LI workforce. Support for services in developing appropriate infrastructures is also important; local and national implementation groups and trainings can provide a structure for developing and sharing good practice in supervision and service development. In England, focus at a national level on the importance of developing systems for professional accreditation and a clear career pathway for the LI workforce is welcomed, and it is hoped this will include recognition of the supervisory role. Finally, it is important to promote the value of the LI workforce as part of a stepped model of CAMHS provision to those funding services and policymakers.

What is the future?

In England, it has become increasingly apparent that the LI workforce is more culturally and socially diverse than some other child mental health training programmes. This might be in part because trainees are in paid employment and released to train through a centrally funded programme. As this workforce progress in their careers, it is important that the same level of diversity is reflected at both supervisor and service lead level, to diversify the whole workforce and be more representative of all communities. Encouraging retention in LI work, as well as offering continuing professional development, including supervision training and accreditation, will be crucial in ensuring this happens. The impact of training courses in developing a new supervisory workforce needs to be incorporated into ongoing evaluation of the LI outcomes, measuring the relationship of investment in supervision to outcomes for young people.

Chapter summary

Frequent good-quality supervision is essential for effective delivery of LI interventions. There is a wealth of research and literature which informs good practice and the consequent training of supervisors for LI practitioners. The implications of this for supervisory practice have been set out, and it is hoped the development of training programmes for supervisors, such as those that exist in the UK, will embed best practice in time. Support for diversifying the child mental health workforce and addressing cultural difference in the supervision process are key areas of focus. It is important that these new roles and trainings are embedded in national delivery and recognized career structures, which is not yet the case in some countries. The ambition of expansion of a trained workforce in England and elsewhere is dependent on sufficient supervisors supporting these new practitioners.

References

Beidas, R. S., Cross, W., & Dorsey, S. (2014). Show me, don't tell me: Behavioural rehearsal as a training and analogue fidelity tool. *Cognitive and Behavioural Practice, 21*(1) 1–11.

Bordin, E. S. (1983). A working alliance based model of supervision. *The Counselling Psychologist, 11*(1), 35–42.

Burnham, J. (2012). Developments in social GRRRAAACCEEESSS: Visible-invisible and voiced-unvoiced. In I.-B. Krause (Ed.), *Culture and reflexivity in systemic psychotherapy: Mutual perspectives* (pp. 139–160). London: Karnac.

Burnham, J., Alvis Palma, D., & Whitehouse, L. (2008). Learning as a context for differences, and differences as a context for learning. *Journal of Family Therapy, 30*(4), 529–542.

Cookson, J., Sloan, G., Dafters, B., & Jahoda, A. (2014). Provision of clinical supervision for staff working in mental health services. *Mental Health Practice, 17*(7), 29–34.

Corrie, S., & Lane, D. A. (2015). *CBT supervision*. London: Sage.

Falender, C. A. (2018). Clinical supervision—the missing ingredient. *American Psychologist, 73*(9), 1240–1250.

Falender, C. A., & Shafranske, E. P. (2017). Competency-based clinical supervision: Status, opportunities, tensions, and the future. *Australian Psychologist, 52*(2), 86–93.

Falender, C. A., Shafranske, E. P., & Ofek, A. (2014). Competent clinical supervision: Emerging effective practices. *Counselling Psychology Quarterly, 27*(4), 393–408.

Ferguson, S., Harper, S., Platz, S., Sloan, G., & Smith, K. (2016). Developing specialist CBT supervision training in Scotland using blended learning: Challenges and opportunities. *The Cognitive Behaviour Therapist, 9*, 1–12.

Fuggle, P., Dunsmuir, S., & Curry, V. (2013). *CBT with children, young people and families*. London: Sage.

Fuggle, P., & Hepburn, C. (2019). *Clinical outcomes for the wellbeing practitioner programme for children, young people and their parents/carers: Update report December 2019*. Report presented to Health Education England prepared by UCL and KCL CWP Workforce Collaborative.

Gonsalvez, C. J., Hamid, G., Savage, N. M., & Livni, D. (2017). The Supervision Evaluation and Supervisory Competence Scale: Psychometric validation. *Australian Psychologist, 52*(2), 94–103.

Hämmig, O. (2017). Health and well-being at work: The key role of supervisor support. *Population Health, 3*, 393–402.

Hawkins, P., & Shohet, R. (2012). *Supervision in the helping professions*. Maidenhead: McGraw-Hill Education (UK).

Inskipp, F., & Proctor, B. (2001). Group supervision. In J. Scaife (Ed.), *Supervision in the mental health professions: A practitioner's guide* (pp. 99–121). Abingdon: Routledge.

Johnston, L. H., Milne, D. L. (2012). How do supervisee's learn during supervision? A grounded theory study of the perceived developmental process. *The Cognitive Behaviour Therapist, 5*(1), 1–23.

Kolb, D. A. (1984). *Experiential learning: Experience as the source of learning and development*. Englewood Cliffs, NJ: Prentice Hall.

Ladany, N. (2014). The ingredients of supervisor failure. *Journal of Clinical Psychology, 70*(11), 1094–1103.

Law, D. (2014). Why bother. In D. Law & M. Wolpert (Eds.), *Guide to using outcomes and feedback Tools with children, young people and families* (pp. 42–44). London: CAMHS Press.

Loades, M. E., & Armstrong, P. (2016). The challenge of training supervisors to use direct assessments of clinical competence in CBT consistently: a systematic review and exploratory training study. *The Cognitive Behaviour Therapist, 9*, e27.

Mastoras, S. M., & Andrews, J. J. (2011). The supervisee experience of group supervision: Implications for research and practice. *Training and Education in Professional Psychology, 5*(2), 102–111.

Milne, D., & Dunkerley, C. (2007). Helpful Aspects of Supervision Questionnaire. Altered by Derek Milne from the Helpful Aspects of Therapy Questionnaire, with permission. Original: Llewellyn, S. (1988). Psychological therapy, as viewed by clients and therapists. *British Journal of Clinical Psychology, 27*, 105–114.

Milne, D., & Dunkerley, C. (2010). Towards evidence-based clinical supervision: the development and evaluation of four CBT guidelines. *The Cognitive Behaviour Therapist, 3*, 43–57.

Milne, D., Aylott, H., Fitzpatrick, H., & Ellis, M. V. (2008). How does clinical supervision work? Using a 'best evidence synthesis' approach to construct a basic model of supervision. *The Clinical Supervisor, 27*(2), 170–190.

Milne, D. L., Reiser, R. P., Cliffe, T., & Raine, R. (2011). SAGE: Preliminary evaluation of an instrument for observing competence in CBT supervision. *Cognitive Behaviour Therapist, 4*(4), 123–138.

Milne, D. L. (2017). *Evidence-based CBT supervision: Principles and practice* (2nd ed.). Chichester: Wiley Blackwell.

O'Donovan, A., Clough, B., & Petch, J. (2017). Is supervisor training effective? A pilot investigation of clinical supervisor training program. *Australian Psychologist, 52*(2), 149–154.

Palomo, M., Beinart, H., & Cooper, M. J. (2010). Development and validation of the Supervisory Relationship Questionnaire (SRQ) in UK trainee clinical psychologists. *British Journal of Clinical Psychology, 49*(Pt 2), 131–149.

Proctor, B. (2008). *Group supervision: A guide to creative practice* (2nd ed.). London: Sage.

Reese, R. J., Usher, E. L., Bowman, D. C., Norsworthy, L. A., Halstead, J. L., Rowlands, S. R., & Chisholm, R. R. (2009). Using client feedback in psychotherapy training: An analysis of its influence on supervision and counsellor self-efficacy. *Training and Education in Professional Psychology*, 3(3), 157–168.

Reiser, R. P., Cliffe, T., & Milne, D. L. (2018). An improved competence rating scale for CBT Supervision: Short-SAGE. *The Cognitive Behaviour Therapist*, 11, e7.

Reiser, R. P., & Milne, D. L. (2016). A survey of CBT supervision in the UK: Methods, satisfaction and training, as viewed by a selected sample of CBT supervision leaders. *The Cognitive Behaviour Therapist*, 9, e20.

Reiser, R. P., Watkins, C. E., & Milne, D. E. (2014). *The Wiley International Handbook of Supervision*. Chichester: Wiley-Blackwell.

Rønnestad, M. H., Orlinsky, D. E., Schröder, T. A., Skovholt, T. M., & Willutzki, U. (2019). The professional development of counsellors and psychotherapists: Implications of empirical studies for supervision, training and practice. *Counselling & Psychotherapy Research*, 19(3), 214–230.

Roth, A. D., Myles-Hooton, P., & Branson, A. (2019). Judging clinical competence using structured observation tools: A cautionary tale. *Behavioural and Cognitive Psychotherapy*, 47(6), 736–744.

Roth, A. D., & Pilling, S. (2008). A competence framework for the supervision of psychological therapies. Retrieved from http://www.ucl.ac.uk/CORE

Richards, D. A., Chellingsworth, M., Hope, R., Turpin, G., & Whyte, M. (2010). ReachOut national programme supervisor materials to support the delivery of training for psychological wellbeing practitioners delivering low intensity interventions. Retrieved from http://www.iapt.nhs.uk/workforce/low-intensity/

Silva, A. E., Newman, D. S., Guiney, M. C., Valley-Gray, S., & Barrett, C. A. (2016). Supervision and mentoring for early career school psychologists: Availability, access, structure, and implications. *Psychology in the Schools*, 53(5), 502–516.

Swift, J. K., Callahan, J. L., Rousmaniere, T. G., Whipple, J. L., Dexter, K., & Wrape, E. R. (2015). Using client outcome monitoring as a tool for supervision. *Psychotherapy*, 52(2), 180–184.

Townend, M., Iannetta, L., & Freeston, M. H. (2002). Clinical supervision in practice: A survey of UK cognitive behavioural psychotherapists accredited by the BABCP. *Behavioural and Cognitive Psychotherapy*, 30(4), 485–500.

Tracey, T. J. G., Wampold, B. E., Lichtenberg, J. W., & Goodyear, R. K. (2014). Expertise in psychotherapy: An elusive goal? *American Psychologist*, 69(3), 218–229.

Vygotsky, L. S. (1986). *Thought and language* (3rd ed.). Cambridge, MA: MIT Press.

Weck, F., Kaufmann, Y. M., & Höfling, V. (2017). Competence feedback improves CBT competence in trainee therapists: A randomized controlled pilot study. *Psychotherapy Research*, 27(4), 501–509.

Weck, F., Kaufmann, Y. M., & Witthöft, M. (2017). Topics and techniques in clinical supervision in psychotherapy training. *The Cognitive Behaviour Therapist*, 10, 3.

Wood, D. J., Bruner, J. S., & Ross, G. (1976). The role of tutoring in problem solving. *Journal of Child Psychology and Psychiatry*, 17(2), 89–100.

Yourman, D. B., & Farber, B. A. (1996). Nondisclosure and distortion in psychotherapy supervision. *Psychotherapy: Theory, Research, Practice, Training*, 33(4), 567–575.

20

Practical applications of implementation science to low intensity cognitive behavioural therapy interventions

Simone Schriger and Rinad Beidas

Learning objectives

- Define implementation science and articulate the rationale for using an evidence-based implementation process.
- Identify what type of research on low intensity cognitive behavioural therapy interventions is urgently needed and why.
- Explain the four phases of implementation and the goal of each phase.
- Articulate the four key factors to consider across each implementation step.
- Be able to apply these concepts to your own setting, using the supplemental checklist to guide you.

Introduction

As demonstrated in prior chapters, low intensity (LI) cognitive behavioural therapy interventions (henceforth referred to as LI interventions) for youth can be used to treat a diverse set of psychological disorders. Broadly, these interventions require less time, cost, and complexity and offer more flexibility and adaptability compared to traditional high intensity interventions. This situates them as a promising solution to the public health crisis of untreated paediatric psychological disorders; in the US, 50% of young people in need of mental health care go without it (Whitney & Peterson, 2019), and this gap is estimated to be even higher in low- and middle-income countries (Patel, Kieling, Maulik, & Divan, 2013). Despite their tremendous potential, few LI interventions have been implemented in routine practice outside the context of research. In this chapter, we will discuss how to implement these interventions in community settings so that their public health potential can be realized.

What is implementation science?

Implementation science (IS) is a field dedicated to understanding how to best facilitate the use of evidence-based practices (EBPs), or interventions with science demonstrating their effectiveness, into routine practice (Eccles & Mittman, 2006). IS can help guide the way in addressing the relative dearth of LI intervention implementation. Given that IS focuses specifically on EBPs, this chapter addresses implementation of LI interventions with strong evidence of effectiveness. We recognize that many LI interventions require further investigation in order to be ready for implementation. This chapter outlines some of the 'greatest hits' in IS (see 'Recommended reading' section for a more comprehensive introduction). By applying insights from IS to LI interventions, these interventions can better reach the youth around the globe who urgently need them.

How to use this chapter

We offer a step-by-step guide to implementing a LI intervention in community settings. Though it may seem intuitive to choose a LI intervention, invest in manuals, train practitioners, and launch, taking an evidence-based approach to implementation will maximize the likelihood of sustained success over the long term and will likely involve less trial and error. This chapter may be particularly relevant to organization leaders and clinic directors (who will likely be involved from Step 1) and to practitioners (who may find Steps 3, 4, and 9 onwards particularly helpful).

We have structured this chapter using the Exploration Preparation Implementation Sustainment (EPIS) framework, a four-phase framework developed for implementation of youth EBPs (Aarons, Hurlburt, & Horwitz, 2011). Although this framework is particularly well-suited to implementation of LI interventions for youth, there are other IS frameworks and models that may be a better fit for you depending on your context (see Nilsen, 2015; Tabak, Khoong, Chambers, & Brownson, 2012). Our 15 practical implementation steps span the four EPIS implementation phases:

- Exploration: understanding your setting and getting the lay of the land.
- Preparation: deciding which LI intervention to implement and planning for implementation.
- Implementation: putting the LI intervention into practice and monitoring outcomes.
- Sustainment: continuing to iterate and improve over time.

At the end of each phase is a brief reflection exercise that we hope will prompt further application of these concepts in your own setting. Across each implementation step, consider the inner context, outer context, intervention characteristics, and intervention–setting fit (Aarons et al., 2011). The inner context includes characteristics of the setting in which you are implementing the LI intervention (a community mental health clinic, primary care centre, school, etc.) that may make it harder or easier to implement. This includes the individuals who work in your setting, the culture of your workplace, and the policies and procedures in place. The outer context includes characteristics of the target population and community that you are working with, government policies, funding mechanisms, and other organizations that you work with that might affect implementation success. It is also important to consider the LI intervention characteristics itself, and the LI intervention–setting fit (see Aarons et al., 2011; Damschroder et al., 2009; Greenhalgh, Robert, Macfarlane, Bate, & Kyriakidou, 2004). For example, if you want to implement a computer-assisted intervention for adolescent depression in a primary care clinic, you might consider the level of support from clinic leaders of this type of intervention, the level of interest of young people in receiving computerized interventions (inner context), and the state and national laws, regulations, and policies that pertain to computerized treatment delivery (outer context). You might also consider intervention characteristics such as the types of technological equipment and expertise required, and factors related to the intervention–setting fit, including how practitioners in the setting feel about interventions delivered via computer, and how digital disparities might affect clients' access to the treatment you select.

In this chapter, we refer to the particular LI intervention of choice as 'the intervention', the specific place that the intervention will be implemented as the 'organization' or 'inner context', and the larger environment of where that organization is positioned as the 'outer context'. We use the term 'setting' to refer collectively to the inner and outer contexts. We refer to the service deliverers as 'practitioners' (with the understanding that some LI interventions are unguided and/or do not have traditional therapists), the individuals receiving these services as 'clients', and the broad group of clients as the 'target population'. We hope that what follows will orient you to the implementation landscape, demystify key IS concepts, serve as a starting point for your implementation process, and whet your appetite for further reading.

The four phases

Step 1: exploration phase

In the exploration phase, you gather information about the needs of your target population and select an unmet need to address. While you may already have a sense of your target problem and LI intervention of choice, we encourage you to engage in this process, as it will make the implementation process more successful.

1. Conduct a needs assessment of your target population and select an unmet need to address

The first step is centred around listening to stakeholders, including clients and their families, community members, administrators, teachers, staff, health system leaders, and others who may be affected by implementation of the LI intervention. The goal of this assessment is to better understand the specific unmet needs and priorities of the target population and the potential impact of addressing these needs, placing particular emphasis on perspectives from individuals within your target population. You may want to ask about previous implementation efforts, both of LI and higher intensity interventions, to understand what has worked and what has not. Through an iterative process, you will begin to refine your understanding of needs. If possible, use an approach that involves both quantitative (e.g. surveys or data from electronic health records) and qualitative (e.g. interviews or focus groups with community members or feedback provided by previous clients) data. You should then select a need that has been prioritized by multiple stakeholders and groups, as you will be relying on many of these stakeholders throughout the implementation process. If you have identified multiple needs, select the one that is most pressing to your target population and most feasibly addressed with the resources that you have.

Reflection exercise: exploration

Can you identify stakeholders from multiple groups who you can involve in a needs assessment? If not, who could you partner with to connect to multilevel stakeholders? Thinking about your target population, are there any needs that have been expressed to date? Which aspects of your inner and outer contexts do you think will make implementation easier and which will make implementation more difficult?

Step 2: preparation phase

In the preparation or pre-implementation phase, you establish a multilevel stakeholder team to lead the implementation process, select a LI intervention, identify necessary adaptations, choose outcomes to measure, and plan for long-term sustainment. It culminates in an implementation blueprint that guides active implementation.

2. Establish a multilevel stakeholder team that includes practitioners, administrators, community members, and clients

Mobilize a subset of the stakeholders that you engaged with in the previous phase to join your stakeholder team. Ensure that there is representation from community members within your target population. Recruit stakeholders who are 'champions' within their respective roles (i.e. individuals particularly dedicated to implementation efforts and motivated to adopt the new intervention) (Miech et al., 2018). A diversity of perspectives will maximize your ability to select an appropriate LI intervention and adapt it to best fit the realities of your setting. If you find that it is difficult to gather a team of motivated stakeholders, you may need to go back to Step 1 and ensure that there is sufficient buy-in to tackle the problem you've identified.

3. Select a LI cognitive behavioural therapy intervention
There may be multiple LI interventions that target the problem you have identified. The ideal intervention will produce the greatest client benefit and have the lowest barriers to use. You may consider factors such as whether your desired intervention will be guided or unguided (i.e. include a practitioner or not), if it will involve technology, if it will involve a single session or multiple sessions, and who will be delivering the intervention. When selecting an intervention, you first must consider the strength of the research evidence (both in terms of quantity and quality of studies). In order to be a good candidate for implementation, the LI intervention should have demonstrated efficacy *and* effectiveness across multiple randomized controlled trials (see Chambless & Ollendick, 2001). Once you have identified interventions that may be appropriate, consider the insights gleaned during the preparation phase. You do not only want to ask 'Is this a good intervention?' but also 'Is this a good intervention for this setting?' Also consider characteristics of the intervention itself, including any aspects of the intervention that may make it easy or difficult to implement, both in the short and long term. As discussed in the exploration phase, it is important that the intervention selected is acceptable not only by a single team member or stakeholder but across stakeholders from different groups.

4. Adapt with intention while maintaining core components
Using the information gathered from the needs assessment and the input from your stakeholder team, identify specific aspects of the intervention that will require adaption to maximize fit with your setting (see Stirman, Baumann, & Miller, 2019). When making adaptations, you will need to balance adapting materials and practices to best fit your setting while maintaining the integrity of the intervention (see Miller, Wiltsey-Stirman, & Baumann, 2020). While some flexibility may be needed, you should follow evidence-based guidelines about which aspects of the intervention can be approached flexibly and which should be carried out with fidelity (i.e. with adherence and competence in intervention delivery) so that the effectiveness of the treatment is not compromised (Georgiadis, Peris, & Comer, 2020). This concept, sometimes called 'flexibility within fidelity', are reviewed in Chapter 9 (see Kendall & Beidas, 2007). Common adaptations include modification of treatment content (e.g. translating to another language, tailoring to a particular culture), treatment delivery modality (e.g. holding sessions virtually rather than in person), and method of training (e.g. shorter in-person trainings with supplemental self-guided components).

5. Select implementation strategies
Implementation strategies are the tools you will use to promote the use of the selected LI intervention in your setting. There are over 70 implementation strategies that can

help with EBP implementation, and these strategies have been grouped into nine clusters, such as supporting practitioners, engaging clients, and financial strategies (see Powell et al., 2015; Waltz et al., 2015). Some of these strategies are built into this implementation checklist (such as the implementation blueprint in Step 8, training in Step 9, and ongoing supervision and consultation in Step 11) (Box 20.1), and others you will select based on the specifics of your setting (see Damschroder et al., 2009; Nilsen & Bernhardsson, 2019). Given the scope of this chapter, we cannot describe all of the relevant factors that affect implementation, but we present several central constructs below that have strong evidence supporting their association with successful implementation (see the Glossary at the end of this book for definitions).

Box 20.1 Low-Intensity Intervention Implementation Checklist

Exploration

1. ☐ Conduct a needs assessment of your target population and select an unmet need to address

Preparation

2. ☐ Establish a multilevel stakeholder team that includes practitioners, administrators, community members, and clients

3. ☐ Select a low intensity cognitive behavioral therapy intervention

4. ☐ Adapt with intention while maintaining the core components

5. ☐ Select implementation strategies

6. ☐ Decide which implementation and clinical outcomes to measure

7. ☐ Plan for sustainment

8. ☐ Create an implementation blueprint to guide implementation

Implementation

9. ☐ Acquire materials, hire personnel, and train all staff involved in implementation of the intervention

10. ☐ Launch your intervention

11. ☐ Provide ongoing clinical supervision and consultation

12. ☐ Measure the outcomes you selected

13. ☐ Establish feedback mechanisms for clinicians and administrators

14. ☐ Carry out intervention fidelity checks

Sustainment

15. ☐ Evaluate, iterate, and improve over time

Consider factors in the inner and outer contexts that may serve to facilitate or impede implementation efforts. In the inner context, this includes organizational culture (Glisson et al., 2008) and organizational readiness for change (Shea, Jacobs, Esserman, Bruce, & Weiner, 2014). In the outer context, this includes sociopolitical factors, such as the presence or absence of external funding, laws, policies, or incentives that may affect implementation efforts, and other networks of care connected to your organization. If you are interested in an intervention that involves lay health workers, you may consider factors related to guilds, licensing, and clinical credentialing, which will vary by your location. You may also consider factors within your organization that may affect the implementation of something new (i.e. a LI intervention), including implementation climate (Weiner, Belden, Bergmire, & Johnston, 2011) and implementation leadership (Aarons, Ehrhart, & Farahnak, 2014).

Taking into account these facilitators and barriers, decide on a set of implementation strategies that will maximize implementation success by leveraging strengths within your setting and addressing any barriers that exist. For example, if you identify that leadership support of your intervention is poor, one implementation strategy could be to increase leadership support. Other strategies that may be particularly relevant to LI interventions include using incentives to promote the use of the LI intervention (and disincentivizing the use of undesired practices), identifying champion practitioners within your setting who can serve as a model for others, writing key implementation tasks into job descriptions of new hires, and using train-the-trainer strategies to create a sustainable workforce.

6. Decide which implementation and clinical outcomes to measure

In order to evaluate the success of implementation efforts, you will need to measure implementation outcomes, which elucidate how much and how well the intervention is used. There are multiple implementation outcomes that may be relevant to your setting (see Glasgow Vogt, & Boles, 1999; Glasgow et al., 2019; Proctor et al., 2011). These should be selected based on priorities and data collection capabilities. Many of these implementation outcomes have validated measures that can be used to capture data (see Allen et al., 2020; Lewis et al., 2015) and include acceptability (the belief among stakeholders that the intervention is satisfactory), appropriateness (the perceived fit of the intervention to the setting), and feasibility (the extent to which the intervention can realistically be implemented in the setting) (Lyon & Bruns, 2019). Additional commonly measured outcomes include fidelity (the extent to which the intervention is being delivered in the way it was designed), penetration (the extent to which the intervention is integrated within a larger service system), and cost (Proctor et al., 2011). Also consider measuring clinical outcomes, which measure how well the intervention works, if you are using the intervention with a novel population or making substantial adaptations (Aarons, Sklar, Mustanski, Benbow, & Brown, 2017) (see Chapter X).

7. Plan for sustainment

Just as you planned ahead for which outcomes you will measure, you should also plan ahead for long-term sustainment of your intervention. Although it is common to think about sustainment as something that comes *after* active implementation, the seeds of sustainment are planted long before implementation. Sustainment is a complex and multifaceted phenomenon that depends upon manifold factors including funding stability, partnerships, and organizational capacity (Shelton, Cooper, & Stirman, 2018). A number of sustainability tools and frameworks have been developed to plan ahead for sustainment, such as the freely available Clinical Sustainability Assessment Tool (CSAT) (Calhoun et al., 2014; Lennox, Maher, & Reed, 2018; Luke Calhoun, Robichaux, Moreland-Russell, & Elliott, 2014; Stirman et al., 2012).

8. Create an implementation blueprint to guide implementation

An implementation blueprint is a living document to be shared between members of your team. It should be updated as needed throughout the implementation process and includes the desired timeframe, important milestones, and metrics you will be using to measure progress. The blueprint should explicitly identify steps needed to facilitate coordination across your inner and outer contexts, including procedures needed to ensure a smooth and organized rollout of the LI intervention. Within this blueprint, you should also outline procedures for measuring desired outcomes, protocols for new practices in workflow and hiring, and processes for dedicating resources to implementation efforts and collaborating with partners (Greenhalgh et al., 2004; Powell, 2015). This document should also include your detailed plans for sustainment.

Reflection exercise: preparation

Are there individuals who you encountered during the exploration phase who you think would be a good fit for your stakeholder team? How will you get in contact with these individuals, and how will you describe what you are requesting from them? Given the characteristics of your setting, what, if any, aspects of the LI intervention you have selected do you think need adaptation? Looking through the list of implementation strategies, which do you think would be most appropriate to use and why? Which outcome measures are most pressing and can they feasibly be measured? Do you plan to measure both implementation and clinical outcomes? Will additional funding be needed to ensure that outcomes are consistently measured? What do you anticipate will be the biggest barriers toward achieving long-term sustainment, and how can you plan ahead to overcome these barriers?

Step 3: implementation phase

Now that you have carried out much of the 'behind the scenes' work, it is time to put your plans into action. This may include purchasing necessary materials, hiring and training staff, launching the intervention, and providing ongoing feedback and support to staff. This stage also involves measuring and evaluating outcomes and carrying out fidelity checks to ensure that the LI intervention is being delivered as planned.

9. Acquire materials, hire personnel, and train all staff involved in implementation of the intervention

You now need to acquire the necessary physical supplies and recruit and hire any additional staff needed. If your intervention relies on technology, this may involve acquiring technological devices or consulting with IT experts. You will then need to train practitioners in the delivery of your LI intervention. If the intervention is un-guided, you will have to prepare written or video-recorded materials. Even if it is not feasible to hold an extensive multi-day training, you will still want to use evidence-based training principles (Beidas & Kendall, 2010; Lyon, Stirman, Kerns, & Bruns, 2011; Stirman et al., 2010; Valenstein-Mah et al., 2020).

10. Launch your intervention

It is finally time to launch your intervention! The specifics of this step will depend on the LI intervention that you have chosen. It may make sense to launch your intervention in a staged manner such that you begin by piloting the intervention and then scale up over time.

11. Provide ongoing clinical supervision and consultation

The initial training carried out in Step 9 is only a starting point. Ongoing clinical supervision and support of practitioners (sometimes called 'consultation') is crucial to implementation success (Edmunds, Beidas, & Kendall, 2013; Nadeem, Gleacher, & Beidas, 2013). These practices are also of vital importance to maintaining fidelity to the intervention and to facilitating long-term sustainment. There are ways to provide consultation even when resources are limited, such as in a group format (Stirman et al., 2017). Best supervision practices involve active strategies (such as role playing and modelling) and a focus on the core EBP elements of the intervention, though these vital elements of supervision are often underutilized (Milne & Reiser, 2017; Schriger, Becker-Haimes, Skriner, & Beidas, 2020).

12. Measure the outcomes you selected

Measuring the outcomes you identified during the preparation phase will help answer in evaluating the success of the intervention and in answering other important questions. For example, what can you learn about the extent to which your intervention is being used, and how well it is being used? What do your outcomes suggest about areas for improvement? Is there anything unexpected? Is the cost of your intervention sustainable over time given your funding? These data will be vitally important to answering these questions and to adapting to changes in your environment over time.

13. Establish feedback mechanisms for practitioners and administrators

Now that you have preliminary implementation outcomes data, you will need to establish and utilize feedback mechanisms to foster continual improvement. Your intervention exists within a dynamic system and will undoubtedly need adjustments as changes in the inner and outer contexts occur. In this step, you will identify mechanisms through which to capture ongoing quantitative and qualitative feedback. This may include soliciting feedback from clients at the end of treatment through quantitative surveys, open-ended comment boxes, focus groups, or informal conversations. You should actively solicit feedback from key stakeholders such as community members and then address the feedback you receive.

14. Carry out intervention fidelity checks

In addition to soliciting feedback from stakeholders, you should systematically assess whether your intervention is being carried out with fidelity. In particular, it is important to determine the extent to which core evidence-based components of the intervention are being delivered as designed and to identify any drift away from these core EBP elements, as such drift can negatively affect client outcomes. Periodic fidelity checks can occur through live supervision, recorded sessions, or other forms of audit that involve careful investigation of what is being delivered. There are also proxy methods that can be used if higher intensity methods of monitoring fidelity are not feasible (Beidas, Cross, & Dorsey, 2014). By engaging in regular fidelity checks, any drift from core EBP elements can be promptly addressed.

Reflection exercise: implementation

Do you have the necessary personnel to implement your intervention? If you need to make additional hires, how will you recruit strong candidates? Who at your organization will need to be trained, and how will the training be structured? Will you be hiring external trainers or using internal personnel? Once your intervention is ready to be launched, how will you recruit clients? Do you anticipate piloting the intervention on a smaller scale prior to full-scale implementation? What is your plan for clinical supervision and consultation? Will you need to allocate additional funds to supervisors, and if so, where will these funds come from? What feedback mechanisms will you use to evaluate your intervention, and how do you plan to carry out fidelity checks? Who will you speak with if you find that aspects of your intervention are not being delivered with fidelity?

Step 4: sustainment phase

Although it is exciting to see your intervention in action after so much planning, the work is not over. While there is no precise definition of when the sustainment phase begins, it is generally conceptualized as beginning no earlier than 2 years after an intervention is launched. Sustainment of your intervention requires continuation of the activities carried out in the implementation phase, such as providing ongoing supervision, measuring outcomes, and carrying out regular fidelity checks. In addition to these key activities, sustainment involves receptivity to changes within the inner and outer contexts. Now begins the iterative process of continuous quality improvement. Continued attention to the intervention–setting fit will maximize long-term sustainment, and thus maximize the public health impact of your intervention.

15. Evaluate, iterate, and improve over time

In order to sustain your intervention success over time, you will have to adjust to dynamic and everchanging ecosystems (Chambers, Glasgow, & Stange, 2013; Shelton, Chambers, & Glasgow, 2020). Organizations able to adapt and change to new developments—sometimes called learning organizations—are best suited to sustain positive client outcomes in the long term (Beidas & Stirman, 2020). Given the rapid advances in technology, the frequent development of new LI interventions, the growing evidence bases for existing interventions, and the changes in the laws affecting delivery of interventions, what is considered best practice at one time may no longer be recommended several years later. What you learned during the initial implementation process will likely need to be updated at regular intervals. It will be important to periodically revisit your sustainment plan and adjust as necessary. You may begin receiving unexpected feedback or surprising data and may even find at some point that your intervention is no longer being implemented successfully. If this happens, consider cycling back to Step 1 and conducting another needs assessment to assess whether transitioning to another intervention is warranted or if changes can be made to enhance the intervention–setting fit. Iteration and changes over time are a good thing, and a sign of success. When it comes to sustainment, the goal is for ongoing *improvement* rather than maintenance of what was first implemented. Given the critical role that LI interventions may play in closing the mental health care gap in youth, such responsiveness to your setting will be vital for improving the lives of youth around the globe.

Reflection exercise: sustainment

Given that there is no precise moment that sustainment begins, how will you know when your intervention has been sustained? Are there any characteristics of your inner and outer contexts that you anticipate will substantially change over the next 5 years? What, if any, characteristics of your intervention do you anticipate may become obsolete? What will you do if you find that, in 2 years, your intervention is no longer fitting well with your setting? Who will you talk with about this, and how will you proceed if some members of your stakeholder group are hesitant to making changes?

Chapter summary

- Implementation and scale up of LI interventions in routine care has been low.
- Key principles from IS can guide implementation of these interventions to realize their public health impact.
- Implementation is a complex process that spans four phases: exploration, preparation, implementation, and sustainment.
- During each step of implementation, consider the inner context, outer context, intervention characteristics, and intervention–setting fit.
- Implementation strategies are the tools used to support successful implementation and should be selected based on the specifics of your setting.
- Planning for sustainment begins prior to implementation and is facilitated by receptivity to changes in the environment over time.

Recommended reading

Albers, B., Shlonsky, A., & Mildon, R. (Eds.). (2020). *Implementation Science 3.0*. New York: Springer.

Beidas, R. S., & Kendall, P. C. (Eds.). (2014). *Dissemination and implementation of evidence-based practices in child and adolescent mental health*. Oxford: Oxford University Press.

Brownson, R. C., Colditz, G. A., & Proctor, E. K. (Eds.). (2017). *Dissemination and implementation research in health: Translating science to practice*. Oxford: Oxford University Press.

Nilsen, P., & Birken, S. A. (2020). *Handbook on implementation science*. Cheltenham: Edward Elgar Publishing.

References

Aarons, G. A., Ehrhart, M. G., & Farahnak, L. R. (2014). The implementation leadership scale (ILS): Development of a brief measure of unit level implementation leadership. *Implementation Science, 9*(1), 45.

Aarons, G. A., Hurlburt, M., & Horwitz, S. M. C. (2011). Advancing a conceptual model of evidence-based practice implementation in public service sectors. *Administration and Policy in Mental Health and Mental Health Services Research, 38*(1), 4–23.

Aarons, G. A., Sklar, M., Mustanski, B., Benbow, N., & Brown, C. H. (2017). 'Scaling-out' evidence-based interventions to new populations or new health care delivery systems. *Implementation Science, 12*(1), 1–13.

Allen, P., Pilar, M., Walsh-Bailey, C., Hooley, C., Mazzucca, S., Lewis, C. C., . . ., & Brownson, R. C. (2020). Quantitative measures of health policy implementation determinants and outcomes: A systematic review. *Implementation Science: IS, 15*(1), 47.

Beidas, R. S., Cross, W., & Dorsey, S. (2014). Show me, don't tell me: Behavioral rehearsal as a training and analogue fidelity tool. *Cognitive and Behavioral Practice, 21*(1), 1–11.

Beidas, R. S., & Kendall, P. C. (2010). Training therapists in evidence-based practice: A critical review of studies from a systems-contextual perspective. *Clinical Psychology: Science and Practice, 17*(1), 1–30.

Beidas, R. S., & Wiltsey Stirman, S. (2020). Realizing the promise of learning organizations to transform mental health care: Telepsychiatry care as an exemplar. *Psychiatric Services, 72*(1), 86–88.

Calhoun, A., Mainor, A., Moreland-Russell, S., Maier, R. C., Brossart, L., & Luke, D. A. (2014). Using the program sustainability assessment tool to assess and plan for sustainability. *Preventing Chronic Disease, 11*, 130185.

Chambers, D. A., Glasgow, R. E., & Stange, K. C. (2013). The dynamic sustainability framework: Addressing the paradox of sustainment amid ongoing change. *Implementation Science, 8*(1), 117.

Chambless, D. L., & Ollendick, T. H. (2001). Empirically supported psychological interventions: Controversies and evidence. In *Annual Review of Psychology, 52*, 685–716.

Damschroder, L. J., Aron, D. C., Keith, R. E., Kirsh, S. R., Alexander, J. A., & Lowery, J. C. (2009). Fostering implementation of health services research findings into practice: A consolidated framework for advancing implementation science. *Implementation Science, 4*(1), 50.

Eccles, M. P., & Mittman, B. S. (2006). Welcome to implementation science. *Implementation Science, 1*(1), 1–3.

Edmunds, J. M., Beidas, R. S., & Kendall, P. C. (2013). Dissemination and implementation of evidence-based practices: Training and consultation as implementation strategies. *Clinical Psychology: Science and Practice, 20*(2), 152–165.

Georgiadis, C., Peris, T. S., & Comer, J. S. (2020). Implementing strategic flexibility in the delivery of youth mental health care: A tailoring framework for thoughtful clinical practice. *Evidence-Based Practice in Child and Adolescent Mental Health, 5*(3), 215–232.

Glasgow, R. E., Harden, S. M., Gaglio, B., Rabin, B., Smith, M. L., Porter, G. C., . . ., & Estabrooks, P. A. (2019). RE-AIM planning and evaluation framework: Adapting to new science and practice with a 20-year review. *Frontiers in Public Health, 7*, 64.

Glasgow, R. E., Vogt, T. M., & Boles, S. M. (1999). Evaluating the public health impact of health promotion interventions: The RE-AIM framework. *American Journal of Public Health, 89*(9), 1322–1327.

Glisson, C., Landsverk, J., Schoenwald, S., Kelleher, K., Hoagwood, K. E., Mayberg, S., . . ., & Palinkas, L. (2008). Assessing the Organizational Social Context (OSC) of mental health services: Implications for research and practice. *Administration and Policy in Mental Health and Mental Health Services Research, 35*(1–2), 98–113.

Greenhalgh, T., Robert, G., Macfarlane, F., Bate, P., & Kyriakidou, O. (2004). Diffusion of innovations in service organizations: Systematic review and recommendations. *Milbank Quarterly, 82*(4), 581–629.

Kendall, P. C., & Beidas, R. S. (2007). Smoothing the trail for dissemination of evidence-based practices for youth: Flexibility within fidelity. *Professional Psychology: Research and Practice, 38*(1), 13–20.

Lennox, L., Maher, L., & Reed, J. (2018). Navigating the sustainability landscape: A systematic review of sustainability approaches in healthcare. *Implementation Science, 13*(1), 27.

Lewis, C. C., Fischer, S., Weiner, B. J., Stanick, C., Kim, M., & Martinez, R. G. (2015). Outcomes for implementation science: An enhanced systematic review of instruments using evidence-based rating criteria. *Implementation Science: IS, 10*, 155.

Luke, D. A., Calhoun, A., Robichaux, C. B., Moreland-Russell, S., & Elliott, M. B. (2014). The program sustainability assessment tool: A new instrument for public health programs. *Preventing Chronic Disease, 11*, 130184.

Lyon, A. R., & Bruns, E. J. (2019). User-centered redesign of evidence-based psychosocial interventions to enhance implementation—hospitable soil or better seeds? *JAMA Psychiatry, 76*(1), 3–4.

Lyon, A. R., Stirman, S. W., Kerns, S. E. U., & Bruns, E. J. (2011). Developing the mental health workforce: Review and application of training approaches from multiple disciplines. *Administration and Policy in Mental Health and Mental Health Services Research, 38*(4), 238–253.

Miech, E. J., Rattray, N. A., Flanagan, M. E., Damschroder, L., Schmid, A. A., & Damush, T. M. (2018). Inside help: An integrative review of champions in healthcare-related implementation. *SAGE Open Medicine, 6*, 2050312118773326.

Miller, C. J., Wiltsey-Stirman, S., & Baumann, A. A. (2020). Iterative decision-making for evaluation of adaptations (IDEA): A decision tree for balancing adaptation, fidelity, and intervention impact. *Journal of Community Psychology, 48*(4), 1163–1177.

Milne, D. L., & Reiser, R. P. (2017). *A manual for evidence-based CBT supervision.* Chichester: John Wiley.

Nadeem, E., Gleacher, A., & Beidas, R. S. (2013). Consultation as an implementation strategy for evidence-based practices across multiple contexts: Unpacking the black box. *Administration and Policy in Mental Health and Mental Health Services Research, 40*(6), 439–450.

Nilsen, P. (2015). Making sense of implementation theories, models and frameworks. *Implementation Science, 10*(1), 53.

Nilsen, P., & Bernhardsson, S. (2019). Context matters in implementation science: A scoping review of determinant frameworks that describe contextual determinants for implementation outcomes. *BMC Health Services Research, 19*(1), 189.

Patel, V., Kieling, C., Maulik, P. K., & Divan, G. (2013). Improving access to care for children with mental disorders: A global perspective. *Archives of Disease in Childhood, 98*(5), 323–327.

Powell, B. J., Waltz, T. J., Chinman, M. J., Damschroder, L. J., Smith, J. L., Matthieu, M. M., . . ., & Kirchner, J. A. E. (2015). A refined compilation of implementation strategies: Results from the Expert Recommendations for Implementing Change (ERIC) project. *Implementation Science, 10*(1), 21.

Proctor, E., Silmere, H., Raghavan, R., Hovmand, P., Aarons, G., Bunger, A., . . ., & Hensley, M. (2011). Outcomes for implementation research: Conceptual distinctions, measurement challenges, and research agenda. *Administration and Policy in Mental Health and Mental Health Services Research, 38*(2), 65–76.

Schriger, S. H., Becker-Haimes, E. M., Skriner, L., & Beidas, R. S. (2020). Clinical supervision in community mental health: Characterizing supervision as usual and exploring predictors of supervision content and process. *Community Mental Health Journal, 57*(3), 552–566.

Shea, C. M., Jacobs, S. R., Esserman, D. A., Bruce, K., & Weiner, B. J. (2014). Organizational readiness for implementing change: A psychometric assessment of a new measure. *Implementation Science, 9*(1), 1–15.

Shelton, R. C., Chambers, D. A., & Glasgow, R. E. (2020). An extension of RE-AIM to enhance sustainability: Addressing dynamic context and promoting health equity over time. *Frontiers in Public Health, 8*, 134.

Shelton, R. C., Cooper, B. R., & Stirman, S. W. (2018). The sustainability of evidence-based interventions and practices in public health and health care. *Annual Review of Public Health, 39*(1), 55–76.

Stirman, S. W., Baumann, A. A., & Miller, C. J. (2019). The FRAME: An expanded framework for reporting adaptations and modifications to evidence-based interventions. *Implementation Science, 14*(1), 58.

Stirman, S. W., Bhar, S. S., Spokas, M., Brown, G. K., Creed, T. A., Perivoliotis, D., . . ., & Beck, A. T. (2010). Training and consultation in evidence-based psychosocial treatments in public mental health settings: The ACCESS model. *Professional Psychology: Research and Practice, 41*(1), 48–56.

Stirman, S. W., Kimberly, J., Cook, N., Calloway, A., Castro, F., & Charns, M. (2012). The sustainability of new programs and innovations: A review of the empirical literature and recommendations for future research. *Implementation science, 7*(1), 17.

Stirman, S. W., Pontoski, K., Creed, T., Xhezo, R., Evans, A. C., Beck, A. T., & Crits-Christoph, P. (2017). A non-randomized comparison of strategies for consultation in a community-academic training program to implement an evidence-based psychotherapy. *Administration and Policy in Mental Health and Mental Health Services Research, 44*(1), 55–66.

Tabak, R. G., Khoong, E. C., Chambers, D. A., & Brownson, R. C. (2012). Bridging research and practice: Models for dissemination and implementation research. *American Journal of Preventive Medicine, 43*(3), 337–350.

Valenstein-Mah, H., Greer, N., McKenzie, L., Hansen, L., Strom, T. Q., Wiltsey Stirman, S., . . ., & Kehle-Forbes, S. M. (2020). Effectiveness of training methods for delivery of evidence-based psychotherapies: A systematic review. *Implementation Science, 15*(1), 40.

Waltz, T. J., Powell, B. J., Matthieu, M. M., Damschroder, L. J., Chinman, M. J., Smith, J. L., . . ., & Kirchner, J. E. (2015). Use of concept mapping to characterize relationships among implementation strategies and assess their feasibility and importance: Results from the Expert Recommendations for Implementing Change (ERIC) study. *Implementation Science, 10*(1), 109.

Weiner, B. J., Belden, C. M., Bergmire, D. M., & Johnston, M. (2011). The meaning and measurement of implementation climate. *Implementation Science, 6*(1), 1–12.

Whitney, D. G., & Peterson, M. D. (2019). US national and state-level prevalence of mental health disorders and disparities of mental health care use in children. *JAMA Pediatrics, 173*(4), 389–391.

21

Service organizations: stepped care

Lauren F. McLellan, Carolyn Schniering, and Viviana Wuthrich

Learning objectives

- To appreciate the various models of stepped care, and the evidence for stepped care in the treatment of youth mental health conditions.
- To gain an awareness of the many considerations required for organizations in implementing stepped care.
- To consider the future of stepped care within organizations.

Introduction

Stepped care is an evidence-based, staged framework for the efficient delivery of clinical services, from the least to the most intensive, matched to the patient's needs. The central principle is that patients move from interventions that require the least therapist time and specialization to interventions that require greater therapist time and specialization, only if required. The early steps of treatment are designed to be less costly and given that a large proportion of patients do not require further steps involving high-intensity interventions, there are significant benefits in terms of waiting times, cost, and effectiveness. This method has been suggested to provide lower cost and greater effectiveness of services compared to treatment as usual, as well as greater flexibility and acceptability of evidence-based interventions across diverse settings in the community (Rapee et al., 2017). The concept of stepped care has been promoted as an essential component of mental healthcare reform (e.g. Australian Government Department of Health, 2016; National Institute for Health and Care Excellence [NICE], 2009), as a means to reduce healthcare costs without compromising on treatment effectiveness. This chapter will focus exclusively on stepped care within the provision of mental health treatment for young people. To date, stepped care interventions have typically occurred within the public health setting or in the context of research studies conducted in specialty clinics. In theory, however, stepped care could be implemented in a range of settings, including education and private settings. It is also possible that stepped care models could occur across settings where educational, public, and private services could be accessed in a stepwise fashion.

Stepped care models vary widely in the way in which steps are structured and what steps contain. There is currently no ideal or empirically validated model of stepped care. Models generally vary steps across the following key dimensions: (1) intensity of a single treatment (e.g. adding more sessions, or advanced techniques), (2) format of a single treatment (e.g. bibliotherapy, internet, or face-to-face), (3) degree of therapist input (e.g. self-help with no therapist input to standard therapy sessions), (4) training level of clinicians employed (e.g. trainee to specialist), and (5) type of treatment used (e.g. cognitive behavioural therapy (CBT) to medication). It is important that stepped care models offer a spectrum of integrated service interventions, rather than operating in individual silos, where there is a lack of communication or continuity across levels.

For example, in a recent stepped care trial for children diagnosed with anxiety conducted through our team's specialty research clinic, Step 1 comprised a therapist-assisted, low intensity (LI) CBT intervention (printed or CD-ROM materials and a maximum of four brief therapy sessions over the phone with a psychology trainee student); Step 2 consisted of the standard manualized Cool Kids group programme face-to-face (run by nationally registered psychologists); and Step 3 comprised up to 12 additional sessions of individually tailored CBT with psychologists holding postgraduate clinical psychology degrees and expertise in working with anxious youth (Rapee et al., 2017). This example demonstrates the way in which stepped care models allow individuals to access the most appropriate evidence-based services for their mental health need at any given time, as they move up or down to different levels of care.

What research exists for stepped care among children and adolescents?

The evidence on stepped care models in child mental health is very limited. Some initial case studies, open trials, and non-randomized trials for treating youth anxiety, depression, and behavioural disorders using a wide range of methodologies in a range of settings report promising results. Most of the research to date has been conducted in anxiety disorders in university clinics and uses various formats of CBT. Only one rigorous randomized controlled trial has been conducted evaluating stepped care, and that was in children and adolescents with a primary anxiety disorder.

Several non-randomized trials have examined the efficacy of stepped care interventions for child anxiety. In a study in the Netherlands, van der Leeden et al. (2011) explored changes in anxiety over time in 133 anxious children (aged 8–12 years) who received face-to-face CBT in university-associated medical clinics, as part of another study. Children were included in the study if they met diagnostic criteria for a primary separation anxiety, social anxiety, specific phobia, or generalized anxiety disorder according to the fourth edition of the *Diagnostic and Statistical Manual of Mental Disorders.* Children with secondary mood or behavioural diagnoses were not excluded. Of the 133 children, at the end of the first phase of CBT, 45% of the sample were free from all anxiety disorders, with the remaining 54% (n = 72) of non-responders offered (56 agreed) an additional five treatment sessions (Step 2), and another additional five sessions (Step 3) as required. They found that the additional sessions provided in Step 2 resulted in an additional 17% (23 of 38) free of all anxiety disorders, and after Step 3, a further 11% (14 of 24) were free from all anxiety disorders. Although participants were not randomized to condition, this study demonstrates the feasibility of stepped care, and that a portion of the sample are likely to benefit from fewer therapy sessions, with others requiring further interventions. Similar findings were found by Pettit et al. (2017) who in an open trial examined the treatment outcomes for 124 children (mean age 9.66 years) with an anxiety disorder who initially received a computer-administered attention bias modification intervention. While secondary anxiety, behavioural, and mood disorders were not exclusionary, participants were not eligible if a clinician severity rating of 7 or more was determined according to the Anxiety Disorders Interview Schedule (Silverman & Albano, 1996). In Step 1, participants completed two sessions of attention bias modification each week over 4 weeks. Each session lasted for a maximum of 15 minutes and included 160 trials of the ABM regime (angry and neutral faces presented for 500 ms with a probe (< or >) in place of the neutral face). Although the intervention was associated with reduced anxiety symptoms for the total sample, 40% of participants chose to move to Step 2 and received 12–14 weeks of face-to-face CBT, which resulted in statistically significant reductions in anxiety symptoms. Participants who discontinued treatment at Step 1 (ABM) had lower anxiety severity ratings on child and clinician reports (but not parent report) and lower levels of attention to threat compared to those who continued to Step 2 (CBT). A recent naturalistic 1-year follow-up study also found similar results (Jolstedt et al., 2021). In this study, 123 children (8–12 years) with an anxiety disorder completed 12-week internet CBT (ICBT) with limited therapist support. Therapist support included asynchronous messages, comments on programme worksheets, and phone support (as needed). On average, therapists spent 20 minutes a week providing support to each family. Participants were assessed at 3- and 12-month follow-up. At 3-month follow-up, 66% of the sample were remitted from their principal diagnosis, and 34% were classed as non-remitters and were offered an additional ten sessions of face-to-face CBT (of which 49% accepted) in Step 2. At the 12-month follow-up, 89% who had ICBT alone were free from their principal anxiety disorder, which was similar to the 83% who had remitted after ICBT plus face-to-face CBT. Finally, a recent case study reported on a new stepped care approach using ICBT (March, Donovan, Baldwin, Ford, & Spence, 2019) in which three non-responders to an initial therapy step (Step 1) consisting of unguided ICBT (five sessions), were stepped up to receive an additional five sessions of therapist-guided ICBT, and reported subsequent positive treatment outcomes. Together, these non-randomized studies in university settings suggest that stepped care models for anxious youth may be acceptable (i.e.

satisfied with the programme and outcomes) and are associated with positive outcomes. A sizable portion of participants reported clinically significant benefits after early steps of treatment, with additional benefits reported for those that receive subsequent therapy steps. This matches the findings from a review that found that, in general, LI interventions (e.g. technology-delivered interventions) are associated with clinically significant effects for anxious youth (Pennant et al., 2015).

Very few studies have examined stepped care models in youth with depression or with behavioural disorders. In a feasibility study, Mufson et al. (2018) randomly allocated 64 depressed adolescents in a primary care paediatric clinic to either a stepped collaborative treatment consisting of eight sessions of brief Interpersonal Psychotherapy for Adolescents (IPT-A) in Step 1 followed by either maintenance treatment (three sessions of IPT-A over 8 weeks) or an additional eight weekly sessions of IPT-A plus antidepressant medication (Step 2) or treatment as usual. Although this feasibility study was not powered to compare clinical effectiveness between interventions, both groups reported significant reductions in symptoms, and about 50% of participants did not require the addition of medication in Step 2. However, there were large study drop-outs with only 37% of the participants in the treatment-as-usual condition engaging in any treatment, compared to 86% in the stepped care intervention condition, and so results are difficult to ascertain. A current study is examining stepped care based on a unified protocol for transdiagnostic presentations in children with internalizing and/or externalizing disorders consisting of two steps of six sessions each delivered via telehealth (Kennedy, Lanier, Salloum, Ehrenreich-May, & Stoch, 2021). The authors report three preliminary case studies using this approach, with two cases not needing any additional support after the first therapy step, and one case progressing to Step 2. This study will be important for informing future directions of models of stepped care for comorbid presentations which are prevalent in real-world settings.

While promising, rigorous studies are needed to truly evaluate the clinical efficacy and cost-effectiveness of stepped care. To date, only two studies have rigorously examined stepped care models in youth. Salloum et al. (2016) randomly allocated 53 children (aged 3–7 years) experiencing post-traumatic stress symptoms to standard face-to-face CBT (12 × 90 minute) or a stepped care intervention. Step 1 consisted of parent-led treatment via a work-at-home manual supported by brief weekly calls, and three therapist sessions (3 × 60 minutes). Step 2 consisted of nine face-to-face CBT sessions with the therapist. The results indicated that both conditions resulted in similar improvements over time between groups; however, the stepped intervention was associated with significantly lower costs primarily due to the lower therapist time needed. In the most rigorous study to date, Rapee et al. (2017) randomly allocated 281 children (aged 7–17 years) with any primary anxiety disorder to individual, standardized, face-to-face ten-session CBT or stepped care. Stepped care consisted of three steps (described above) with participants choosing whether they wanted to receive subsequent steps. At 12-month follow-up, the clinical benefits of both interventions were similar, although stepped care was associated with significantly less therapist time. Similar to the findings from the uncontrolled studies, Step 1 was associated with 40% of the sample being satisfied with their improvements and declining further treatment; after Step 2, a total of 80% of the sample were satisfied with their improvements and declined further treatment. At 12-month follow up, remission from the primary disorder did not differ significantly between groups (stepped care remission = 67%, single treatment = 69%), although the stepped approach was associated with significantly less therapist time (2 hours). The full economic analysis (Chatterton et al., 2019) revealed that stepped care was associated with significantly less societal costs but not health costs. In summary, there is emerging evidence that stepped care is associated with significant and lasting improvements with lower intensity steps for some participants, but others require additional therapy in order to achieve the same outcomes. Ideally, models that could predict who will benefit from lower intensity interventions could provide further cost benefits to mental health delivery.

The key to stepped care success is the demonstration that stepped care is feasible, acceptable, and at least equivalent to standard care in terms of clinical and cost-effectiveness in real-world settings. Limited research has examined this issue. One study examined the use of stepped care for child anxiety in a case study conducted in a child and adolescent mental health service in the UK (Wuthrich & McLachlin, 2015). An adolescent girl (aged 15) with a generalized anxiety disorder-type presentation completed computerized CBT (10 weeks) supported by five brief phone calls from her therapist, followed by face-to-face CBT for ten sessions. The adolescent and therapist reported improvements in symptoms post computerized CBT, and additional improvements post face-to-face sessions, as well as positive feedback regarding the stepped approach. More recently, a similar stepped care approach for treating adolescent anxiety in community mental health settings ('headspace') in Australia has been evaluated in a small randomized controlled trial (Wuthrich et al., 2021). Fifty-three adolescents presenting with anxiety as their main problem at two headspace sites randomized to condition received either treatment as usual or a stepped care intervention consisting of ICBT with guided therapist calls (Step 1) followed by face-to-face CBT (Step 2) if needed. The findings indicated similar clinical benefits between conditions; however, feasibility was problematic as only 56% of adolescent allocated to stepped care engaged with the guided therapist calls despite utilizing the internet modules, and 46% of the sample did not complete follow-up assessments. This makes conclusions about the true effectiveness of the stepped care intervention difficult to determine, although this real-world trial does highlight the feasibility and acceptability issues related to using stepped care models in which adolescents are not seen face-to-face.

Overall, while promising, very limited information is available about the true clinical and cost benefits of stepped care approaches in youth. There is some limited evidence that stepped care models are at least as efficacious as standard care, and are likely to use less therapist time (Rapee et al., 2017; Salloum et al., 2016), but the evidence on whether they are more cost-effective as well is mixed

(Chatterton et al., 2019; Salloum et al. 2016). Overall, the results suggest that lower resource-intensive therapy steps are associated with treatment success for a reasonable number of youth, with rough estimates suggesting about 40–50% of youth experience clinically significant benefits from a range of lower cost interventions. Furthermore, there is emerging evidence that further therapy steps provide additional benefits for the remaining participants. However, very few studies have been conducted in real-world settings, and findings from those studies demonstrate clear challenges to applying stepped care models outside university research settings (Wuthrich et al, in press).

Challenges and potential solutions

The motivation for stepped care is to increase access to crucial mental health services—an important mission. Yet, there is still much that needs to be understood to ensure stepped care can be implemented successfully within organizations. The successful implementation of stepped care within an organization is likely to benefit from careful planning and training and the provision of substantial infrastructure and financial investment over an extended period of time.

Organizations considering stepped care should consider the following:

Increased scale

By its very design, stepped care intends to facilitate large numbers of youth accessing care. The flow-on effects of a dramatic increase in patient numbers needs to be carefully considered and managed.

The steps (and pathways—assessment, eligibility, triaging, monitoring)

Careful consideration is required when deciding on the number and nature of steps within a stepped care service. There is still limited evidence about what delivery method, format, and duration each step should include. NICE guidelines provide some recommendations for the treatment of depression (Richards et al., 2012), and as a result, clinical guidelines for related emotional disorders, including anxiety, have following suit, recommending stepped care.

Part and parcel with this consideration are the questions of how assessments will be conducted, who will be eligible for stepped care, which step an individual should be recommended to begin with, when/how an individual progresses through steps, how clients who fail to respond or who discontinue treatment will be detected and managed, and whether client preferences will be considered. Many of these considerations rely on the premise of regular (every session) monitoring of symptoms and/or functioning. There are many important considerations that relate to outcome monitoring of this nature—for example, how will an organization get accurate and regular data, how quickly will decisions need to be made based on this data, what/how much will clients agree to (and accurately) complete? Decisions about triaging clients into stepped care systems and managing their care across steps has the potential to quite dramatically change pathways to care. Even when huge investment is made to support the implementation of a prescribed stepped care system, as was the case in the UK Improving Access to Psychological Therapies system (albeit for adults), variability in how stepped care was implemented across sites (e.g. where clients start, how they are stepped along the system, and how quickly this occurs) led to dramatically different experiences for clients (Richards et al., 2012).

Support systems and processes

With large numbers of patients being managed by services delivering stepped care, there needs to be sufficient administrative capacity and systems to handle clients before, during, and as they potentially step between engagements with services. This includes considerations related to information technology systems, for example, security of patient information especially if LI steps involve electronic delivery methods, and updating and upgrading systems over time to function appropriately. Consideration needs to be paid to the appropriateness of the physical space available within an organization—can it accommodate telehealth and in-person consultations while maintaining confidentiality?

Clearly documented policies and processes need to be in place to increase efficiency and ensure appropriate governance and clinical care, especially in the case of risk or emergency situations. Such processes are particularly important for managing clinical interactions in LI steps, where patient and clinician may not be meeting in person, or may not even reside in close geographical proximity.

Practitioner qualifications

Typically, early steps are usually more structured using internet modules, workbooks, and so on. When clinician guidance is provided alongside these structured programmes they can potentially be delivered by a broader range of practitioners, as has been the case in some research evaluating stepped care models (e.g. Rapee et al., 2017). Training and supervision of these clinicians warrants careful consideration, as does the nature of the support that is to be provided.

Overall recommendations

When reflecting on the above considerations for implementing stepped care for youth mental health, we recommend that organizations prioritize the following when making decisions: (1) emerging evidence informs practice, (2) client perspectives and choice be valued and considered, (3) factors related to the local context be considered so that resulting services meet the potentially variable needs of the local communities they serve, and (4) organizations monitor and evaluate in real time so that we can better understand and evaluate many of the question that we are currently unable to answer based on scientific data. Beyond these key overarching recommendations, we encourage organizations to provide clear information and education to their clients about treatment recommendations so that they appreciate the credibility of the service they are receiving and their pathways of subsequent care. Chapter 20 describes how services may use implementation science to support with this decision-making process.

What is the future? How we see stepped care in service organizations into the future

While stepped care is a popular policy in many countries, there is still limited empirical evidence about the efficacy of stepped care, especially among youth, and even fewer evaluations of stepped care in real-world settings. With demand for mental health services only likely to increase, and greater flexibility in service delivery likely to be a necessity (e.g. as a result of the impact of COVID-19), stepped care models are likely to continue to offer an attractive solution for service organizations.

Preliminary data point to several key areas for future development in stepped care models for youth. Where stepped care approaches have been evaluated in real-world settings, there have been reports of patients who refuse to engage in the therapy as they held a strong preference for a particular mode of delivery (e.g. face-to-face versus internet) (see Wuthrich et al., 2021). These findings suggest that stepped care interventions may be more effective and acceptable to clients if individual preferences and client perspectives are taken into account.

In addition, if stepped care is to be successfully implemented in service organizations, we expect that workforce-readiness campaigns including targeted education for general practitioners, practice managers, allied healthcare providers, and others engaged in primary mental health service delivery will be required. Effective governance will be central to the success of stepped care models. A high level of specification will be required for the service elements under the model, and each element will need appropriate levels of clinical governance, including quality assessment and risk management. Therefore, more specific and highly funded policies will be required with the expectation for ongoing evaluation and redesign.

As pressures continue to lend themselves to stepped care service models, we expect (and hope) that research evaluating such models will exponentially increase. Such research must address the optimal number and composition of steps for the treatment of disorders in youth and evaluate better methods for individually tailoring stepped care approaches according to a client's unique profile (e.g. target disorders, comorbidity/severity, other risk factors/vulnerabilities, geographical location) and the service delivery setting (e.g. available workforce, funding, organization structure/policies, local needs).

Chapter summary

Stepped care has been widely embraced as an ideal model of service delivery; however, as a healthcare approach for children and adolescents with mental illness, the field is in its infancy and substantial further development and research is required. A growing body of evidence suggests that under controlled conditions in university settings, stepped models are as efficacious as standard care and are likely to use less therapist time; however, the clinical and cost-effectiveness of stepped care models in real-world settings has been minimally evaluated. There is currently no gold standard model of stepped care, and the ideal combination of steps will depend on the unique features of both the patient and the service delivery site. Service organization will be central to the effective delivery of LI interventions to youth in primary mental health settings. The successful implementation of stepped care models will require a healthcare framework that includes high-level policy specifications, effective governance of service elements including assessment and risk management, engagement of various stakeholders, implementation via a workforce-readiness campaign, and ongoing monitoring, evaluation, and modification. Finally, preliminary evidence on the cost-effectiveness of this approach for childhood emotional disorders has been mixed, and further economic evaluations across multiple settings are recommended (see Chapter 5 for further detail on health economic evaluations of stepped care).

Recommended reading

Rapee, R. M., Lyneham, H. J., Wuthrich, V. M., Chatterton, M.-L., Hudson, J. L., Kangas, M., & Mihalopoulos, C. (2017). Comparison of stepped care delivery against a single, empirically validated CBT program for anxious youth: A randomized clinical trial. *Journal of the American Academy of Child and Adolescent Psychiatry*, 56(10), 841–848.

Richards, D. A., Bower, P., Pagel, C., Weaver, A., Utley, M., Cape, J., . . ., & Vasilakis, C. (2012). Delivering stepped care: An analysis of implementation in routine practice, *Implementation Science, 7*, 3.

References

Australian Department of Health. (2016). PHN primary mental health care flexible funding pool implementation guidance: Stepped care. Retrieved from http:// www.health.gov.au

Chatterton, M.-L., Rapee, R. M., Catchpool, M., Lyneham, H. J., Wuthrich, V., Kangas, M., & Mihalopoulos, C. (2019). Economic evaluation of stepped care for the management of childhood anxiety disorders: Results from a randomised trial. *Australian and New Zealand Journal of Psychiatry*, 53(7), 673–682.

Jolstedt, M., Vigerland, S., Mataix-Cols, D., Ljótsson, B., Wahlund, T., Nord, M., . . ., & Serlachius, E. (2021). Long-term outcomes of internet-delivered cognitive behaviour therapy for paediatric anxiety disorders: Towards a stepped care model of health care delivery. *European Child & Adolescent Psychiatry*, 30(11), 1723–1732.

Kessler, R. C., Berglund, P., Demler, O., Jin, R., Merikangas, K. R., & Walters, E. E. (2005). Lifetime prevalence and age-of-onset distributions of DSM-IV disorders in the National Comorbidity Survey Replication. *Archives of General Psychiatry*, 62(6), 593–602.

Kennedy, S. M., Lanier, H., Salloum, A., Ehrenreich-May, J., & Stoch, E. A. (2021). Development and implementation of a transdiagnostic, stepped-care approach to treating emotional disorders in children via telehealth. *Cognitive and Behavioral Practice*, 28(3), 350–363.

March, S., Donovan, C. L., Baldwin, S., Ford, M., & Spence, S. H. (2019). Using stepped-care approaches within internet-based interventions for youth anxiety: Three case studies. *Internet Interventions*, 18, 100281.

Mufson, L., Rynn, M., Yanes-Lukin, P., Choo, T. H., Soren, K., Stewart, E., & Wall, M. (2018). Stepped care interpersonal psychotherapy treatment for depressed adolescents: A pilot study in pediatric clinics. *Administration and Policy in Mental Health*, 45(3), 417–431.

Pennant, M. E., Loucas, C. E., Whittington, C., Creswell, C., Fonagy, P., Fuggle, P., . . ., & Kendall, T. (2015). Computerised therapies for anxiety and depression in children and youth people: A systematic review and meta-analysis. *Behaviour Research and Therapy*, 67, 1–18.

Pettit, J. W., Reya, Y., Bechora, M., Melendeza, R., Vaclavika, D., Buitrona, V., . . ., & Silverman, W. K. (2017). Can less be more? Open trial of a stepped care approach for child and adolescent anxiety disorders. *Journal of Anxiety Disorders*, 51, 7–13.

Rapee, R. M., Lyneham, H. J., Wuthrich, V. M., Chatterton, M.-L., Hudson, J. L., Kangas, M., & Mihalopoulos, C. (2017). Comparison of stepped care delivery against a single, empirically validated CBT program for anxious youth: A randomized clinical trial. *Journal of the American Academy of Child and Adolescent Psychiatry*, 56(10), 841–848.

Richards, D. A., Bower, P., Pagel, C., Weaver, A., Utley, M., Cape, J., . . ., & Vasilakis, C. (2012). Delivering stepped care: An analysis of implementation in routine practice. *Implementation Science*, 7, 3.

Salloum, A., Wang, W., Robst, J., Murphy, T. K., Scheeringa, M. S., Cohen, J. A., & Storch, E. A. (2016). Stepped care versus standard trauma-focused cognitive behavioral therapy for young children. *Journal of Child Psychology and Psychiatry*, 57(5), 614–622.

Silverman, W. K., & Albano, A. M. (1996). *The anxiety disorders interview schedule for children and parents— DSM-IV version*. New York: Graywind.

van der Leeden, A. J. M., van Widenfelt, B. M., van der Leeden, R., Liber, J. M., Utens, E. M. W. J., & Treffers, P. D. A. (2011). Stepped care cognitive behavioural therapy for children with anxiety disorders: A new treatment approach, *Behavioural and Cognitive Psychotherapy*, 39(1), 55–75.

Wuthrich, V. M., & McLachlan, N. (2015). Application of the cool teens computerized CBT program with an anxious adolescent in a community mental health center. *Contemporary Behavioral Health Care*, 1, 28–32.

Wuthrich, V. M., Rapee, R. M., McLellan, L., Wignall, A., Jagiello, T., Belcher, J., & Norberg, M. (2021). Psychological stepped care for anxious adolescents in community mental health services: A pilot effectiveness trial. *Psychiatry Research*, 303, 114066.

Wuthrich, V.M., Rapee, R. M., McLellan, L., Wignall, A., Jagiello, T., Norberg, M., & Belcher, J. (in press). Psychological Acceptability and Feasibility of Stepped-care for Anxious Adolescents in Community Mental Health Services: A Secondary Analysis, *Child Psychiatry & Human Development*. Doi: 10.1007/s10578-021-01291-7

22

Overview of training and implementation considerations

Jonathan Parker and Catherine Gallop

Learning objectives

- To outline the context of mental health needs within children and young people.
- To describe the key workforce initiatives and roles working within early intervention and their scope of practice and service contexts.
- To provide an outline of the training models that underpin the new workforce.
- To consider key implementation principles and process supporting the development and sustainability of these early intervention roles.

Children and young people: mental health and political context

The context of need in children and young people (CYP)

There is strong substantiation that 50% of mental health problems are established by age 14 and 75% by age 24 (Kessler et al., 2005). Further research indicates that adolescent mental health problems can be linked to difficulties in later life Clayborne, Varin, & Colman, 2019). A 2015 meta-analysis of mental health difficulties affecting children and adolescents concluded the world-wide pooled prevalence was 13.4% (Polanczyk, Salum, Sugaya, Caye, & Rhde, 2015). A 2017 national survey conducted in England by the Department of Health and NHS England (NHS Digital, 2018), reported that one in eight (12.8%) of young people aged between 5 and 19 years had at least one mental health disorder when assessed. Of these, anxiety was reported in 7.2% of young people aged 5–19 and depression 2.1% (Table 22.1). Data from this, and the preceding survey series, reveal an increase over time in the prevalence of mental disorders in England for those aged 5–15 years, rising from 10.1% in 2004, to at least 11.2% in 2017 (NHS Digital, 2018). Most recently, a follow-up for the Mental Health Survey for Children and Young People (2020) indicated that results of probable mental health disorder at any given time have increased from one in nine (10.8%) to one in six (16%) in children aged 5–16 years.

Table 22.1 Emotional disorder prevalence (anxiety, depression and behavioural difficulties) for CYP in England

Mental disorders	All		
	Boys (%)	Girls (%)	All (%)
Any disorder	12.6	12.9	12.8
Any disorder (trends)	12.6	12.4	12.5
Emotional disorders	6.2	10.0	8.1
Emotional disorders (trends)	6.1	9.4	7.7
Anxiety disorders	5.4	9.1	7.2
Anxiety disorders (trends)	5.4	8.3	6.8
Separation anxiety disorder	0.7	0.6	0.7
Generalized anxiety disorder	1.3	1.8	1.5
Obsessive–compulsive disorder	0.5	0.4	0.4
Specific phobia	0.7	0.9	0.8
Social phobia	0.5	1.1	0.8
Agoraphobia	0.2	0.8	0.5
Panic disorder	0.5	1.7	1.1
Post-traumatic stress disorder	0.3	0.9	0.6
Body dysmorphic disorder	0.3	1.8	1.0
Other anxiety disorder	1.3	1.9	1.6
Depressive disorders	1.4	2.8	2.1
Major depressive episode	1.0	2.0	1.5
Other depressive episode	0.4	0.8	0.6
Bipolar affective disorder	0.0	0.1	0.0
Behavioural disorders	5.8	3.4	4.6
Oppositional defiant disorder	3.6	2.2	2.9
Conduct disorder confined to family	0.1	0.1	0.1
Unsocialized conduct disorder	0.4	0.3	0.4
Socialized conduct disorder	1.0	0.4	0.7
Other conduct disorder	0.7	0.3	0.5

Data from NHS Digital (2018).

Policy context: key workforce initiatives and roles

In an effort to address unmet need and modernize existing provision, the CYP Improving Access to Psychological Therapies (IAPT) programme in England was guided by a set of key principles (NHS England, 2016) that targeted the sustainable transformation of child and adolescent mental health services (CAMHS) across England (Fonagy & Clark, 2015). At its core was the requirement to train existing clinical staff within CAMHS in evidenced-based practice approaches (NHS England, 2017). More recently, with the CYP-IAPT initiative approaching 100% national coverage, it formally disbanded and transitioned into an expected standard of delivery from 2019. However, national policy guidance in England has continued to emphasize the need for the expansion of the CYP mental health workforce in an effort to improve access rates for CYP experiencing the most common mental health difficulties (NHS England, 2016). Furthermore, World Health Organization (2019) guidance recommends comprehensive, integrated, and responsive mental health services in community-based settings for early recognition and evidence-based management of childhood mental health difficulties. It was acknowledged that within the existing core training portfolio, there had been insufficient provision for brief, evidence-based early intervention for CYP and families (Health Education England, 2017). This has facilitated the funding of supplementary training pathways for new, specialist mental health workers in addition to the upskilling of existing staff, with the need for low intensity (LI) cost-effective interventions from highly trained staff a key consideration (Fonagy, et al., 2016). As a result, two LI workforce roles working with CYP have been developed in England, which may serve as models for workforce development initiatives in other countries.

Children's well-being practitioner (CWP)

The CWP is a CYP mental health workforce development initiative (Health Education England, 2017). Recognizing the achievements of the adult IAPT LI psychological well-being practitioner programme (Clark, 2011) and the shortage of accessible, evidence-based early intervention within existing services (NHS England, 2015), the CWP programme was commissioned in 2017 and aims to support the delivery of an additional level of evidence-based provision at a stage of early intervention.

The CWP programme provides a pathway into a career within CYP mental health for a cohort of potential applicants otherwise restricted by entry requirements for more established roles and training routes. As a result, it was anticipated a platform would be provided to support workforce expansion and positively impact both the availability of support and the related local access target requirements (NHS England, 2017). The CWP role provides an additional resource to support and intervene with CYP and families experiencing the most common low-level mental health difficulties, specifically targeting the needs of those who do not currently receive a service. These posts are not commissioned as a new, stand-alone service, but are integrated into an existing locality-based provision and intended to provide brief, evidence-based interventions at an early stage of need to improve outcomes and reduce the requirement for future, more costly specialist interventions.

Education mental health practitioner (EMHP)

The EMHP role stems from the UK government's *Transforming Children and Young People's Mental Health: A Green Paper* (Department of Health and Social Care & Department for Education, 2017). 'Green Papers' are documents produced by the UK government setting out proposals that invite feedback from members of parliament and consultation from the public before being finalized as legislation or policy. Building on the 2015 NHS publication, *Future in Mind* (NHS England, 2015), and the ongoing expansion of NHS-funded CYP mental health provision, the Green Paper set out an ambition to ensure that CYP showing early signs of distress are able to access the right help, in the right settings, at their time of need. The paper was informed by existing best practice in the education sector and a systemic review of evidence on the best ways to promote positive mental health within education settings. It aims to support early intervention, to prevent problems escalating, and to ensure all CYP have access to high-quality mental health and well-being support linked to their school or college. The paper outlined three core components of the approach: designated senior leads for mental health within education settings to oversee the approach to mental health and well-being, the trialling of a 4-week waiting time for access to specialist NHS CYP mental health services, and the funding of new mental health support teams (MHSTs) to provide extra capacity for early intervention. The EMHP role signified a further workforce expansion initiative and represents a core component of the MHST service. In the first year of deployment, the EMHP undertakes a 12-month graduate or postgraduate diploma training programme that builds on the foundational LI curriculum of the CWP before undertaking additional specialist training in whole-school approaches to well-being and education-specific support, liaison, and consultation. These additional education-facing modules are reflected in the EMHP training having a diploma level status in contrast to the certificate level of the CWP programme.

Scope of practice and service context

The CWP role in practice

CWPs provide additional resources to support and intervene with CYP offering targeted support with CYP experiencing low-level/mild to moderate anxiety, low mood, and behavioural difficulties. The role is not intended to support those services that are working with serious and enduring mental health problems or to work with those with high levels of risk to themselves or others, or who need a more specialist level of care. It is important that all work is suitably supervised and managed (see Chapter 7 on assessment and Chapter 19 on supervision).

The CWP delivers interventions face-to-face, by phone, and online. One-to-one support usually includes between four and eight sessions but this may vary according to need; the flexibility to adapt intervention timescales is a key aspect of the CWP role. This reflects the lower level of complexity anticipated and the brief, focused, but flexible nature of intervention. The primary objectives of the role are therefore to facilitate access to support from community services, offer evidence-based help to CYP with mild to moderate difficulties, and reduce waiting lists to specialist CAMHS.

CWP interventions are based on evidence-based approaches either through supported self-help or clinically evidenced materials used directly to support face-to-face sessions as well as health technologies such as online programmes or smartphone applications (Donker et al., 2013). To improve the effectiveness of LI interventions, CWPs receive guidance in the use of self-help materials and undertake training focused on the competencies required to support LI interventions (Roth & Pilling, 2015). This guidance is focused on supporting CYP and parents/carers to effectively engage with the intervention process, including helping them to problem-solve any difficulties faced and provide motivation and encouragement to work through the materials.

National guidance is clear; regardless of the employing agency, CWPs can be deployed from any relevant organization working with CYP. It is recognized that different areas have differing service requirements and environments, resulting in day-to-day CWP operational flexibility across localities. Within their organization and locality, consideration should be given as to where the CWP will best receive the required level of service integration and role advocacy. These are important considerations in order to help avoid role dilution and/or the role substituting for existing services; it is important for the CWP role to be a specific and independently recognized provision. CYP services are encouraged to actively consider the deployment of the CWPs into universal community services, youth settings, and general practitioner practices. It has been recognized that within these settings, low-level mental health difficulties are most likely to be first identified and that those with early indications of mental health difficulties may not seek to access support within more traditional, clinic-based settings.

The flexibility to implement the CWP role according to local context is an important component of the programme and shared learning and good practice examples between areas continue to support role development. However, it is critical for the CWP role to maintain the remit of working with referrals at a stage of early intervention. The challenge of this is acknowledged with the demand for support from more complex presentations well reported across the sector. However, both the efficacy of the CWP role and the feasibility of managing a high caseload likely rely on working with an appropriate cohort of referrals.

The challenges associated with being part of a new project—a new role in what is often a well-established system and culture—can be difficult and can require additional resilience from trainee practitioners as the role develops and establishes itself. Being part of a service development initiative inevitably requires managing anxieties and possible opposition arising from the change process. Supporting the needs of the new CWP role within this context has been important, with role awareness and advocacy from colleagues and across senior leadership structures essential. As part of this process, consistent and supportive supervision is central to the safe and effective practice of CWPs—nurturing their theory-to-practice development and ensuring appropriate delivery flexibility within clinical fidelity across both the training year and post qualification.

The EMHP role in practice

In alliance with NHS England, the Department for Education, and Health Education England, the EMHP roles are overseen by local MHSTs who in collaboration with local education providers and key stakeholders ascertain where these posts can be implemented and will operate most effectively. Launched in 2019, the MHSTs are designed to help meet the mental health needs of CYP in education settings. They are made up of senior clinicians and specialist CAMHS practitioners in additions to EMHPs. Each MHST works within and across the existing local mental health support systems already and work to ensure that the offer reflects the needs of the CYP and the education settings they support. The new EHMPs form part of these MHSTs, alongside other mental health practitioners and specialist supervisors.

The primary objectives of the EMHP role are to provide targeted mental health support within educational settings. They offer evidence-based help to CYP and families with mild to moderate mental health difficulties. In conjunction with the wider MHST, EMHPs support the delivery of a whole-school approach to well-being in response to the local context and current provision. As well as supporting a whole-school approach to mental health, EMHPs work directly with CYP with mild to moderate common mental health difficulties, specifically anxiety, low mood, and behavioural difficulties. EMHPs should not work with those with high levels of risk to themselves or others, or who need a more specialist level of care, and it is important that all work is suitably supervised and managed. The initiative aims to deliver improved outcomes, reduce access waiting times, and decrease the need for future, more costly specialist interventions. The support and interventions offered by EMHPs in schools and colleges acknowledge the broad range of difficulties felt by many CYP, including adverse experiences and common problems experienced within an education setting. EHMPs are trained to work within a model of CYP that recognizes both the effects of adversity on children and the limits of their autonomy. They promote the well-being of CYP by supporting their cognitive, emotional, social, and physical development in the context of their family, school, and other systems.

Core outline of training models

The CWP in training

The CWP undertakes a 12-month graduate or postgraduate certificate training programme. Access onto the CWP training is gained through a successful application and interview process within a participating young people's mental health service, who are the employer throughout the duration of the 12-month training programme. Interest in these roles is often high and therefore competitive, with a good level of previous CYP mental health experience and/or related qualifications often necessary to reach the interview stage. This curriculum is designed to enable mental health professionals to gain skills and knowledge in delivering brief, CBT-informed LI interventions. The CWP trainee undertakes three core modules, beginning with a foundational understanding of undertaking the role of a professional practitioner within the context of CYP mental health services. Within these initial stages of the programme, the CWP develops the knowledge and understanding relating to legal and professional issues, local and national services context and principles, multi-agency working, as well as an overview of CYP MH therapies and the evidence base. Building from this core contextual understanding, the trainee CWP begins to establish the skills to assess CYP and families presenting with a range of mental health difficulties. The CWP is trained to undertake a CYP-centred assessment in support of identifying the presenting difficulties, strengths, goals, and available resources as well as identifying any risk to self or others (see Chapter 7). They are required to understand the child in their context and consider developmental, physical, and other psychological factors. Effective engagement and the development of a therapeutic alliance are core aspects of the training with the requirement to gather information from a range of appropriate sources. From this foundation, the CWP is able to collaboratively engage with the young person/family so as to develop a shared understanding of the difficulty and the options of what evidence-based interventions are likely to be appropriate. The final module supports the trainee CWP with the development of the knowledge and skills across a range of LI interventions for mild to moderate anxiety, low mood, and behavioural difficulties (see Chapters 10–12). Often with the use of written self-help materials and manualized workbooks they are informed by cognitive behavioural and social learning principles and include behavioural activation, graded exposure, cognitive restructuring, problem-solving,

CBT-informed sleep management, and parent training as well as supporting phys-ical activity. Support is specifically designed to enable CYP and parents/carers to optimize the use of self-management techniques. Interventions can be delivered through face-to-face work, telephone, email, or video call individually to CYP, through group workshops, or in collaboration with parents/carers.

A CWP undertakes a range of assessments during their training including the submission of clinical practice assessments and intervention recordings. They are required to evidence a range of competencies and undertake 80 hours of clinical practice including eight completed LI intervention cases across a spread of difficulties to include working with anxiety, low mood, behavioural difficulties, and direct work with parents/carers. Across the 12-month training programme, the CWP must also undertake a minimum total of 40 hours of clin-ical supervision: 20 hours of case management, and 20 hours of clinical skills supervision.

The EMHP in training

The EMHP role is accessed by application directly to the local MHST service, with recruitment usually taking place on an annual basis. EMHP trainees under-take a 12-month graduate or postgraduate diploma programme designed to de-velop the clinical competencies and knowledge of trainees in order to proficiently practise as an EMHP, as determined by the relevant national curriculum for the programme. Specifically, these include developing skills in assessment and LI evidence-based interventions alongside the core competencies required to work with CYP presenting with anxiety, low mood, and behavioural difficulties. The EMHP will also learn the key skills in auditing and consultation within an edu-cational setting to help promote whole-school well-being and participation. The programme also focuses on an understanding of ways to adapt clinical practice with CYP and parents/carers to accommodate diversity and increase access to evidence-based psychological therapies. A strong emphasis throughout the pro-gramme is placed upon the personal and professional development of the EMHP. While on the training course, similar to CWPs, EMHPs need to achieve 80 hours of clinical work in education settings, and a minimum of 40 hours of supervision (20 hours of clinical skills and 20 hours of case management). In conjunction with the wider MHST, EMHPs contribute to the understanding and development of whole-school approaches (Weare, 2015) during their training. As part of the process, the EMHP will propose and then conduct an educational audit within a school or college setting. This audit is a collaborative process and enables an understanding of existing educational well-being support as well as areas of im-provement. The specific audit tool/framework is agreed locally under guidance from the course taught material.

Implementation and support considerations

Underpinning principles

Careful consideration should be given to the delivery model for these roles. The *Future in Mind* (NHS England, 2015) report says that:

> Services need to be outcomes focused, simple and easy to access, based on best evidence, and built around the needs of children, young people and their families rather than defined in terms of organisational boundaries.

Collaboratively facilitated regional steering groups are a helpful platform to review implementation progress and work towards core principles and support clarity on the model adopted, shaping subsequent decisions on how and where these posts are best implemented and accessed. The model adopted should reflect the ethos and established principles of CYP mental health delivery, with an emphasis on:

- Improved access with a focus on young people and their families being able to approach services and support directly (i.e. self-referral).
- Greater collaboration with an emphasis on shared decision-making.
- Outcomes-informed practice and working in such a way as to define the goal or endpoint of all work with CYP and their families.
- Transformation: the role should provide something different but complementary to the way in which existing mental health provision is currently provided and—in the case of the EMHP—facilitating an expansion of provision for CYP within educational settings.
- The central role of the CYP and parent/carer and educational staff in the participation of design, delivery, and development of the programme across localities.

Access, referral, and assessment

With the increase in availability of mental health support, a core objective of the CYP mental health programme in England, the CWP and EMHP roles are designed to significantly contribute to this policy priority. Locally, mental health services are expected to agree to work towards appropriate and accessible referral routes for the EMHP and CWP roles. Service providers work in collaboration with a range of stakeholders, including young people and families, to ensure participation is at the centre of the service design and delivery structures. In line with *Future in Mind* guidance (NHS England, 2015), an emphasis on ease of access is critical; particular attention is given to the availability of support in areas and through mediums that encourage inclusivity and diversity of access while prioritizing the early intervention remit of the roles. It is important to effectively integrate the roles into the local health and educational infrastructure with local professionals being clear where and how the new roles can assist and operate. A collaborative forum can enable full consideration, learning, and development of any additional concerns regarding risk and safeguarding management.

Referral criteria for one-to-one LI practice

Given both roles are designed to support CYP with common low-level mental health difficulties, with an emphasis on early intervention, they do not take on work which should be addressed in specialist CAMHS services. This means the agreed referral criteria should be different from existing CAMHS referral criteria. Table 22.2 represents a guide to the specific difficulties the role could be expected to address via one-to-one LI interventions in line with the training curricula. It also summarizes those presenting difficulties that are beyond their scope of practice, and those situations where discretion is required and a case-by-case decision made through the use of appropriate supervision.

Table 22.2 Guide to presenting difficulties

Common mental health difficulties that may respond to early intervention	Conditions which may respond to early intervention but require discretion	Significant levels of need/ complex conditions which are not suitable for brief early intervention
Low mood/mild to moderately severe depression	Anger difficulties	Pain management
Panic disorder	Low self-esteem	Post-traumatic stress disorder
Panic disorder and agoraphobia	Mild social anxiety disorder	Bipolar disorder
Generalized anxiety disorder/ worry	Some compulsive behaviours	Psychosis
Simple phobia (but not blood, needle, vomit)	Mild health anxiety	Personality disorders
Sleep problems	Assertiveness/interpersonal challenges (e.g. with peers)	Eating disorders
Stress management	Self-harm is disclosed but is assessed as linked to low mood but *is not assessed as enduring and high risk* in nature	Chronic depression/anxiety
Behavioural difficulties	Obsessive–compulsive disorder	Established health anxiety
		Historical or current experiences of abuse or violence
		Complex interpersonal challenges
		Bereavement
		Active, enduring, and significant self-harm
		Relationship problems

Signposting and liaison work

Advising young people and families where they can access the right sort of early support is an important element of the CWP and EMHP roles. It is therefore very important that they have current information on the range of services available locally. In addition, the postholder needs to ensure that local services and teams develop a good understanding of the new roles and how they fit into the network of mental health support and services available to CYP and their families. Should needs escalate during the work provided by EMHPs and CWPs, or more complex needs emerge, it is appropriate to facilitate access to a more appropriate worker within the CYP mental health service or MHST. This may include social care provision or specialist mental health services and such cases should be discussed as a priority within supervision and in line with the local agreements, policies, procedures, and care pathways.

Case management and responding to need

When qualified, EMHPs and CWPs work with a high volume of CYP. This reflects the expected relatively low level of need that will be addressed and the brief nature of the work that is intended. During their training year, they are expected to increase from a caseload of around four to eight CYP at the beginning of the training to a caseload of 25–30 when they are fully operational. This involves working with up to 25 client contacts per week over 40 weeks (1000 contacts per year); undertaking six sessions per case (between four and eight sessions are anticipated); and one-to-one session length lasting up to 1 hour for assessments but between 15 and45 minutes for intervention sessions (allowing for flexibility if needed for developmental and contextual adaptations). It is, however, recognized that different areas and educational settings have different needs and operating environments, meaning the way the posts are deployed varies. Each CYP mental health service or MHST therefore needs to establish its own caseload requirements in line with the stated expectations. Where one-to-one intervention is required, CYP and their families should be seen/contacted on a weekly or fortnightly basis depending on the level of assessed need. Interventions are expected to be completed within 4–6 weeks. Flexibility of intervention and contact is a critical aspect of the roles with case load supervision guiding this process (see Chapters 9 and 19).

Supervision

Specialist CWP and EMHP supervisor roles are in place to provide safe and effective practice during both the training year and once qualified (see Chapter 19 for further detail). Supervisors are mental health professionals with a substantive depth of experience in working within CYP mental health settings and the relevant clinical knowledge and qualifications, such as CBT-informed practice. Based within the same organization as the practitioners, EMHP and CWP supervisors are selected and/or recruited in collaboration between the training provider and the service and are required to undertake a postgraduate certificate in clinical supervision.

LI supervision involves weekly caseload management supervision in which the supervisee's complete caseload is reviewed and managed, with individual cases being prioritized as necessary. In caseload management supervision, the focus is on discussing risk, changes in presentation, clinical outcomes, and appropriate care planning (discharge, continued work on clear goals, step up or down to alternative intervention). Alongside this, fortnightly clinical skills supervision, which is usually delivered within a group format, supports further practice proficiencies and clinical competence. The focus of clinical skills supervision is on clinical skills delivery and treatment fidelity. Clinical skills supervisors are responsible for assessing supervisees' clinical competences in accordance with the course curriculum outcomes and role descriptors. EMHPs and CWPs engage in clinical skills preparation and practice with their supervisor through, for example, use of role plays and review of their practice utilizing video recordings.

Routine outcome monitoring

The interventions and support CWPs and EMHPs provide should be outcome focused and they need to be able to demonstrate that the course of support and interventions are decided through collaboratively agreed goals. Session-by-session routine outcome monitoring is therefore a core aspect of both EMHP and CWP practice with the effective administration and monitoring of these outcome tools central to effective delivery. Table 22.3 outlines current recommended practice in relation to one-to-one assessment, outcome, and feedback measurement tools. Alongside this, and in line with local service procedures and agreements, for each CYP that engages with an EMHP or CWP, it will likely be required that key demographic and care pathway information will be collected.

An ongoing priority for the CWP and EMHP programmes is to progress understanding for the capacity of these new roles to deliver effective support to CYP and families. If this is not achieved, the programme is at risk of refutation from existing staff, managers, and commissioners, and consequently would be at risk of achieving little towards the improvement of outcomes for CYP and families. In addition, the rising prevalence of mental health difficulties and subsequent growth of national investment generate access target requirements and the requisite to effectively monitor and understand the impact of workforce development programmes and service delivery initiatives. Evaluating the impact of the new roles will be a central component of its success, spread, and sustainability. In order to help support this element of the

Table 22.3 Outcome and feedback tools

Presenting problem	Assessment	Treatment sessions	Final session
Depression	Current view		
	RCADS (full) self-reported, 8+	RCADS (depression subscale) self-reported, 8+	RCADS (full) self-reported, 8+
	RCADS (full) parent reported, under 8 (This may also be collected if feasible/desirable for young people 8+)	RCADS (depression subscale) parent reported, under 8	RCADS (full) parent reported, under 8
	ORS (13+)	ORS (13+)	ORS (13+)
	CORS (6–12)	CORS (6–12)	CORS (6–12)
	Goal-based outcomes (to be set in assessment)	Goal-based outcomes	Goal-based outcomes
	SFQ	SFQ	SFQ
Anxiety	Current view		
	RCADS (full) self-reported, 8+	RCADS (anxiety disorder-specific subscale) self-reported, 8+	RCADS (full) self-reported, 8+
	RCADS (full) parent reported, under 8 (This may also be collected if feasible/desirable for young people 8+)	RCADS (anxiety disorder-specific subscale) parent reported, under 8	RCADS (full) parent reported, under 8
	ORS (13+)	ORS (13+)	ORS (13+)
	CORS (6–12)	CORS (6–12)	CORS (6–12)
	Goal-based outcomes (to be set in assessment)	Goal-based outcomes	Goal-based outcomes
	SFQ	SFQ	SFQ
Parenting/ behaviour	Current view		
	SDQ-Parental	SDQ-Parental	SDQ-Parental
	SDQ-Child (if possible) (11–17)	SDQ-Child (if possible) (11–17)	SDQ-Child (if possible) (11–17)
	ODDp	ODDp	ODDp
	BP-SES	BP-SES	BP-SES
	SFQ	SFQ	SFQ

BP-SES, Brief Parent Self Efficacy Scale; CORS, Child Outcome Rating Scale; ODDp, Oppositional defiant disorder, parent reported; ORD, Outcome Rating Scale; RCADS, Revised Child Anxiety and Depression Scale; SFQ, Session Feedback Questionnaire.

programme, it is the expectation that all CYP mental health and MHST services capture outcome data as part of standard practice and then securely transfer the collated service data to the NHS mental health services data set. NHS England provides further guidance and examples in relation to specific requirements and best practice in regard to data flow.

Chapter summary

Given the growing prevalence of mental health problems in CYP, the government in England has responded by expanding the CYP's mental health workforce, with a particular focus on offering support at a stage of early intervention. New roles have been developed with associated specialist training to support the delivery of LI, evidenced-based interventions for emerging mental health difficulties in CYP and families. These new roles have aimed to improve access to early intervention mental health support, through the effective implementation and integration into community-based and education-facing settings. Key principles and processes (e.g. referral criteria and pathways, supervision, the use of routine outcomes measures) have been key to their successful implementation and will be an important consideration for sustainability and continued effectiveness of these roles.

Recommended reading

Burton, M., Pavard, E., & Williams, B. (2014). *An introduction to child and adolescent mental health*. London: Sage.

Cooper, M., Hooper, C., & Thompson, M. (2005). *Child and adolescent mental health: Theory and practice*. London: Hodder Arnold.

Department of Health and Social Care, & Department for Education. (2017). *Transforming children and young people's mental health provision: A green paper*. Retrieved from https://assets.publishing.service.gov.uk/government/uploads/system/uploads/attachment_data/file/664855/Transforming_children_and_young_people_s_mental_health_provision.pdf

Public Health England. (2015). *Promoting children and young people's emotional health and wellbeing: A whole school and college approach*. Retrieved from https://assets.publishing.service.gov.uk/government/uploads/system/uploads/attachment_data/file/1020249/Promoting_children_and_young_people_s_mental_health_and_wellbeing.pdf

Roth, A., & Fonagy, P. (2006). *What works for whom? A critical review of psychotherapy research* (2nd ed.). London: Guildford Press.

References

Clark, D. M. (2011). Realizing the mass public benefit of evidence-based psychological therapies: The IAPT program. *Annual Review of Clinical Psychology, 23*(4), 159–183.

Clayborne, Z. M., Varin, M., & Colman, I. (2019). Systematic review and meta-analysis: Adolescent depression and long-term psychosocial outcomes. *Journal of the American Academy of Child and Adolescent Psychiatry, 58*(1), 72–79.

Department for Health and Social Care, & Department for Education. (2017). Transforming children and young people's mental health provision: A green paper. Retrieved from https://assets.publishing.service.gov.uk/government/uploads/system/uploads/attachment_data/file/664855/Transforming_children_and_young_people_s_mental_health_provision.pdf

Donker, T., Petrie, K., Proudfoot, J., Clarke, J., Birch, M. R., & Christensen, H. (2013). Smartphones for smarter delivery of mental health programs: A systematic review. *Journal of Medical Internet Research*, *15*(11), e247.

Fonagy, P., & Clark, D. (2015). Update on the Improving Access to Psychological Therapies programme in England: Commentary on children and young people's improving access to psychological therapies. *British Journal of Psychiatry*, *39*(5), 248–251.

Fonagy, P., Cottrell, D., Phillips, J., Bevington, D., Glaser, D., & Allison, E. (2016). *What works for whom: A critical review of treatments for children and adolescents*. London: Guilford Press.

Health Education England. (2017). *Headline plan and process for the establishment of the CYP PWP role*. London: Health Education England.

Kessler, R. C., Berglund, P., Demler, O., Jin, R., Merikangas, K. R., & Walters, E. E. (2005). Lifetime prevalence and age-of-onset distributions of DSM-IV disorders in the National Comorbidity Survey Replication. *Archives of general psychiatry*, *62*(6), 593–602. https://doi.org/10.1001/archpsyc.62.6.593

Mental Health of Children and Young People in England, 2020: Wave 1 follow up to the 2017 survey. Retrieved from NHS Digital: https://digital.nhs.uk/data-and-information/publications/statistical/mental-health-of-children-and-young-people-in-england/2020-wave-1-follow-up#

NHS Digital. (2018). Mental health of children and young people in England. Retrieved from https://files.digital.nhs.uk/A6/EA7D58/MHCYP%202017%20Summary.pdf

NHS Digital. (2020). Mental health services data set. Retrieved from https://digital.nhs.uk/data-and-information/data-collections-and-data-sets/data-sets/mental-health-services-data-set

NHS England. (2015). *Future in mind*. London: Department of Health. Retrieved from https://assets.publishing.service.gov.uk/government/uploads/system/uploads/attachment_data/file/414024/Childrens_Mental_Health.pdf

NHS England. (2016). Children and young people's Improving Access to Psychological Therapies programme. Retrieved from https://www.england.nhs.uk/mental-health/cyp/iapt/

NHS England. (2017). CYP-IAPT. Children and young people's Improving Access to Psychological Therapies programme. Retrieved from https://www.england.nhs.uk/mental-health/cyp/iapt/

Polanczyk, G. V., Salum, G. A., Sugaya, L. S., Caye, A., & Rhde, L. A. (2015). Annual research review: A meta-analysis of the worldwide prevalence of mental disorders in children and adolescents. *Journal of Child Psychology and Psychiatry*, *56*(3), 345–365.

Roth, A. D., & Pilling, S. (2015). *A competence framework for the supervision of psychological therapies*. London: UCL.

Weare, K. (2015). What works in promoting social and emotional well-being and responding to mental health problems in schools? Retrieved from https://www.walworth.durham.sch.uk/wp-content/uploads/sites/59/2017/09/Promoting-Social-Emotional-Well-being-etc-NCB.pdf

World Health Organization. (2019). Child and adolescent mental health. Retrieved from https://www.who.int/news-room/fact-sheets/detail/mental-disorders

SECTION 4

BRIEF AND LOW INTENSITY INTERVENTIONS FOR THE TWENTY-FIRST CENTURY

23

Single-session interventions for children and adolescents

Isaac Ahuvia and Jessica L. Schleider

Learning objectives

- To overview the definition and utility of single-session interventions (SSIs) for mental health problems in children and young people.
- To identify the types of SSIs available for use with this population, along with the evidence base supporting their efficacy and effectiveness.
- To understand potential mechanisms of change in evidence-based SSIs.
- To learn strategies for administering a well-tested, web-based SSI for youth internalizing distress (e.g. anxiety, depressive symptoms).

Introduction

Single-session interventions (SSIs) are defined as 'specific, structured programs that intentionally involve just one visit or encounter with a clinic, provider, or program' (Schleider, Dobias, Sung, & Mullarkey, 2020). Like low intensity interventions generally, the need for SSIs is driven by the lack of access to and underutilization of traditional forms of mental health support. Nearly 80% of youth in need of mental health services do not successfully access care (Kataoka, Zhang, & Wells, 2002). Even those who do access care often do not engage with it for the intended duration of treatment. Ironically, even among longer interventions for youth, the modal number of sessions attended is only one (Hoyt, Bobele, Slive, Young, & Talmon, 2018).

There are many structural barriers that contribute to the underutilization of mental healthcare services, including logistical barriers for families and high treatment costs, which are particularly burdensome for those who lack health insurance in countries such as the US (Reardon et al., 2017; Rowan, McAlpine, & Blewett, 2013; Walker, Cummings, Hockenberry, & Druss, 2015). SSIs offer promise to fill this 'treatment gap' with more accessible, and often more affordable, interventions. SSIs may also make it easier to reach 'hard-to-reach' populations who face additional barriers to care (Sung, Dobias, & Schleider, 2020). In short, SSIs create a new treatment access pathway for youth experiencing mental illness, carrying particular benefits for those who might otherwise go without support entirely.

The apparent potential of SSIs has led to the development of many new interventions in recent years, many of which have been rigorously evaluated. A systematic review of SSIs for youth found a significant benefit of SSIs relative to comparison conditions, with an overall small to medium effect size post intervention (Hedge's g effect size of g = 0.32; Schleider & Weisz, 2017). The meta-analysis found the largest effects on anxiety (g = 0.59) and smallest on substance abuse (g = 0.08). In the 5 years since that first review was conducted, already many more SSIs have been evaluated (Schleider, Dobias, et al., 2020). Although the contents of evidence-based SSIs for youth mental illness vary in many ways, we find it useful to divide these interventions into two categories: guided and unguided.

Guided SSIs

Guided SSIs are those that require facilitation from a trained practitioner. As such, guided SSIs are generally face-to-face. However, they can also be administered remotely (e.g. over video chat or email). Guided SSIs take many forms, and there is no consensus on what makes one effective. We therefore aim to give a sense of the emerging evidence base by highlighting specific interventions that have been evaluated.

One intervention used a modified version of behavioural activation treatment for depression (Gawrysiak, Nicholas, & Hopko, 2009), condensing traditional behavioural activation methods into a single session. Whereas traditional behavioural activation encourages participants to engage in an increasing number of activities over time (designed to elicit a sense of pleasure as a way to combat depressive symptoms), this intervention targeted a much greater number of activities all at once. When administered in a sample of high-symptom older adolescents (mean age = 18.4 years), it showed strong effects on depression symptoms versus a waiting-list control. Another evaluation studied a brief suicide prevention intervention administered in high schools to students deemed at suicide risk (Randell, Eggert, & Pike, 2001). The intervention utilized a 1.5–2-hour assessment interview followed by a brief motivational counselling session and a social network intervention in which participants were personally connected to a case manager or teacher in the school (to foster communication between the youth and school personnel) and via phone to the parent/guardian of their choice (to further enhance support networks and the future accessibility of help). The intervention yielded significant decreases in depressive symptoms compared to baseline—though only slightly superior to 'treatment as usual' (here, a minimally intensive safety assessment followed by the notification of parents and a school counsellor).

Effective guided SSIs also exist for anxiety disorders; one-session treatment for specific phobias has been demonstrated to be effective with children (Ollendick et al., 2009). This intervention uses *in vivo* exposure to challenge catastrophic beliefs about the target of the child's phobia. As opposed to more long-term graduated exposure techniques, this treatment is maximized to 3 hours. This intervention was shown to be superior to both a waiting-list control and an education support treatment in terms of clinician-rated phobia severity.

Transdiagnostic SSIs have also been evaluated. One, a 2-hour solution-focused family therapy intervention, found statistically and clinically significant improvements in the major presenting problem as well as effects on internalizing and externalizing symptoms (Perkins, 2006). Notably, this study drew in a broad sample of adolescents, enrolling 90% of all 5- to 15-year-old clients accepted into a public clinic over a 14-month period (10% were ineligible). Thus, a variety of provider-guided SSI LI intervention approaches—from behavioural activation to psychoeducation to motivational interviewing—hold promise to ameliorate mental illness in youth. Further, larger trials are needed to gauge the potential clinical superiority of any single approach.

Unguided SSIs

Unguided SSIs are those that require no provider facilitation, supervision, or check-ins. They leverage online or other remote mediums (e.g. websites, self-help booklets) to maintain structure in an intervention without the presence of a facilitator, which can allow youth to access and engage with them more flexibly, and at a far lower cost than provider-delivered options. Like guided SSIs, unguided SSIs have used a wide range of clinical approaches, and have been designed to target diverse mechanisms of change. We highlight a few well-tested interventions here.

Many unguided SSIs are administered via online modules that young people interact with directly. One such intervention, called 'Project Personality', aims to teach a 'growth mindset'—the belief that personal traits are malleable. In a recent randomized controlled trial of 96 high-risk early adolescents, this 30-minute SSI predicted significant reductions in a variety of symptoms (parent-reported depressive and anxiety symptoms and youth-reported depressive symptoms) across a 9-month follow-up relative to an active, supportive therapy control (Schleider & Weisz, 2018). A second web-based SSI based on the Project Personality intervention, delivered to (and self-administered by) adolescent girls in rural US public schools, also produced significant depressive symptom reductions 4 months later relative to an active, unguided comparison programme (teaching healthy relationship skills; Schleider, Burnette, Widman, Hoyt, & Prinstein, 2020). Previous research (Schleider & Weisz, 2016) has indicated that growth mindset interventions such as these may work by strengthening participants' perceived control: 'a belief an individual holds about the nature of control over situational factors and events' (Weems & Silverman, 2006, p. 117). The model these interventions follow is discussed in greater detail in the following section.

Self-guided online interventions are not the only unguided SSIs, however. One evaluation examined a parent-directed psychoeducation SSI intended to communicate evidence-based parenting practices (Cardamone-Breen et al., 2018). However, the evaluation did not demonstrate significant effects on child symptoms. On the whole, there is promising evidence for many unguided SSIs. This evidence base is primed to develop rapidly in the coming years as more SSIs are developed and tested.

Project Personality: an unguided SSI for youth depression

Multiple single-session approaches may mitigate depression in young people. Here, we introduce a single-session, evidence-supported, self-guided intervention—Project Personality—that is freely accessible online for adolescents and clinicians to use (see http://www.schleiderlab.org/yes). This intervention is intended for self-administration by youths themselves; providers are not needed for programme delivery. When offering Project Personality to youth, particularly via our open, online platform for youth mental health support ('Project YES'), family members or providers may frame it as 'an online activity that lets you learn new ways to cope with stress, while helping others to do the same' (indeed, within the Project YES platform, young people are invited to share anonymous coping advice with others as part of the programme experience; Schleider, Dobias, et al., 2020).

Considerable research suggests that viewing one's traits as malleable (called a 'growth mindset'), as opposed to immutable (called a 'fixed mindset'), predicts increased depressive symptoms in youth (Schleider & Schroder, 2018). Drawing on this research, Project Personality instils the belief that personal characteristics and experience—including depression symptoms and coping—are inherently amenable to change, given personal effort and support. In multiple trials, Project Personality has strengthened youths' sense of control over their own behaviours and emotions (Schleider & Weisz, 2016), decreased hopelessness (Schleider, Dobias, et al., 2020), and reduced depression up to 9 months later in both high-symptom (Schleider & Weisz, 2018) and non-referred adolescents (Schleider, Burnette, et al., 2020). Across these trials, Project Personality has been rated as acceptable by youth aged 11–17 years, suggesting appropriateness for younger and older adolescents.

Project Personality follows four evidence-based design principles within SSI research, previously summarized as the 'B.E.S.T. Principles' for SSI development (Schleider, Dobias, et al., 2020) and rooted in basic social-psychological research (Lewin, 1944):

1. B: *Brain* science to normalize concepts in the programme.
2. E: *Empower* youths to a 'helper' or 'expert' role.
3. S: *Saying*-is-believing exercises to solidify learning.
4. T: *Testimonials* and evidence from valued others.

Brain science to normalize concepts

To enhance message credibility and to encourage youths to perceive their experiences as normative, Project Personality incorporates ideas from brain science to support its message that people can change. More specifically, the programme recruits the concept of neuroplasticity to explain why our symptoms and coping skills are modifiable, via practice and support. In addition to piquing youths' interest, this explanation helps render the programme's message easier for youth to trust as universally true, despite personal challenges they might have experienced. For instance, one programme section reads as follows:

> Scientists say it's like the connections in our brains are made with *pencil*, not permanent marker. That means it's possible for us to erase old connections and write new ones. Of course, changing brain connections is not as easy as making a pencil drawing. We need patience and effort, and we need to be kind to ourselves if things don't change right away. It takes lots of practice using new ways of thinking. But with the right help, anyone can change over time.

Thus, Project Personality orients youth to understand their inherent capacity to alter the course of their own emotional difficulties.

Empower youths to a 'helper' or 'expert' role

To optimize acceptability of youth-directed interventions, it is helpful to recruit and respond to young people's perspectives and expertise—particularly with respect to self-directed SSIs. Beyond strengthening youths' investment in a given activity, this approach can help bolster youths' active involvement and contributions within a programme by strengthening their feelings of competence, agency, and relatedness—all of which are important to positive social-emotional outcomes (Samdal & Rowling, 2015). Thus, Project Personality treats youth as experts rather than passive treatment recipients. For example, the programme begins as follows:

> We need your help! We are scientists from Stony Brook University. Every day, we work with young people who are going through challenges and changes in their lives, like starting at a new school, making new friends, or learning to cope with difficult emotions and life events. We also study personality and the brain, and how these things relate to dealing with challenges in everyday life. We ask questions like 'Can people change?' and 'If they can change, how do they do it?' Young people often tell us that this science is interesting, and that it may help kids who are going through difficult times in their lives. But we need your help explaining it in a better way to help more people like you. Please help us and others by completing this activity carefully.

In our research on Project Personality, as well as in our open-access programme evaluation of the intervention (http://www.schleiderlab.org/yes), youths' responses and advice to peers throughout the programme are used to update its content. We believe this feature helps bolster youths' sense of agency and ownership during programme completion.

Saying-is-believing activities to solidify learning

'Saying-is-believing' activities are designed to promote internalization of novel beliefs or ideas via self-persuasive writing exercises. They are drawn from social psychological theory (Aronson, 1999) and have been included in numerous educational interventions for adolescents (e.g. targeting achievement motivation; Aronson, 1999; Yeager & Walton, 2011). The activity consists of two parts. First, the youth is asked to write in detail about a setback, stressor, or struggle relevant to a given intervention's main message, following within-programme prompts. Next, the youth is asked to offer advice to a hypothetical peer who is now facing that same stressor, explaining to the peer how they might use newly gleaned knowledge from the intervention to cope with the stressor at hand, or view it in a new, more helpful light. In Project Personality's final saying-is-believing activity, youths are first provided with a hypothetical scenario describing peer rejection and asked to respond, in writing, to the following prompt: 'How do you think you would feel if this happened to you? What kinds of thoughts do you think you would have?' Afterwards, youths are asked to 'imagine that the same event you just wrote about happened to another kid just like you. What could you say to help them understand they can change, or things that are happening to them could change? When writing your answer, think about what you learned today about personality and the brain.' In a recent trial of Project Personality's effects on youth experiencing depressive symptom, two youths shared different perspectives on the latter prompt:

1. 'I would tell them to remember that even though it feels like these things will never end, nothing is forever. Maybe by being nice to the kid, you can make him realize that he is being mean and his neurons will help him change for the better.'
2. 'People got different brains. Everybody's brain is constantly growing and changing. That friend of yours probably got some struggle going on in theirs and they may just need time, but even if they don't come back to be your friend, they're not the only person who would care about you.'

Per basic psychological research on saying-is-believing activities, advocating for a persuasive message to a personally relevant audience—like a peer—can strengthen one's own belief in that message.

Testimonials and evidence from valued others

The usefulness of testimonials (personal narratives) has received considerable attention among health communication researchers (Hamby, Daniloski, & Brinberg, 2015). By engaging readers both cognitively and emotionally, they can increase the persuasiveness of mental health-related messaging (Johnson et al., 2017). For young people, the persuasive power of testimonials appears more pronounced when narratives come from peers or 'experts' in a given domain (Borah & Xiao, 2018). As such, Project Personality includes several stories from older peers and 'experts' (typically scientists) to illustrate its core ideas.

Implementation challenges and potential solutions

SSIs, including but not limited to Project Personality, are designed for ease of implementation: youth are empowered to complete online SSIs independently. However, Project Personality and other online SSIs may be used *either* as a stand-alone unguided mental health support, *or* as a low intensity element of longer-term treatment. Although online, self-guided SSIs may be sufficient to meaningfully reduce mental health difficulties in some youth, many will require additional clinical support, and it is not yet possible to precisely forecast *which* youth are likely to benefit from unguided SSIs alone versus *in adjunct to* further treatment. Thus, in cases where longer-term treatment is an option, we suggest assessing short-term response to SSIs to guide subsequent clinical decision-making around further treatment. In our own work, we often assess whether youth report improvements in *hopelessness* or *perceived agency* (see 'Recommended measures' at the end of this chapter) from immediately before to after completion of an SSI. Given early evidence that these short-term changes may predict odds of longer-term response (Schleider, Abel, & Weisz, 2019), the *absence* of short-term gains in these domains may indicate a low likelihood of future depression symptom reductions—and as such, a potential need for further treatment.

Chapter summary

Many SSIs show promise as low-cost alternatives and adjuncts to traditional youth mental health interventions. We have highlighted some promising interventions, described a single-session, unguided activity that has reduced depression in youth, and outlined design principles for developing future unguided SSIs. However, more work remains to be done towards matching SSIs' *potential* with their *impact* to alleviate mental illness in youth. Future work should also focus on improving accessibility by moving SSIs into community settings, encouraging larger-scale testing of interventions that show promise, and investigating promising programs' effects in new populations. A focus not only on research, but also on implementation, will help SSIs meet their promise in the future.

Recommended measures

- Four-item Beck Hopelessness Scale and three-item State Hope Scale—Agency Subscale—useful to assess pre-to-post change in hopelessness when administered with single-session online interventions (Forintos, Rózsa, Pilling, & Kopp, 2013; Snyder et al., 1996).
- Perceived Control Scale for Children—useful to assess pre-to-post change in perceived control when administered with single-session online interventions (Weisz, Southam-Gerow, & McCarty, 2001).
- Revised Children's Anxiety and Depression Scale-25 (RCADS-25)—a free and brief measure of youth depression and anxiety symptoms; useful for symptom tracking and assessment (Chorpita, Ebesutani, & Spence, 2015).

Additional materials

Project YES website. Retrieved from http://www.schleiderlab.org/yes

Recommended reading

Burnette, J. L., Knouse, L. E., Vavra, D. T., O'Boyle, E., & Brooks, M. A. (2020). Growth mindsets and psychological distress: A meta-analysis. *Clinical Psychology Review, 77*, 101816.

Gawrysiak, M., Nicholas, C., & Hopko, D. R. (2009). Behavioral activation for moderately depressed university students: Randomized controlled trial. *Journal of Counseling Psychology, 56*(3), 468–475.

Merry, S. N., Stasiak, K., Shepherd, M., Frampton, C., Fleming, T., & Lucassen, M. F. G. (2012). The effectiveness of SPARX, a computerised self help intervention for adolescents seeking help for depression: Randomised controlled non-inferiority trial. *BMJ, 344*(7857), e2598.

Schleider, J. L., Dobias, M. L., Sung, J. Y., & Mullarkey, M. C. (2020). Future directions in single-session youth mental health interventions. *Journal of Clinical Child & Adolescent Psychology, 49*(2), 264–278.

Schleider, J. L., Dobias, M., Sung, J., Mumper, E., Mullarkey, M. C. (2020). Acceptability and utility of an open-access, online single-session intervention platform for adolescent mental health. *JMIR Mental Health, 7*(6), e20513.

Schleider, J., & Weisz, J. (2018). A single-session growth mindset intervention for adolescent anxiety and depression: 9-month outcomes of a randomized trial. *Journal of Child Psychology and Psychiatry and Allied Disciplines, 59*(2), 160–170.

References

Aronson, E. (1999). The power of self-persuasion. *The American Psychologist, 54*(11), 875. doi:10.1037/h0088188

Borah, P., & Xiao, X. (2018). The importance of "Likes": The interplay of message framing, source, and social endorsement on credibility perceptions of health information on facebook. *Journal of Health Communication, 23*(4), 399–411. doi:10.1080/10810730.2018.1455770

Cardamone-Breen, M. C., Jorm, A. F., Lawrence, K. A., Rapee, R. M., Mackinnon, A. J., & Yap, M. B. H. (2018). A single-session, web-based parenting intervention to prevent adolescent depression and anxiety disorders: Randomized controlled trial. *Journal of Medical Internet Research*, 20(4), e148.

Chorpita, B. F., Ebesutani, C., & Spence, S. H. (2015). Revised children's anxiety and depression scale. Retrieved from https://www.childfirst.ucla.edu/wp-content/uploads/sites/163/2018/03/RCADS25-Youth-English-2018.pdf

Forintos, D. P., Rózsa, S., Pilling, J., & Kopp, M. (2013). Proposal for a short version of the Beck Hopelessness Scale based on a national representative survey in Hungary. *Community Mental Health Journal*, 49(6), 822–830.

Gawrysiak, M., Nicholas, C., & Hopko, D. R. (2009). Behavioral activation for moderately depressed university students: Randomized controlled trial. *Journal of Counseling Psychology*, 56(3), 468–475.

Hamby, A., Daniloski, K., & Brinberg, D. (2015). How consumer reviews persuade through narratives. *Journal of Business Research*, 68(6), 1242–1250.

Hoyt, M. F., Bobele, M., Slive, A., Young, J., & Talmon, M. (2018). Single-session/one-at-a-time walk-in therapy. In M. F. Hoyt, M. Bobele, A. Slive, J. Young, & M. Talmon (Eds.), *Single-session therapy by walk-in or appointment: Administrative, clinical, and supervisory aspects of one-at-a-time services* (pp. 3–24). New York: Routledge.

Johnson, J. M. Q., Quintero Johnson, J. M., Yilmaz, G., & Najarian, K. (2017). Optimizing the presentation of mental health information in social media: The effects of health testimonials and platform on source perceptions, message processing, and health outcomes. *Health Communication*, 32, 1121–1132. doi:10.1080/10410236.2016.1214218

Kataoka, S. H., Zhang, L., & Wells, K. B. (2002). Unmet need for mental health care among U.S. children: Variation by ethnicity and insurance status. *American Journal of Psychiatry*, 159(9), 1548–1555.

Lewin, G. W. (1944). Constructs in field theory. In Cartwright, D. (Ed.), *Resolving social conflicts and field theory in social science* (pp. 191–199). New York, NY: Harper and Brothers.

Ollendick, T. H., Ost, L.-G., Reuterskiöld, L., Costa, N., Cederlund, R., Sirbu, C., . . ., & Jarrett, M. A. (2009). One-session treatment of specific phobias in youth: A randomized clinical trial in the United States and Sweden. *Journal of Consulting and Clinical Psychology*, 77(3), 504–516.

Perkins, R. (2006). The effectiveness of one session of therapy using a single-session therapy approach for children and adolescents with mental health problems. *Group Dynamics: Theory, Research, and Practice*, 79(2), 215–227.

Randell, B. P., Eggert, L. L., & Pike, K. C. (2001). Immediate post intervention effects of two brief youth suicide prevention interventions. *Suicide & Life-Threatening Behavior*, 31(1), 41–61.

Reardon, T., Harvey, K., Baranowska, M., O'Brien, D., Smith, L., & Creswell, C. (2017). What do parents perceive are the barriers and facilitators to accessing psychological treatment for mental health problems in children and adolescents? A systematic review of qualitative and quantitative studies. *European Child & Adolescent Psychiatry*, 26(6), 623–647.

Rowan, K., McAlpine, D. D., & Blewett, L. A. (2013). Access and cost barriers to mental health care, by insurance status, 1999–2010. *Health Affairs*, 32(10), 1723–1730.

Samdal, O., Rowling, L. (2015). Implementation strategies to promote and sustain health and learning in school. In: Simovska, V., Mannix McNamara, P. (Eds.), *Schools for Health and Sustainability*. Dordrecht, The Netherlands: Springer.

Schleider, J. L., Abel, M. R., & Weisz, J. R. (2019). Do immediate gains predict long-term symptom change? Findings from a randomized trial of a single-session intervention for youth anxiety and depression. *Child Psychiatry and Human Development*, 50, 868–881. doi:10.1007/s10578- 019-00889-2

Schleider, J. L., Burnette, J. L., Widman, L., Hoyt, C., & Prinstein, M. J. (2020). Randomized trial of a single-session growth mind-set intervention for rural adolescents' internalizing and externalizing problems. *Journal of Clinical Child and Adolescent Psychology*, 49(5), 660–672.

Schleider, J. L., Dobias, M. L., Sung, J. Y., & Mullarkey, M. C. (2020). Future directions in single-session youth mental health interventions. *Journal of Clinical Child and Adolescent Psychology*, 49(2), 264–278.

Schleider, J. L., & Weisz, J. R. (2016). Reducing risk for anxiety and depression in adolescents: Effects of a single-session intervention teaching that personality can change. *Behaviour Research and Therapy*, 87, 170–181.

Schleider, J. L., & Weisz, J. R. (2017). Little treatments, promising effects? Meta-analysis of single-session interventions for youth psychiatric problems. *Journal of the American Academy of Child and Adolescent Psychiatry, 56*(2), 107–115.

Schleider, J. & Weisz, J. (2018). A single-session growth mindset intervention for adolescent anxiety and depression: 9-month outcomes of a randomized trial. *Journal of Child Psychology and Psychiatry, and Allied Disciplines, 59*(2), 160–170.

Snyder, C. R., Sympson, S. C., Ybasco, F. C., Borders, T. F., Babyak, M. A., & Higgins, R. L. (1996). Development and validation of the State Hope Scale. *Journal of Personality and Social Psychology, 70*(2), 321–325.

Sung, J., Dobias, M., & Schleider, J. L. (2020). Single-session interventions: Complementing and extending evidence-based practice. Retrieved from https://doi.org/10.31234/osf.io/z7bw2

Walker, E. R., Cummings, J. R., Hockenberry, J. M., & Druss, B. G. (2015). Insurance status, use of mental health services, and unmet need for mental health care in the United States. *Psychiatric Services, 66*(6), 578–584.

Weems, C. F., & Silverman, W. K. (2006). An integrative model of control: Implications for understanding emotion regulation and dysregulation in childhood anxiety. *Journal of Affective Disorders, 91*(2–3), 113–124.

Weisz, J. R., Southam-Gerow, M. A., & McCarty, C. A. (2001). Control-related beliefs and depressive symptoms in clinic-referred children and adolescents: Developmental differences and model specificity. *Journal of Abnormal Psychology, 110*(1), 97–109.

Yeager, D. S., & Walton, G. M. (2011). Social-psychological interventions in education. *Review of Educational Research, 81*, 267–301. doi:10.3102/0034654311405999

24

Playing anxiety and depression away

Serious games for mental health problems
in children and adolescents

Mathijs F. G. Lucassen, Theresa M. Fleming, Matthew J. Shepherd,
 Karolina Stasiak, and Sally N. Merry

Learning objectives

- To outline the benefits of serious games for children and adolescents with mild to moderate mental health problems.
- To summarize the benefits and challenges of using serious games to support children and adolescents with mental health problems.
- To briefly describe the evidence base for serious games for child and adolescent mental health problems.

Introduction

Games and play are as old as time, with play being especially important in helping to facilitate healthy development (Yogman et al., 2018). However, computer technology over the recent decades has dramatically changed the world of play (Paulus, Ohmann, Von Gontard, & Popow, 2018) and computer games have become part of everyday life. It is now estimated that more than 90% of children and adolescents engage with this popular form of media (Children's Commissioner for England, 2019; Gentile et al., 2017), but computer games are more than pure entertainment. For instance, commercial computer games are thought to potentially enhance cognitive skills (e.g. spatial skills), social functioning (e.g. they frequently encourage teamwork), and motivational styles (e.g. they can cultivate a persistent and optimistic motivational approach) (Granic, Lobel, & Engels, 2014). Computer games are utilized for a range of serious reasons, including for educational purposes (Hainey, Connolly, Boyle, Wilson, & Razak, 2016) and to support the mental health of children and adolescents. For example, applied games such as serious games (i.e. computerized games for serious purposes) and gamification (i.e. gaming elements used outside of commercial games) have the ability to increase treatment adherence by making learning in a therapeutic context enjoyable (Fleming et al., 2017). Serious games can also lead to more effective mental health interventions, because they provide opportunities for both conventional and non-traditional processes for learning and behaviour change (Fleming et al., 2017). Furthermore, a systematic review and meta-analysis of serious games for mental health (including the treatment of depression), reported that these interventions had a moderate effect on symptom improvements ($g = 0.55$) (Lau, Smit, Fleming, & Riper, 2017).

In this chapter, we present the case study of a serious game in computerized cognitive behavioural therapy (cCBT) format called SPARX (Smart, Positive, Active, Realistic, X-factor thoughts) (Merry et al., 2012). SPARX is one of only three forms of evidence-based cCBT recommended for adolescents with mild depression in the most recent National Institute for Health and Care Excellence (2019, p. 30) guidelines for depression in children and young people, the other two interventions being Stressbusters and Grasp the Opportunity. To date, these three evidence-based cCBT interventions are not freely available in the UK.

The case study of SPARX

SPARX is a seven-module intervention designed for the treatment of mild to moderate depressive symptoms in adolescents aged 12–19 years old (Figures 24.1 and 24.2). The intervention uses visually appealing graphics and a range of interactive exercises to engage adolescents. Each of SPARX's seven modules is designed to take 20–30 minutes to complete and modules have a direct teaching

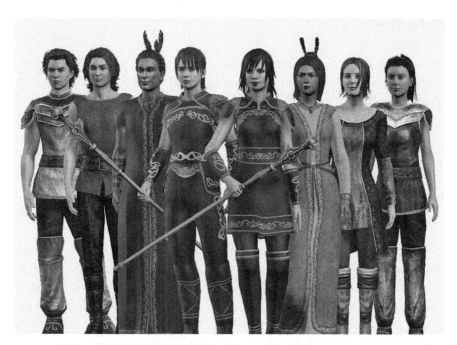

Figure 24.1 The main characters in SPARX (the male and female avatars are the two characters in the middle holding staffs).

used with permission of the copyright owner © Auckland UniServices Limited.

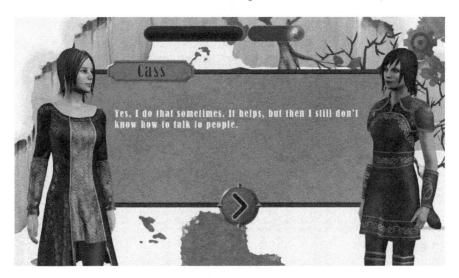

Figure 24.2 An avatar (on the right) attempting to negotiate with a character (Cass) in the 'Ice Province'.
used with permission of the copyright owner © Auckland UniServices Limited.

component, to demonstrate how skills from SPARX's fantasy world can be applied to an adolescent's real life.

SPARX is based on core cognitive behavioural therapy (CBT) skills, and homework tasks are set with adolescents to allow practice and support skill generalization. Adolescents earn a 'power gem' after they complete a module, each of which brings the fantasy world closer to being in balance, after the user's avatar fights GNATs (Gloomy, Negative, Automatic Thoughts) and catches SPARXs. The main CBT skills covered are physically represented by 'the shield against depression'. This shield consists of six power gems based on CBT content, in particular:

1. 'Relax' (relaxation training).
2. 'Do it' (e.g. behavioural activation).
3. 'Sort it' (e.g. social skills training).
4. 'Spot it' (recognizing or naming common cognitive distortions).
5. 'Solve it' (problem-solving).
6. 'Swap it' (e.g. cognitive restructuring).

In the first randomized controlled trial of SPARX, the intervention was found to be non-inferior to treatment as usual (i.e. it was at least as good as the interventions usually offered) for adolescents (n = 187) seeking help for their depression. Treatment as usual mostly consisted of face-to-face counselling (mean number of sessions 4.8) with more than half of the sessions being 45 minutes or longer and delivered by qualified counsellors in schools or primary care settings (Merry et al., 2012). Since 2014, under funding from the New Zealand Ministry of Health, SPARX has been made freely available to anyone in New Zealand via https://www.sparx.org.

nz/home. In the first 5 years of its national roll-out over 13,000 adolescents (aged 12–19 years old) accessed the intervention (Lucassen et al., 2021), representing approximately 2% of the adolescent population in the country (where there are just over 600,000 young people aged 10–19 years; Statistics New Zealand, 2020). Strengths of the intervention's national roll-out have included its free access, wide access geographically, and the provision of back-up support for SPARX users, from contracted providers, 24 hours a day 7 days a week. SPARX has been used by a diverse cross-section of male and female adolescents from across New Zealand, with over 15% being Māori (i.e. indigenous young people), 8% being Asian, and 4% being adolescent users of Pacific heritage (Lucassen et al., 2021).

Case example

Tui is a 15-year-old girl who goes to see her school guidance counsellor, Jen, because she is 'stuck feeling stink' about herself. During their initial meeting, Jen finds out that Tui likes reading fantasy-based books and that she played a lot of computer games when she was younger. Due to the high demand for Jen's services (where young people in crisis are prioritized), she decides to offer Tui SPARX with the addition of two or three check-ins, either face-to-face or over the phone. Jen is aware of SPARX's content, so after Tui completes Modules 1 and 2 of SPARX and learns about progressive muscle relaxation and using controlled breathing, Jen and Tui discuss how to apply relaxation exercises in real life during their initial check-in. Tui later reports finding the SPARX content in Modules 3 and 4 fairly straightforward, in particular problem-solving using 'STEPS' (i.e. Say what the problem is, Think of solutions, Examine these ideas, Pick one and try it, See what happens). But during their second check-in, Tui highlights that she has found other SPARX content more challenging, especially in terms of recognizing the 'Sparks' (i.e. positive or helpful thoughts about her future) in her own life. As a result, Tui and Jen spend the second check-in talking about Tui's negative thoughts and how to find ways to combat them (e.g. how to potentially take 'Another view' as suggested in SPARX). In their final check-in, Jen asks Tui to 'rate' SPARX. Tui says that it was useful but not as much fun as other computer games and that she probably would not have completed SPARX if Jen had not encouraged her to do so. Jen thanks her for this feedback and resolves to be more explicit to other clients that SPARX is a 'serious game' and therefore different to commercial games when using the intervention with adolescents in the future.

Challenges

Despite the advantages associated with SPARX, and other forms of cCBT for children and adolescents with mild to moderate mental health problems, notable challenges remain. Keeping pace with technology is an issue, given the time required to ensure that interventions are effective and then made available to users outside of a research context (Stasiak et al., 2016). Moreover, adaptations are likely to be required for underserved populations, such as gender-diverse adolescents (Lucassen et al., 2021). Finally, as with many psychosocial interventions, completion rates are an issue when moving from randomized controlled trials to real-world implementation (Fleming et al., 2018).

In addition to the challenges specifically associated with cCBT interventions, there is concern more generally about children's and adolescents' overexposure to screens. However, gamified cCBT interventions lack the intensely immersive and interactive nature of commercial games and online entertainment (e.g. games like World of Warcraft). Therefore, by their very nature, cCBT interventions are usually time limited and not as appealing as commercial games, thus overuse is unlikely. Nonetheless, when using computer games in a therapeutic context, it is important to consider their possible negative impacts, as computer game usage can be conceptualized as a continuum, from an enjoyable leisure activity at one end to a pathological or addictive behaviour at the other of the spectrum (Paulus et al., 2018).

Potential solutions

Future work is needed on ways to support engagement or retention in cCBT interventions in serious game format for a diverse range of children and adolescents. Potential ways forward include the use of more personalized support or automated reminders; improved game mechanics, game narrative, and immersive game play; and increased use of persuasive design and appealing interfaces (Arigo et al., 2019). The time lag between the development of evidence-based tools and their implementation could be addressed by trial designs which allow for rapid testing and comparisons to other tools, previously identified as evidence based (Arigo et al., 2019; Fleming et al., 2016). Serious games could be used to meet the needs of underserved populations with high mental health needs, including indigenous adolescents (Shepherd et al., 2015), and sexual and gender minority youth (Lucassen et al., 2018; Lucassen et al., 2021). SPARX was developed by a company led by a Māori director, and included co-design work facilitated by a Māori clinician (i.e. Dr Matthew Shepherd) among Māori rangatahi (adolescents). This work was all overseen by a Kaumātua (i.e. respected Māori elder) and a cultural advisory group. However, other underserved populations, including transgender adolescents, need particular attention. Recent analyses suggest transgender users of SPARX have not benefited from the same levels of symptom improvements as their non-transgender (i.e. cisgender) peers (Lucassen et al., 2021). Possible solutions to the issues include planning the inclusion of underserved groups from the start; adapting existing interventions, as in work undertaken in Australia to enhance SPARX specifically for transgender adolescents (Strauss et al., 2019); or using more flexible formats than serious games.

For instance, developing a chatbot (i.e. where a computer simulates a conversation via online messages that is independent from any human operator) specifically for transgender adolescents.

What is the future?

We anticipate therapists will increase their use of commercial computer games therapeutically. For instance, Wii Sports and games such as Pokémon GO (i.e. where a game interfaces with the real world and requires physical activity) could be used more regularly as tools for behavioural activation. We also hope that alongside commercial computer games, technology will be harnessed more generally so that cCBT is much more than a 'manual online' (Stasiak et al., 2016). Doing so can result in opportunities for children and adolescents to engage freely with immersive experiences to develop skills and address problems in non-threatening, scalable, and safe ways (Stasiak et al., 2016) and potentially help address the needs of underserved or 'at-risk' populations.

Chapter summary

In summary, serious games have demonstrated considerable potential in terms of supporting the mental health of children and adolescents. However, only a handful of such interventions are currently available to children and adolescents outside of formal research projects.

Recommended reading

The following open-access paper provides a useful summary of serious games and gaming in the mental health field:

Fleming, T. M., Bavin, L., Stasiak, K., Hermansson-Webb, E., Merry, S. N., Cheek, C., . . ., & Hetrick, S. (2017). Serious games and gamification for mental health: Current status and promising directions. *Frontiers in Psychiatry*, *7*, e215.

References

Arigo, D., Jake-Schoffman, D. E., Wolin, K., Beckjord, E., Hekler, E. B., & Pagoto, S. L. (2019). The history and future of digital health in the field of behavioral medicine. *Journal of Behavioral Medicine*, *42*(1), 67–83.

Children's Commissioner for England. (2019). *Gaming the system*. London: Children's Commissioner for England.

Fleming, T. M., Bavin, L., Lucassen, M., Stasiak, K., Hopkins, S., & Merry, S. (2018). Beyond the trial: Systematic review of real-world uptake and engagement with digital self-help interventions for depression, low mood, or anxiety. *Journal of Medical Internet Research*, *20*(6), e199.

Fleming, T. M., Bavin, L., Stasiak, K., Hermansson-Webb, E., Merry, S., Cheek, C., . . ., & Hetrick, S. (2017). Serious games and gamification for mental health: Current status and promising directions. *Frontiers in Psychiatry*, *7*, e215.

Fleming, T. M., De Beurs, D., Khazaal, Y., Gaggioli, A., Riva, G., Botella, C., . . ., & Riper, H. (2016). Maximizing the impact of e-therapy and serious gaming: Time for a paradigm shift. *Frontiers in Psychiatry*, *7*, e65.

Gentile, D. A., Bailey, K., Bavelier, D., Brockmyer, J. F., Cash, H., Coyne, S. M., . . ., & Young, K. (2017). Internet gaming disorder in children and adolescents. *Pediatrics*, *140*(Suppl 2), S81–S85.

Granic, I., Lobel, A., & Engels, R. C. M. E. (2014). The benefits of playing video games. *American Psychologist*, *69*(1), 66–78.

Hainey, T., Connolly, T. M., Boyle, E. A., Wilson, A., & Razak, A. (2016). A systematic literature review of games-based learning empirical evidence in primary education. *Computers & Education*, *102*, 202–223.

Lau, H. M., Smit, J. H., Fleming, T. M., & Riper, H. (2017). Serious games for mental health: Are they accessible, feasible, and effective? A systematic review and meta-analysis. *Frontiers in Psychiatry*, *7*, e209.

Lucassen, M. F. G., Samra, R., Iacovides, I., Fleming, T., Shepherd, M., Stasiak, K., & Wallace, L. (2018). How LGBT+ young people use the internet in relation to their mental health and envisage the use of e-therapy: Exploratory study. *JMIR Serious Games*, *6*(4), e11249.

Lucassen, M. F. G., Stasiak, K., Fleming, T., Frampton, C. M., Perry, Y., Shepherd, M., & Merry, S. (2021). Computerised cognitive behavioural therapy for gender minority adolescents: Analysis of the real-world implementation of SPARX in New Zealand. *Australian and New Zealand Journal of Psychiatry*, *55*(9), 874–882.

Merry, S. N., Stasiak, K., Shepherd, M., Frampton, C., Fleming, T., & Lucassen, M. F. G. (2012). The effectiveness of SPARX, a computerised self help intervention for adolescents seeking help for depression: Randomised controlled non-inferiority trial. *BMJ*, *344*(e2598), 1–16.

National Institute for Health and Care Excellence. (2019). *Depression in children and young people: Identification and management* [NICE Guideline NG134]. London: National Institute for Health and Care Excellence.

Paulus, F. W., Ohmann, S., Von Gontard, A., & Popow, C. (2018). Internet gaming disorder in children and adolescents: A systematic review. *Developmental Medicine & Child Neurology*, *60*(7), 645–659.

Shepherd, M., Fleming, T., Lucassen, M., Stasiak, K., Lambie, I., & Merry, S. N. (2015). The design and relevance of a computerized gamified depression therapy program for indigenous Māori adolescents. *JMIR Serious Games*, *3*(1), e1.

Stasiak, K., Fleming, T., Lucassen, M., Shepherd, M., Whittaker, R., & Merry, S. N. (2016). Computer-based and online therapy for depression and anxiety in children and adolescents. *Journal of Child and Adolescent Psychopharmacology*, *26*(3), 235–245.

Statistics New Zealand. (2020). Age and sex by ethnic group (grouped total response), for census usually resident population counts, 2006, 2013, and 2018 Censuses (urban rural areas). Retrieved 4 November 2020 from http://nzdotstat.stats.govt.nz/wbos/

Strauss, P., Morgan, H., Wright Toussaint, D., Lin, A., Winter, S., & Perry, Y. (2019). Trans and gender diverse young people's attitudes towards game-based digital mental health interventions: A qualitative investigation. *Internet Interventions*, *18*, e100280.

Yogman, M., Garner, A., Hutchinson, J., Hirsh-Pasek, K., Golinkoff, R. M., & Committee on Psychosocial Aspects of Child and Family Health. (2018). The power of play: A pediatric role in enhancing development in young children. *Pediatrics*, *142*(3), e20182058.

25

New ideas: one-at-a-time therapy

Windy Dryden

Learning objectives

- To understand the nature and goals of one-at-a-time therapy (OAATT).
- To understand the mindset of OAATT and how it challenges conventional thinking about the practice of therapy.
- To understand what constitutes good practice in OAATT.
- To understand the issues that need to be considered concerning the delivery of OAATT and its dissemination.

What is one-at-a-time therapy and what are its goals?

The terms 'single-session therapy' and 'one-at-a-time therapy' (OAATT) are used interchangeably in the literature; in this chapter we will refer to OAATT throughout.[1] We define OAATT as a single session of therapy where therapist and client agree to meet to address the client's most pressing concern in that session, but with the understanding that further help is available if the client needs it. This help may be another single session or whatever other support the therapist and client decide the client needs.

The goals of OAATT are mainly to help the client as much as possible with their most pressing concern and with a plan of how they can implement this solution in their everyday life. Here, the therapist adopts a solution-focused helping stance. Where possible, this solution may be shared with the client's caregivers if they can help the client implement the solution. Sometimes, however, all the client needs is a listening ear and an opportunity to talk about what has been on their mind. In this case, the therapist adopts a more exploratory helping stance. OAATT is not a specific therapeutic approach. Instead, it is a mindset and a mode of delivering therapy.

---

[1] In this chapter, we will discuss therapeutic interventions which occur interactively between therapist and client and in real time (e.g. face-to-face, over an online platform, or over the telephone). We will not discuss the pioneering work of Jessica Schleider and her team at Stony Brook University in the US which focuses on self-administered single-session interventions (see Sung, Dobias, & Schleider, submitted).

Box 25.1 Components of the OAATT mindset

- Recognizing that clients are less interested in therapy than therapists and tend to prefer brief therapeutic encounters, often attending only one (Hoyt & Talmon, 2014).
- Approaching the first session 'as if' it could be the last, irrespective of diagnosis, complexity, or severity.
- Beginning therapy in the first moment with a minimum of assessment, history taking, and case formulation, and forming an alliance quickly.
- Focusing on what can be achieved in the *now* by focusing on what the client wants to focus on and walk away with by the end of the session.
- Searching for one meaningful point that the client can implement after the session has finished and which can make a difference to their life.
- Effecting closure and clarifying next steps.

There are no papers investigating the use of OAATT as defined in this chapter in child and adolescent services. Why then are we including this in a book about children and young people? Previous chapters have demonstrated a clear need for novel approaches within child and adolescent mental health services in order to cope with the current demands worldwide. There are numerous advantages of this innovative approach. While the approach is typically used and has been researched within adult services, the mindset and practice can and should be translated into mental health settings for children and young people.

The OAATT mindset

The therapist needs to adopt the OAATT mindset if they are going to help the client get the most from the session. The main components of this mindset are described in Box 25.1.

The OAATT mindset challenges conventional thinking about clinical practice in a number of ways. First, it questions the idea that certain clinical activities need to be carried out before treatment can begin. While such activities (e.g. a full assessment of the child or adolescent, history taking, and case formulation) are valuable in other modes of therapy delivery, they interfere with OAATT's emphasis on the importance of beginning therapy at first contact. Second, OAATT challenges conventional wisdom that the therapeutic relationship needs time to develop. While this may be the case in certain instances, experience and research have shown that the therapeutic alliance can be developed quickly and influences outcome in OATT (Simon, Imel, Ludman, & Steinfeld, 2012).

Good practice in OAATT

The following is deemed to be good practice in OAATT. Of course, not all points need to be present in every session:

- Develop the working alliance at the outset and maintain it throughout.
- Be clear with the client concerning the purpose of the session and what can and cannot be achieved.
- Ask the client how they think they can best be helped and give examples if necessary.
- Elicit the client's goal for the session, rather than from therapy.
- Ask what the client is prepared to sacrifice to achieve their goal.
- Be focused and encourage the client to stay focused.
- If the practitioner is both problem and solution focused, elicit and understand the problem from the client's perspective.
- Assess the problem using whatever concepts are generally employed in problem assessment.
- Bridge to the future whenever possible.
- Use questions constructively. Here it is important that the therapist gives the client time to answer questions and ensures that the client answers the questions they are asked.
- Be clear. This includes, whenever practicable, explaining interventions, checking the client's understanding of substantive points, and making clear how the client can access further help if needed.
- Encourage the client to be as specific as possible but be mindful of opportunities for generalization.
- Identify and encourage the client to use salient strengths.
- Identify previous attempts to solve their problem, encouraging the client to capitalize on successful attempts and discouraging the client from using unsuccessful attempts.
- Undertake solution-focused work.
- Offer the client expertise without assuming the role of expert.
- Look for ways of making an emotional impact without pushing for it.
- Encourage the client to select a solution that they are most likely to implement.
- Encourage the client to rehearse the solution in the session.
- Encourage the client to take away just one thing.
- Have the client summarize the session.
- Help the client to develop an action plan.
- Encourage the client to identify and problem-solve potential obstacles to change.
- Identify and respond to the client's doubts, reservations, and objections.
- Tie up any loose ends. This involves reminding the client of how they may access future help if needed (e.g. encouraging them to reflect and digest what they

learned from the session, taking appropriate action then waiting before making a decision about further help), inviting the client to ask any last-minute questions, or to tell the therapist something that they need to say before the close of the session.
- Seek feedback from the client.

Issues in the implementation and dissemination of OAATT

OAATT can be delivered through walk-in services or by appointment-based services (see Hoyt, Bobele, Slive, Young, & Talmon, 2018). There are several advantages of OAATT by walk-in. The main advantage for the therapy agency is that it eliminates the problem of people not showing up for appointments since none are required. For clients, the advantages are outlined by Slive, McElheran, and Lawson (2008, p. 6) who say that 'walk-in therapy enables clients to meet with a mental health professional at their moment of choosing. There is no red tape, no triage, no intake process, no waiting list, and no wait. There is no formal assessment, no formal diagnostic process, just one hour of therapy focused on clients' stated wants.'

Despite the advantages to both services and clients, walk-in services are less common in the UK than OAATT delivered by appointment. In this latter delivery system, it is important that an appointment is offered to clients very quickly since the therapeutic potency of OAATT rests on the principle of 'help provided at the point of need' rather than 'help at the point of availability', the latter being the more common in low intensity psychological services for children and young people. Given this, whether OAATT services can be integrated into the service delivery system of agencies providing therapeutic help for children and adolescents will depend on a number of factors. These include flexibility to respond speedily to requests for OAATT interventions, support for OAATT among professional administrative staff in the agency, and widespread acceptance of the OAATT mindset.

Once an agency has decided to offer OAATT then it needs to decide how to bring the existence of this service to the attention of both potential clients and fellow professionals. Issues of OAATT concern *what* is disseminated, *how* it is to be disseminated, and to *whom*. The foundation for dissemination should be the target audience. The way OAATT is disseminated to professionals will be very different to the way that it is disseminated to children and adolescents and their caregivers. Having said that, the following issues should be addressed when disseminating OAATT:

- A clear description of what OAATT is.
- How clients can access OAATT.
- The reasons why a person might choose OAATT.
- Example of typical issues people bring to OAATT.

- What OAATT involves.
- Who provides OAATT.

OAATT is usually disseminated on an agency's website where the above issues are clearly outlined. Alternatively, flyers covering the same material can be printed and distributed to places where they are likely to be seen and read. With children and adolescents, caregivers and teachers should also receive this information.

Finally, a good way of describing OAATT in a vivid way is through the medium of videos and whiteboard animations (e.g. https://www.youtube.com/watch?v=wIcu OVOABRw&t=7s and http://www.bristol.ac.uk/students/wellbeing/services/stud ent-counselling-service/).

What is the future?

The mental health consequences of the COVID-19 pandemic are likely to involve increasing numbers of children and adolescents seeking help from mental health services. Some are likely to require long-term interventions, but the majority in our view are likely to benefit from a single session of focused help offered at the point of need with further help available as needed. OAATT has the potential to deliver such help in a variety of formats. Such flexibility may well suit children and adolescents and the future challenge for OAATT practitioners is to modify service delivery to meet the treatment preferences of this client group. See Dryden (2021) for a discussion of the future of OAATT. There is a need for further research on the clinical and economic outcomes of OAATT in comparison to more traditional blocks of sessions for children and young people and their families.

Wider implementation: training and supervising therapists in OAATT

For this clinical need to be properly met, therapists will need proper training and supervision in OAATT. As OAATT is a mindset and a way of delivering services rather than a specific approach, such training and supervision can be open to practitioners from a diverse range of therapeutic modalities who are prepared to embrace this mindset.

Chapter summary

- OAATT is a mindset and a way of delivering therapy services. It is not a discrete approach to therapy.
- The potency of OAATT rests on the principle of help provided at the point of need rather than at the point of availability.

- OAATT reflects the behaviour of many clients who often seek and are satisfied with brief therapy, often provided in a single session.
- OAATT can be integrated into an agency where there is a variety of services.
- Therapists from a broad range of therapeutic approaches who are willing to embrace the OAATT mindset can be trained to deliver this service.

Recommended reading

Dryden, W. (2020). *The single-session therapy primer: Principles and practice.* Monmouth: PCCS Books.

References

Dryden, W. (2021). *Single-session therapy and its future: What SST leaders think.* Abingdon: Routledge.

Hoyt, M. F., Bobele, M., Slive, A., Young, J., & Talmon, M. (Eds.). (2018). *Single-session therapy by walk-in or appointment: Administrative, clinical, and supervisory aspects of one-at-a time services.* New York: Routledge.

Hoyt, M. F., & Talmon, M. F. (2014). What the literature says: An annotated bibliography. In M. F. Hoyt & M. Talmon (Eds.), *Capturing the moment: Single session therapy and walk-in services* (pp. 487–516). Bethel, CT: Crown House Publishing.

Slive, A., McElheran, N., & Lawson, A. (2008). How brief does it get? Walk-in single session therapy. *Journal of Systemic Therapies, 27*(4), 5–22.

Simon, G. E., Imel, Z. E., Ludman, E. J., & Steinfeld, B. J. (2012). Is dropout after a first psychotherapy visit always a bad outcome? *Psychiatric Services, 63*(7), 705–707.

Sung, J. Y., Dobias, M. L., & Schleider, J. L. (2020). Single-session interventions: Complementing and extending evidence-based practice. *Advances in Cognitive Therapy.* Retrieved from: https://www.academyofct.org/page/AdvancesinCT/Advances-in-Cognitive-Therapy-Newsletter.htm

26

The power of peer support

Sophie D. Bennett, Lauren Croucher, Ann Hagell, Elif Mertan,
Wendy Minhinnett, and Roz Shafran

Learning objectives

- To understand how difficulties in accessing evidence-based interventions for children and young people leads parents and young people to turn to alternative sources of support and advice.
- To understand what these alternative sources and support may be, particularly considering online and peer support groups for parents of children with mental health problems.
- To consider how peer-mediated support groups may be used as an adjunct to current services.

Introduction: challenges facing young people with mental health problems and their parents/carers

While evidence-based treatments for mental health disorders in children and young people exist, including self-help (see Chapter 3), access to such interventions is challenging. Mental health services are overstretched and often have increasingly tight inclusion criteria and long waiting lists. Delays to treatment can lead to worsening mental health and many families are left struggling without. In the UK, for those able to access child and adolescent mental health services (CAMHS), more than one in five wait over 6 months (NHS Digital, 2017) and national survey data from the third sector reported that two-thirds of parents are not being signposted to appropriate forms of support during this wait (Young Minds, 2019).

Parents consider that in addition to long waiting lists, one of the main barriers to accessing support is knowledge and understanding of mental health problems and the help-seeking process (Reardon et al., 2017). Where can families go for this advice and information? What other options might there be in the absence of a trained therapist? How can parents learn about what self-help options are available? This chapter considers how peer support may be used in addition to traditional support delivered by mental health professionals.

There are various ways of conceptualizing peer support. Mead et al. (2001) define peer support as 'a system of giving and receiving help founded on key principles of respect, shared responsibility, and mutual agreement of what is helpful'. It is 'not one particular programme or method that can be applied in any context' (Cowie, 2020). Davidson et al. (1999) suggested three overarching types of peer support within mental health: informal/naturally occurring peer support, peers participating in peer-run programmes, and the employment of service users to provide support in traditional services. Since Davidson's review, one of the biggest advances in peer support has been the introduction of online groups and fora. This chapter considers two examples of online peer support. These examples are of support for *parents* of children and young people with mental health difficulties. Many other forms of peer support exist within the area of children and young people's mental health, including support directed at the young people themselves.

Online peer support

Social media transcends educational, cultural, and racial barriers to allow a community environment in which people can share their knowledge (Ahmed et al., 2019; Chou, Hunt, Beckjord, Moser, & Hesse, 2009). A unique benefit of utilizing online communities is anonymity. Many online communities allow users to discuss potentially sensitive information under the guise of a self-created username or pseudonym. Anonymity provides users with the ability to discuss their issues freely in a way that would be considered unacceptable if the information were identifiable (De Choudhury & De, 2014) and this may be particularly important for stigmatizing issues such as concerns about mental health (Lawlor & Kirakowski, 2014; Sayal et al., 2010). The anonymity within online communities gathers emotionally involved and engaging feedback from other users (De Choudhury & De, 2014).

The benefits of online peer support and social media use in mental health may include a feeling of greater social connectedness and group belonging as well as learning 'strategies for coping with day-to-day challenges of living with a mental illness' (Naslund, Aschbrenner, Marsch, & Bartels, 2016). It may also be a containing place for parents to express feelings and obtain advice and information from experts by experience.

Example 1: Rollercoaster parent support group via closed Facebook groups and face-to-face meetings

Rollercoaster is a support service in the North East of England for parents/carers who are supporting a child or young person with any kind of emotional or mental health problem including anxiety, low mood, depression, self-harm, eating disorders, sleep problems, suicidal thoughts, or obsessions and compulsions. It was named 'Rollercoaster' as living with a child or young person with emotional or mental health issues can be challenging, isolating, and like riding an emotional rollercoaster. Rollercoaster was set up by two parents of young people experiencing mental health problems, in partnership with the Tees, Esk and Wear Valley Trust CAMHS service. In addition to a face-to-face group, there is an e-network, and closed and open Facebook groups (not anonymous). The project was initially delivered on a voluntary basis and is now in the third year of delivering as a commissioned service. The group is moderated by its founder. Feedback from users of the Facebook group as reported in an unpublished report of the service, referred to the 24/7 nature of the group, for example, 'Great to be able to reach out when at crisis', 'Always someone to listen, even if you just want to scream!!!'. The importance of 'quick answers' was stressed, 'even in the middle of the night when you might be at a real low point'. The Facebook page complements the work of face-to-face groups and a report from Rollercoaster included the following quote, provided by a parent in session feedback: 'Great support especially in between support groups or if you just need some info as someone generally can point you in the right direction. Or for when you just need a little virtual hug.'

Example 2: Mumsnet—an open internet forum

In contrast to Rollercoaster, which combines internet and face-to-face support, Mumsnet is the largest internet parenting forum in the UK (Pederson & Lupton, 2016) which provides a user-driven online community (Pederson & Smithson, 2010). Mumsnet includes a discussion forum named 'Talk'. Talk offers an open platform for discussions organized around over 200 established topics, one of which is child mental health, and receives over 1 million visits per month (Pederson & Smithson, 2013).

Previous research on Mumsnet has highlighted the site's ability to provide a lifeline for struggling parents (Pederson & Smithson, 2013). The Mumsnet Talk discussion forum can be viewed by any internet user, but only Mumsnet account holders can participate in the discussion. In a study of the content posted under the Talk discussion page titled 'Child Mental Health', the reasons parents posted on the forum were grouped into three main themes: emotional support, emotional expression, and advice and information (Croucher, Mertan, Shafran, & Bennett, 2020). Posts expressed a need for emotional support and provided emotional support, with many saying that they did not get support from other sources: 'I'm not really talking to real people about this.' Parents were supported and praised by other parents, commenting that 'your son is lucky to have you on side and it's great that you're seeking advice'. Many parents used the forum as a place to express their difficulties, for example, 'I'm just going to use this as a place to vent and write everything down', 'I've admitted I'm not coping very well with it'. Importantly, a number of parents asked for advice or information about their child's difficulties and/or how to navigate the health system to access support: 'Anybody got any ideas on how I help and support her?', 'Has anyone gone private for a child psychiatrist? CAMHS have an 18wk waiting list and my son is really struggling with anxiety', 'Is it something that points to potentially a condition that is diagnosable and anything I can do to improve it?' Other parents responded with advice: 'Ask your GP for a referral to your local CAMHS service', 'You could ask for the medication to be prescribed so he can manage school well but doesn't take the rest of the time'. The advice offered was compared to evidence-based guidance such as those from the UK National Institute for Health and Care Excellence (NICE). Over 58% of the knowledge exchange on the Mental Health page of the Talk forum was congruent with evidence-based clinical guidelines and only 2.9% of advice directly contradicted guidance. While this is promising, such fora have not been formally evaluated regarding their impact on child and/or parent mental health.

Challenges in implementing peer support interventions

While studies regarding peer support for parents of children with mental health problems are promising, there is a lack of quantitative evidence supporting their efficacy. There are three main concerns regarding their implementation, particularly for those groups that are not facilitated. Many of the challenges may be mitigated by offering facilitated groups with access to qualified mental health professionals, as in the Rollercoaster support group:

1. *The extent to which advice from other parents is congruent with evidence.* Although the internet forum study suggested that only a very small proportion of advice offered was not evidence based, this small percentage is important if such advice is dangerous. Many families will not know if advice is evidence based and may find it difficult to evaluate the accuracy of information.
2. *The lack of in-depth assessment.* Families accessing these peer support networks may not have had an in-depth assessment and therefore it is possible that important aspects of the child's mental health difficulties will not be detected. Low intensity interventions are typically offered by CAMHS in the UK and elsewhere following a detailed assessment with practitioners under close supervision. For example, parents in clinical practice often report 'obsessions' and the evidence-based options for assessment and treatment are very different if these are related to obsessive–compulsive disorder compared to strong interests seen in children with autism spectrum disorder.
3. *The lack of facilitated support.* In addition to concerns about the accuracy of advice offered, there may be other risks to unfacilitated groups. Parents and young people may make close bonds with other members in the group. In fora designed to support children with mental health problems or their parents, it is likely that very difficult situations may arise. For example, there may be

safeguarding issues, young people may feel suicidal, may self-harm, or be admitted to inpatient care. In such situations, other parents may feel responsible for supporting the family, or may feel guilty that they did not provide the right advice at the right time. Parents may frighten each other and worry more about their own child's circumstances, which could in turn have an adverse effect on their own health and well-being. This issue may be compounded in fora such as Mumsnet in which users are anonymous and therefore where it is more difficult for services to be alerted if required.

4. *Other difficulties.* As in other therapies, peer support may have adverse effects (see Chapter 6). It may be that other difficulties arise particularly relating to the format of online peer support, for example, conflicts may arise, which may escalate with no facilitation. Some of these difficulties may be mitigated by having professional support.

What is the future?

Considering the lack of in-depth assessment and concerns around the accuracy of information offered, it is likely that these types of support should be offered in addition to, and not in place of, traditional mental health services. They may be offered while young people are on the waiting list for treatment, for example. A brief questionnaire while on the waiting list may help families access the right support from the right peer support groups for them. Further research is needed to investigate the extent to which families agree with and/or act on any advice provided in the peer support networks and to investigate how they understand and process difficult situations arising in the groups. There is little research into either the effectiveness of such groups in improving child and/or parent mental health, the implications of different ways of delivery (online versus in person), and mechanisms of action and these should all be explored further.

Chapter summary

There is a clear need for support for families outside of traditional formal mental health services, given significant problems accessing interventions and navigating mental health services. Peer support groups, particularly those online, may have a number of advantages and are well received by parents who participate. They can be used for emotional support and expression as well as places to receive and provide advice, and research should investigate their efficacy in supporting parents while children are on waiting lists for assessment and/or intervention. However, the evidence base is very limited, and we need more research to identify the key mechanisms by which peer support best helps parents to achieve good outcomes for themselves and their children. We also need more guidance on the key elements and underlying principles that should shape peer support in these circumstances.

Recommended reading

Croucher, L., Mertan, E., Shafran, R., & Bennett, S. D. (2020). The use of Mumsnet by parents of young people with mental health needs: Qualitative investigation. *JMIR Mental Health, 7*(9), e18271.

Hagell, A. (2022). Key findings from an evaluation of rollercoaster: a parent support group for parents and carers of children and young people with mental health difficulties. London: Association for Young People's Health https:/ayph.org.uk/wp-content/uploads/2022/05/AYPH_Rollercoaster-Briefing-Paper.pdf

Naslund, J. A., Aschbrenner, K. A., Marsch, L. A., & Bartels, S. J. (2016). The future of mental health care: Peer-to-peer support and social media. *Epidemiology and Psychiatric Sciences, 25*(2), 113–122.

References

Ahmed, Y. A., Ahmad, M. N., Ahmad, N., & Zakaria, N. H. (2019). Social media for knowledge-sharing: A systematic literature review. *Telematics and Informatics, 37*, 72–111.

Berry, N., Lobban, F., Belousov, M., Emsley, R., Nenadic, G., & Bucci, S. (2017). #WhyWeTweetMH: Understanding why people use Twitter to discuss mental health problems. *Journal of Medical Internet Research, 19*(4), e107.

Chou, W. Y., Hunt, Y. M., Beckjord, E. B., Moser, R. P., & Hesse, B. W. (2009). Social media use in the United States: Implications for health communication. *Journal of Medical Internet Research, 11*(4), e48.

Choudhury, M. D., & De, S. (2014). Mental health discourse on reddit: Self-disclosure, social support, and anonymity. *Proceedings of the 8th International Conference on Weblogs and Social Media, 8*(1), 71–80.

Cowie, H. (2020). Peer Support. In Hupp S and Jewell J (Eds). The Encyclopedia of Child and Adolescent Development. New Jersey: Wiley.

Crenna-Jennings, W., & Hutchinson, J. (2020). *Access to child and adolescent mental health services in 2019*. London: Education Policy Institute.

Croucher, L., Mertan, E., Shafran, R., & Bennett, S. D. (2020). The Use of Mumsnet by parents of young people with mental health needs: Qualitative investigation. *JMIR Mental Health, 7*(9), e18271.

Davidson, L., Chinman, M., Kloos, B., Weingarten, R., Stayner, D., & Tebes, J. K. (1999). Peer support among individuals with severe mental illness: A review of the evidence. *Clinical Psychology Science and Practice, 6*, 165–187.

Lawlor, A., & Kirakowski, J. (2014). Online support groups for mental health: A space for challenging self-stigma or a means of social avoidance? *Computers in Human Behavior, 32*, 152–161.

Lowe, P., Powell, J., Griffiths, F., Thorogood, M., & Locock, L. (2009). Making it all normal: The role of the internet in problematic pregnancy. *Qualitative Health Research, 19*(10), 1476–1484.

Mead, S., Hilton, D., & Curtis, L. (2001). Peer support: a theoretical perspective. *Psychiatric rehabilitation journal, 25* (2), 134.

Naslund, J. A., Aschbrenner, K. A., Marsch, L. A., & Bartels, S. J. (2016). The future of mental health care: Peer-to-peer support and social media. *Epidemiology and Psychiatric Sciences, 25*(2), 113–122.

NHS Digital. (2017). Adult Psychiatric Morbidity Survey: Survey of Mental Health and Wellbeing, England, 2014. Retrieved from: https://digital.nhs.uk/data-and-information/publications/statistical/adult-psychiatric-morbidity-survey/adult-psychiatric-morbidity-survey-survey-of-mental-health-and-wellbeing-england-2014

O'Connor, E. E., & Langer, D. A. (2019). I heard it through the grapevine: Where and what parents learn about youth mental health treatments. *Journal of Clinical Psychology, 75*(4), 710–725.

Pedersen, S., & Smithson, J. (2013). Mothers with attitude—how the Mumsnet parenting forum offers space for new forms of femininity to emerge online. *Women's Studies International Forum, 38*, 97–106.

Pedersen, S., & Lupton, D. (2016). 'What are you feeling right now?' Communities of maternal feeling on Mumsnet. *Emotion, Space and Society, 26*, 57–63.

Pedersen, S., & Smithson, J. (2010). Membership and activity in an online parenting community. In R. Taiwo (Ed.), *Handbook of Research on Discourse Behavior and Digital Communication: Language Structures and Social Interaction* (pp. 83–103). Hershey, PA: IGI Global.

Reardon, T., Harvey, K., Baranowska, M., O'Brien, D., Smith, L., & Creswell, C. (2017). What do parents perceive are the barriers and facilitators to accessing psychological treatment for mental health problems in children and adolescents? A systematic review of qualitative and quantitative studies. *European Child & Adolescent Psychiatry, 26*(6), 623–647.

Repper, J., & Carter, T. (2011). A review of the literature on peer support in mental health services. *Journal of Mental Health, 20*(4), 392–411.

Rude, S. S., Gortner, E.-M., & Pennebaker, J. W. (2004). Language use of depressed and depression-vulnerable college students. *Cognition and Emotion, 18*(8), 1121–1133.

Saha, S. K., Prakash, A., & Majumder, M. (2019). 'Similar query was answered earlier': processing of patient authored text for retrieving relevant contents from health discussion forum. *Health Information Science and Systems, 7*(1), 4.

Sayal, K., Tischler, V., Coope, C., Robotham, S., Ashworth, M., Day, C., . . ., & Simonoff, E. (2010). Parental help-seeking in primary care for child and adolescent mental health concerns: Qualitative study. *British Journal of Psychiatry, 197*(6), 476–481.

Shilling, V., Morris, C., Thompson-Coon, J., Ukoumunne, O., Rogers, M., & Logan, S. (2013). Peer support for parents of children with chronic disabling conditions: A systematic review of quantitative and qualitative studies. *Developmental Medicine & Child Neurology, 55*(7), 602–609.

Young Minds. (2019). Three-quarters of young people seeking mental health support become more unwell during wait for treatment—new report. Retrieved from https://youngminds.org.uk/media/2619/ three-quarters-of-young-people-seeking-mental-health-support-become-more-unwell-during-wait-for-treatment.pdf

Zufferey, M., & Schulz, P. (2009). Self-management of chronic low back pain: An exploration of the impact of a patient-centered website. *Patient Education and Counseling, 77*, 27–32.

27

Apps for mental health problems in children and young people

Paul Stallard

Learning objectives

- To define and summarize the rationale for the use of technologically delivered mental health interventions.
- To review the use of mental health apps with children and young people and to summarize key issues in app development, content, and effectiveness.
- To highlight how mental health apps can be integrated into clinical work.

Introduction

Why do we need technologically delivered interventions (TDIs)?

Improving the mental health of children and adolescents is a global priority. While effective psychotherapeutic interventions are available, child and adolescent mental health services have limited capacity resulting in many children failing to seek, or receive, the help they require. Alternative approaches to delivering evidence-based mental health interventions at scale are required with technologically delivered interventions offering a potential way of bridging the mental health treatment gap (Bhugra et al., 2017). This may be particularly appealing to children and adolescents who are typically early adopters and vociferous users of technology.

What is a TDI?

TDI is a broad term defined as 'interventions that provide information, support and therapy (emotional, decisional, behavioural and neurocognitive) for physical and/or mental health problems via a technological or digital platform (e.g. website, computer, mobile phone application (app), SMS, email, videoconferencing, wearable device)' (Hollis et al., 2017). This definition encapsulates 'mhealth', that is, where healthcare is supported by mobile devices such as smartphones and tablets and 'ehealth' (electronic health) which includes the use of electronic patient records and electronic communication such as SMS, text, and video consultations. This review will focus on the most common TDI, mental health smartphone apps.

Apps

The number of apps available has expanded exponentially over the past 5 years. It is estimated that there are over 300,000 health apps available and of these over 10,000 are concerned with mental health. The overwhelming majority have been developed for use with adults and unfortunately few have been specifically developed for use by children and young people (Grist, Porter, & Stallard, 2017). Typically, they focus on one specific technique such as psychoeducation, assessment, or skill development and rarely contain the range of techniques which would be included in most evidence-based, multi-component interventions (Wasil, Venturo-Conerly, Shingleton, & Weisz, 2019).

Apps offer many benefits. Given the almost universal nature of the internet and smartphone usage, apps can be easily accessed by those who experience difficulties accessing traditional mental health services. Apps are a familiar technology for children and young people which can be directly accessed without necessitating a referral or registering personal information. They offer convenience, and can be used when and where the child would like, and are available 24/7.

Apps can be directly accessed and used without additional professional support. They might focus on specific techniques, such as emotional expression (e.g. Cove, an app for creating music to express feelings), controlled breathing (e.g. Chill Panda, which uses smartphone cameras to capture heart rate, asks children and adults to rate their mood, and supports people to take part in 'playful tasks and activities, including breathing and light exercise'), or emotional management (e.g. Smiling Mind, a meditation app with tailored programmes for different age groups), or teach skills to help children become more resilient (e.g. ThinkNinja, an app based on CBT principles including a chatbot 'virtual coach', goal setting, mood rating, and cognitive and behavioural strategies to manage stress, negative thoughts, difficult feelings, and to learn to relax and improve sleep). They can also be used as part of a professionally guided mental health intervention, providing a readily accessible tool to use at times of crisis (e.g. BlueIce, an app to help young people manage their emotions and reduce urges to self-harm through a mood diary, toolbox of evidence-based techniques to reduce distress, and automatic routing to emergence numbers if urges to harm continue). Apps can also be used for assessment, for example, to monitor mood (Daylio), or to offer support/contact with others (e.g. For Me, the UK Childline app).

The ubiquitous nature of mobile phones and the internet alongside the ready availability of mental health apps will result in their widespread use, particularly among adolescents. This highlights three key implications for clinicians.

Firstly, apps and internet usage need to be discussed during assessment. Be curious and ask what apps the young person has used, what they found helpful/unhelpful and whether there are any others they would like to use? This allows any shortfalls or inaccuracies to be corrected and offers opportunities to suggest apps with robust content or stronger evidence.

Secondly, apps can be integrated within clinical practice to provide a blended care approach that utilizes the benefits of TDIs within the context of a responsive therapeutic relationship. They can be particularly helpful for introducing and practising particular skills such as mindfulness (e.g. Headspace) or distress management (e.g. Calm Harm).

Thirdly, a discussion about apps can be used as a relationship-strengthening activity, providing the adolescent with the opportunity to share their knowledge. Given the huge number of apps that are available, it will be impossible for clinicians to keep up to date with what young people are using. Take the opportunity to empower adolescents and learn from them about the apps they find helpful.

Challenges of smartphone apps

While offering many benefits, there are a number of concerns about app content, privacy, responsiveness, effects on subsequent help seeking, usage, and effectiveness.

In terms of content, the overwhelming majority have been developed by the media industry for commercial reasons, often without any user or clinical input. Apps are not regulated, with reviews finding that some contain inaccurate or indeed harmful content (Anthes, 2016; Huckvale, Nicholas, Torous, & Larsen, 2020). Concerns have also been identified about security and how personal data is saved, transmitted, and used, with many apps breaching the users' privacy. In addition, there are concerns about safety and how apps might respond to adverse events such as suicidal ideation or self-harm. Most are based on standard algorithms and do not respond flexibly and safely to such events.

In terms of help-seeking, the use of apps could delay this, a particular concern if problems are chronic or severe. Their use may also adversely affect future help-seeking and engagement. An app may profess to be based on a particular approach but contain limited therapeutic content, potentially tarnishing attitudes towards future engagement with such an approach.

A further challenge is the usage of apps with many being used only one or twice, usually after download. The majority are self-directed and require motivation and commitment. This may be challenging for children and young people particularly if they are ambivalent about acknowledging a difficulty or embarking on a process of change.

However, most importantly, the development of apps has significantly outpaced the evidence to demonstrate their effectiveness. Despite thousands of apps being available, only a handful have any evidence to demonstrate their benefits and at present it is only possible to conclude that they appear promising (Gist, Porter, & Stallard, 2017; Punukollu & Marques, 2019; Wang, Varma, & Prosperi, 2018).

Finally, while access to digital technologies is almost universal, some people and age groups lack confidence or digital literacy, may not have access to the internet, or may choose not to engage with technology. The clinician needs to be mindful of the digital divide.

Potential solutions

In terms of safety, in the UK, the NHS app library provides a thorough assessment of apps and online programmes although relatively few have gone through this process. Alternatively, app review sites such as ORCHA (https://www.orcha.co.uk), Health Navigator (https://www.healthnavigator.org.nz/apps/m/mental-health-and-wellbeing-apps/) or PsyberGuide (https://psyberguide.org/), offer independent reviews although they may not necessarily check the accuracy of app content.

The proliferation of commercially developed apps has highlighted the need to include professionals and end users in the development and design process. This would ensure that the content is evidence based and that apps meet end users' needs (Bevan-Jones et al., 2020: Wang et al., 2018). An example of a self-harm app that has met these criteria is BlueIce (Stallard, Porter, & Grist, 2018). BlueIce was co-designed with young people with a lived experience of self-harm. A series of workshops explored the concept, design, and appearance while workshops with clinicians ensured that content was evidence based.

In terms of effectiveness, given that many apps focus on one specific technique, if the content is accurate, it is debatable whether a robust, costly, time-consuming scientific evaluation is required. However, this would be essential for those that claim to be 'mental health interventions'. Nonetheless, at the very least it is important for apps to demonstrate that they are safe, do no harm, are acceptable, and are helpful for users.

What is the future?

Mental health apps are here to stay. It is important that clinicians embrace their use and find ways to integrate them into their clinical work. The blended approach, whereby apps are used alongside face-to-face interventions to augment and teach specific skills works well for those with more significant mental health problems. From a public health perspective, those with robust content and user appeal could be widely promoted. In the future, apps will inevitably become more sophisticated with, for example, the use of real-time sensors being able to independently monitor changes in mood or behaviour. While such developments offer the opportunity to be responsive to those in need, it also highlights the need to address the privacy, security, and safety issues identified earlier.

Chapter summary

Smartphone apps are the most accessible of all the TDIs and yet the evidence for their impact on mental health is scant. Given their widespread use, professionals should routinely ask what apps a young person has used, highlight any limitations, and correct any inaccuracies of content. Apps can be integrated within traditional clinical practice and are particularly useful for sharing information and introducing skills.

Recommended reading

Anthes, E. (2016). Mental health: There's an app for that. *Nature*, 532(7597), 20.

Grist, R., Porter, J., & Stallard, P. (2017). Mental health mobile apps for preadolescents and adolescents: A systematic review. *Journal of Medical Internet Research*, 19(5), e176.

References

Bevan Jones, R., Stallard, P., Agha, S. S., Rice, S., Werner-Seidler, A., Stasiak, K., . . ., & Evans, R. (2020). Practitioner review: Co-design of digital mental health technologies with children and young people. *Journal of Child Psychology and Psychiatry*, 61(8), 928–940.

Bhugra, D., Tasman, A., Pathare, S., Priebe, S., Smith, S., Torous, J., . . ., & Ventriglio, A. (2017). The WPA-Lancet Psychiatry Commission on the future of psychiatry. *Lancet Psychiatry*, 4(10), 775–818.

Grist, R., Croker, A., Denne, M., & Stallard, P. (2019). Technology delivered interventions for depression and anxiety in children and adolescents: A systematic review and meta-analysis. *Clinical Child and Family Psychology Review*, 22(2), 147–171.

Hollis, C., Falconer, C. J., Martin, J. L., Whittington, C., Stockton, S., Glazebrook, C., & Davies, E. B. (2017). Annual research review: Digital health interventions for children and young people with mental health problems—a systematic and meta-review. *Journal of Child Psychology and Psychiatry*, 58(4), 474–503.

Huckvale, K., Nicholas, J., Torous, J., & Larsen, M. E. (2020). Smartphone apps for the treatment of mental health conditions: Status and considerations. *Current Opinion in Psychology*, 36, 65–70.

Punukollu, M., & Marques, M. (2019). Use of mobile apps and technologies in child and adolescent mental health: A systematic review. *Evidence-Based Mental Health*, 22(4), 161–166.

Stallard, P., Porter, J., & Grist, R. (2018). A smartphone app (BlueIce) for young people who self-harm: Open phase 1 pre-post trial. *JMIR mHealth and uHealth*, 6(1), e32.

Wang, K., Varma, D. S., & Prosperi, M. (2018). A systematic review of the effectiveness of mobile apps for monitoring and management of mental health symptoms or disorders. *Journal of Psychiatric Research*, 107, 73–78.

Wasil, A. R., Venturo-Conerly, K. E., Shingleton, R. M., & Weisz, J. R. (2019). A review of popular smartphone apps for depression and anxiety: Assessing the inclusion of evidence-based content. *Behaviour Research and Therapy*, 123, 103498.

FIRST

An efficient intervention for youths with multiple mental health problems

Olivia Fitzpatrick, Abby Bailin, Katherine Venturo-Conerly, Melissa Wei, and John Weisz

Learning objectives

- To understand examples of research on youth psychiatric disorder comorbidity.
- To consider how efficient interventions can be adapted to address the needs of youths with multiple mental health problems, with a focus on FIRST.
- To identify benefits and challenges—and potential solutions to these challenges—in implementing FIRST.

Introduction

Across recent decades, numerous evidence-based psychotherapies (EBPs) for children and adolescents (herein 'youths') have been developed, with many demonstrating beneficial effects in research trials (Weisz, Bearman, Santucci, & Jensen-Doss, 2017; Weisz, Vaughn-Coaxum, et al., 2020). Most of these EBPs for youth mental health difficulties are *focal treatments*—designed to address one specific disorder or problem domain (e.g. obsessive–compulsive disorder, conduct problems). These focal EBPs offer important advantages, providing an avenue through which specialty mental healthcare can be provided to young people with specific treatment needs (Comer & Barlow, 2014). Along with these benefits, focal treatments may have limitations for youths with multiple mental health problems, like many who are treated in community-based settings (Merikangas et al., 2010). A number of the focal EBPs are also rather linear in design, with a sequence of sessions designed to be delivered in a relatively consistent, prescribed order. This can be a valuable approach for some youths, but perhaps less so for the substantial number for whom mental health problems and treatment needs fluctuate frequently. An additional challenge faced by some EBPs may be the number of sessions required to complete treatment. Across the array of tested youth psychotherapy protocols, the average number of prescribed sessions is 16 (Weisz,

Kuppens, et al., 2017). In contrast, episodes of care tend to be briefer, with some evidence indicating that youths in treatment attend an average of 3.9 sessions (Harpaz-Rotem, Leslie, & Rosenheck, 2004). To be clear, there are key advantages to focused, linear, and sometimes lengthy treatments, and their development has substantially improved intervention science. However, there may also be a need to complement these approaches with treatments designed for youths with multiple mental health problems and frequently fluctuating treatment needs, and who may not stay in treatment very long.

Transdiagnostic and multi-diagnostic interventions

One such complementary approach is seen in protocols that target *multiple* mental health problems among youths (e.g. Chorpita & Weisz, 2009; Ehrenreich, Goldstein, Wright, & Barlow, 2009; Weisz & Bearman, 2020). This strategy aligns with psychotherapies that are considered *multi-diagnostic*—featuring a modular menu of different therapeutic skills for multiple disorders (e.g. cognitive restructuring for depression, rewards-based behaviour management for conduct problems)—or *transdiagnostic*—featuring a menu of therapeutic skills that can be flexibly applied across various disorders (e.g. relaxation skills for anxiety, depression, or conduct problems). In recent years, several multi-diagnostic and transdiagnostic protocols have been developed for youth mental health difficulties and have shown clinical benefits in research studies, including Modular Approach to Therapy for Children with Anxiety, Depression, Trauma, or Conduct Problems (MATCH; Chorpita et al., 2017; Chorpita & Weisz, 2009; Weisz et al., 2012; but see also Merry et al., 2020; Weisz, Bearman, et al., 2020) and the Unified Protocols for Transdiagnostic Treatment of Emotional Disorders in Children & Adolescents (UP-C/A; Ehrenreich et al., 2009; Ehrenreich-May et al., 2017; García-Escalera et al., 2020). Although these and other multi-diagnostic and transdiagnostic protocols are important additions to the array of available treatment options, and there is evidence supporting their benefits, there may be advantages to further adjustments in treatment design.

In the case of MATCH, for example, we have wondered if the level of complexity might pose an implementation challenge for some clinicians, particularly those who are unfamiliar with EBPs or have relatively little clinical experience (Weisz, Ng, & Bearman, 2014). This question is highlighted by the findings of two recent MATCH trials (Merry et al., 2020; Weisz, Bearman, et al., 2020), in which the level of weekly expert consultation provided to therapists implementing MATCH was reduced from the weekly *individual* consultation provided in the two initial and successful trials (Chorpita et al., 2017; Weisz et al., 2012) to weekly *group* supervision. In the trials with reduced implementation support, MATCH did not outperform usual clinical care on most clinical outcomes. Taken together, results of the four MATCH trials suggest the possibility that MATCH can work well when it has rather intensive implementation support, but perhaps not as well when support is reduced to a level closer to what might be available in everyday clinical care. It is possible that a transdiagnostic treatment protocol that is briefer, simpler in structure, and designed for efficiency in clinician training and uptake, might improve prospects for effective implementation by some clinicians in practice settings. We think it would be ideal for such a protocol to address both internalizing and externalizing problems, as MATCH does, given evidence that youths often present with both types of difficulties (Merikangas et al., 2010); protocols that are equipped to flexibly target challenges across these domains might offer benefits for a wider range of youths. We now shift to describing a treatment protocol that aims to address these challenges: FIRST (Weisz & Bearman, 2020).

Description of and evidence for FIRST

FIRST, which is the main focus of this chapter, is a transdiagnostic, individual intervention that targets depression, anxiety, post-traumatic stress, and misbehaviour in children and young people. FIRST is guided by five empirically supported principles of therapeutic change. Each of these principles is represented by a letter in FIRST: Feeling calm, Increasing motivation, Repairing thoughts, Solving problems, and Trying the opposite (Weisz & Bearman, 2020). These principles, which are described below, were selected in the design of FIRST because they have been included in multiple tested psychotherapies for various problems and disorders, and each has shown significant effects when used as a standalone treatment (Weisz, Hawley, & Jensen-Doss, 2004; Weisz & Bearman, 2020).

- *Feeling calm* includes self-calming and relaxation techniques (e.g. progressive muscle relaxation, deep breathing).
- *Increasing motivation* captures the use of environmental contingencies (e.g. differential attention, praise) to reward adaptive behaviour more than maladaptive behaviour.
- *Repairing thoughts* focuses on the identification and modification of biased, distorted, and unhelpful cognitions (e.g. self-blaming thoughts, overestimations of threat).
- *Solving problems* involves learning and practising sequential problem-solving (e.g. identify the problem, identify solutions, weigh the pros and cons of each solution).
- *Trying the opposite* captures engagement in activities that directly counter the behavioural problem (e.g. graduated exposure, behavioural activation, practising adaptive responses to interpersonal conflicts).

FIRST has been tested in three open trials in community settings. In the initial trial, Weisz, Bearman, et al. (2017) tested FIRST in community outpatient clinics with clinically referred youths (ages 7–15) presenting with an array of mental health difficulties. Clinicians employed in the clinics participated in 2 days of training, followed by weekly group consultation meetings. On average, youths attended 18.63 (standard deviation (SD) = 13.05, range = 2–59) sessions. Two additional open benchmarking trials were conducted by Cho, Bearman, Woo, Weisz, and Hawley (2021) in an outpatient clinic staffed by trainees, with treatment duration limited to six sessions. On average, youths attended 5.68 (SD = 0.89) and 5.00 (SD = 1.81) sessions, respectively. The slopes of change in outcome measures in the FIRST trials were benchmarked against slopes for MATCH (Chorpita et al., 2017; Weisz et al., 2012); FIRST slopes were quite similar to those of MATCH, with MATCH outcomes stronger on standardized checklist measures, and FIRST outcomes stronger than MATCH on our functional measure severity ratings (Top Problems Assessment (TPA); Weisz et al., 2011) and on percentage reduction in number of diagnoses based on standardized assessments (60% reduction via FIRST; 51% via MATCH). In a follow-up study with FIRST therapists in our initial trial, 92% reported that understanding the FIRST principles increased their clinical confidence and competence and made them want to continue using the intervention with patients on their own. In a follow-up study of clinicians in the second two trials, 67% reported continuing to use FIRST after the research had ended (Bearman, Bailin, Terry, & Weisz, 2020). See Box 28.1 for a case study of FIRST.

Implementation challenges: FIRST

Despite the promise of FIRST and other transdiagnostic treatments, there are several challenges in delivering these protocols, some of which are unique to transdiagnostic interventions and some of which are universal across psychotherapies. As with all treatments, one challenge is that clinicians must decide which presenting problem(s) to address, and in which order, during therapy; this can be particularly difficult when youths endorse a range of mental health difficulties. Next, given the flexibility of FIRST, especially compared to protocols that require treatment techniques to be delivered in a prescribed sequence, clinicians are faced with selecting the principle(s), and the order in which these principle(s) are presented, that might be most helpful in addressing the problems for which families are seeking treatment. As with most psychotherapies, not all youths respond to the FIRST principles in the same way. With this in mind, clinicians are often tasked with determining how to address unexpected responses to the FIRST principle(s) that they assigned a given patient (e.g. the assigned principle does not result in symptom improvement; the patient does not like or is unwilling to engage with the principle). Lastly, another common challenge faced by clinicians across treatment protocols, but which might be enhanced by the flexibility of FIRST, is deciding when to terminate treatment. More specifically, treatment timelines are baked into protocols that feature a set number of sessions, whereas FIRST enables clinicians to flexibly decide how many sessions might

---

Box 28.1 Case study: FIRST

Luke was an 11-year-old white, Hispanic boy who presented with his mother to outpatient services in an urban area of the US. He presented with internalizing (e.g. irritability, depressed mood, and withdrawal from family) and externalizing (e.g. verbal aggression, disobedience, and non-compliance with house rules/chores) problems. During the 45-minute intake, the licensed marriage and family therapist collected a broad symptom measure from Luke and his mother (i.e. Child Behavior Checklist; Achenbach & Rescorla, 2001) and conducted a semi-structured interview that included an assessment of the problems that Luke and his mother each wanted to address in therapy (i.e. TPA; Weisz et al., 2011). Monitoring of Luke's response to treatment was assessed prior to each weekly 45-minute session via youth and caregiver ratings of the severity of top problems and a brief assessment of internalizing and externalizing symptoms (i.e. Behavior and Feelings Survey (BFS); Weisz, Vaughn-Coaxum, et al., 2020). The FIRST decision tree for misbehaviour with a caregiver focus was initiated to establish an environment that reinforced desired behaviours. Following rapport-building and psychoeducation with Luke's mother, the therapist introduced *Increasing motivation*, teaching and practising strategies to increase desired behaviours, including youth-led interaction, active attending (i.e. noticing/praising desired behaviours like completing chores), differential attention (i.e. active attending to desired behaviours like using 'appropriate language' combined with removal of attention from undesired behaviours like 'talking back'), and tangible rewards. After six sessions, Luke's mother reported decreased externalizing symptoms (e.g. talking back/arguing) and increased compliance (e.g. completion of house chores), as well as ongoing internalizing symptoms (e.g. irritability, withdrawal). These data informed the therapist's decision to switch the focus of treatment to address Luke's comorbid depression. The therapist initiated the FIRST decision tree for depression and began meeting weekly with Luke, with ongoing check ins with his mother. The therapist implemented *Trying the opposite*, highlighting the goal to engage in activities that countered his behavioural problems (i.e. withdrawal from family, avoiding homework) via behavioural activation and positive activity scheduling. In the next three 45-minute weekly sessions, Luke practised mood monitoring and in-session mood boosters and built a hierarchy of activities that he had been avoiding (e.g. homework, family dinners). Activities were scheduled and assigned for between-session practice. Concurrently, the therapist supported Luke's mother in using positive attention and tangible rewards to reinforce completion of these activities. By the 11th and 12th sessions, Luke reported improvements in internalizing symptoms, including feeling less irritable and depressed. He and his mother also reported increased homework completion, reduced time spent alone in his room, and reduced familial conflict. With progress towards Luke's top problems and a reduction in both externalizing and internalizing symptoms, treatment concluded after 12 sessions.

be feasible and necessary for their patients. With this flexibility comes additional opportunities for clinical decision-making, to which we now turn.

Potential solutions

There are several ways in which clinicians can address the implementation challenges outlined above and, ultimately, these decisions must be guided by clinical judgement. However, we provide broad recommendations stemming from the FIRST protocol below:

Which problems need to be addressed and in which order?

We recommend administering the TPA (Weisz et al., 2011) and the BFS (Weisz, Vaughn-Coaxum, et al., 2020), which are freely available on our website, prior to and weekly throughout therapy to determine which problems are most pressing for families. Through the TPA (an idiographic measure), youths and their caregivers are separately asked, at baseline, to identify up to three of the top problems that they would like to target during therapy and then rate each problem on a scale from 0 (not a problem) to 4 (a very big problem). The TPA can be complemented with the BFS, which is a brief, 12-item, standardized instrument that captures the severity (0 = not a problem; 4 = a very big problem) of internalizing and externalizing problems among youths. Using these tools in tandem, clinicians can better understand which problems might be most important to prioritize during treatment.

Which principle(s) can be used to address these problems and in which order?

Although each patient is different and treatment should be personalized accordingly, we recommend a general treatment sequence for youths based on their primary presenting problem. For youths with depression, we advise beginning with, or working toward, *Trying the opposite* (behavioural activation). For youths of all ages with primary misbehaviour, we advise beginning with, or working towards, *Increasing motivation* if caregivers are involved, or *Solving problems* if caregivers are not involved. For youths with anxiety or post-traumatic stress, we advise beginning with, or working toward, *Trying the opposite*. Of note, not every patient will be ready to start treatment with the recommended principle; this is why we use the language *beginning with or working towards*. For some youths, it will be most effective to begin with a principle that serves as the foundation for future principles, is more quickly mastered, and/or targets a specific aspect of the presenting problem (e.g. a youth seeking treatment for misbehaviour, and who experiences anger arousal, may benefit from learning quick-calming skills before problem-solving). These decisions ultimately require clinical judgement, and it is helpful to remember that each of the principles can be flexibly applied to a variety of presentations and at different points throughout treatment.

What if a patient does not respond to a given principle as desired?

Sometimes, patients may not respond as expected to the assigned principle, in which case clinicians can try a few options. For example, if the patient does not like the principle or is unwilling to try it, clinicians might consider employing motivational interviewing techniques to increase engagement or, if that does not work, revisiting the decision tree to find an alternative principle that might fit, or revisiting the TPA completed at the beginning of treatment to identify another top problem that might be addressed via a different principle. If the patient is open to using a principle, but it doesn't seem to be improving symptoms and functioning, clinicians might consider presenting the principle in a different way to enhance patient understanding and flexible use of the strategies. Any time a patient does not respond as expected to the assigned principle, clinicians are encouraged to use the TPA as a tool to help patients understand concrete ways in which they can apply the principle being discussed to the specific problems they would like to address in therapy. A continuing challenge, for which better empirical guidance is needed, is deciding—when a youth is not responding to a particular principle—whether to persevere and try different methods of making that principle work or shift to another principle.

When should treatment be terminated?

Given that FIRST is intentionally flexible, with no set end date, clinicians can decide, in collaboration with families, when to terminate treatment based on the needs of each patient. Ending treatment is often not completed in just one meeting, and it can be helpful to identify specific goals that will indicate when the youth is ready to end treatment (e.g. mastery of skills learned, reduced symptoms). Administering the TPA and BFS consistently throughout treatment (e.g. weekly) is one way to track patient progress, ultimately offering information on whether symptoms and functioning appear to be improving across the course of therapy. It is important to note that some patients may be ready to end treatment after learning just one principle, whereas others may require a few more tools in their toolbox before terminating treatment. Regardless of the number of principles used, it can be helpful for clinicians to terminate treatment when caregivers and youths show expertise, mastery, and confidence in the strategies necessary to maintain gains autonomously.

Future directions

Future research may focus on increasing access to and improving clinician decision-making in transdiagnostic mental health interventions. Several recent studies have shown that brief, transdiagnostic interventions delivered via digital platforms may be effective for youths with multiple mental health problems (e.g. Osborn et al., 2020; Schleider & Weisz, 2018). Additionally, some efficient interventions have been developed for alternative delivery settings, such as in schools (e.g. Michelson et al., 2019), and using alternative delivery methods, such as employing lay-providers instead of mental health professionals (e.g. Osborn et al., 2019). Future research may refine and extend these approaches to make interventions for youths with multiple mental health problems more widely accessible. Additionally, clinicians must make many decisions throughout intervention (e.g. which problem to target first, which module to apply, when to switch to another module, when to terminate treatment), especially in modular treatments (e.g. FIRST). Future research should empirically investigate how different treatment decisions affect clinical outcomes.

Chapter summary

Most youths receiving community-based mental healthcare have multiple difficulties and will terminate treatment early. Thus, interventions that can efficiently target several, frequently fluctuating treatment needs might be appropriate for these youths. One such approach is FIRST, an efficient, transdiagnostic intervention grounded in evidence-based principles of therapeutic change. The current chapter outlines some benefits, challenges, and potential solutions to these challenges of delivering FIRST.

Recommended measures

We recommend two measures ideal for frequent (e.g. weekly) assessments:

- TPA (Weisz et al., 2011).
- BFS (Weisz, Vaughn-Coaxum, et al., 2020).

Both of these measures are freely available on our website (https://weiszlab.fas.harv ard.edu/measures), along with supporting materials (e.g. the TPA administration manual).

Recommended reading

Articles outlining the FIRST trials

Cho, E., Bearman, S. K., Woo, R., Weisz, J. R., & Hawley, K. M. (2021). A second and third look at FIRST: Testing adaptations of a principle-guided youth psychotherapy. *Journal of Clinical Child and Adolescent Psychology*, 50(6), 919–932.

Weisz, J. R., Bearman, S. K., Santucci, L. C., & Jensen-Doss, A. (2017). Initial test of a principle-guided approach to transdiagnostic psychotherapy with children and adolescents. *Journal of Clinical Child & Adolescent Psychology*, 46(1), 44–58.

The FIRST manual

Weisz, J. R., & Bearman, S. K. (2020). *Principle-guided psychotherapy for children and adolescents: The FIRST treatment program for behavioral and emotional problems*. New York: Guilford Press.

References

Achenbach, T. M., & Rescorla, L. A. (2001). *Manual for the ASEBA school-age forms & profiles*. Burlington, VT: University of Vermont, Research Center for Children, Youth, and Families.

Bearman, S. K., Bailin, A., Terry, R., & Weisz, J. R. (2020). After the study ends: Sustaining evidence-based practices for youth in services as usual settings. *Professional Psychology: Research and Practice*, 51(2), 134–144.

Cho, E., Bearman, S. K., Woo, R., Weisz, J. R., & Hawley, K. M. (2021). A second and third look at FIRST: Testing adaptations of a principle-guided youth psychotherapy. *Journal of Clinical Child and Adolescent Psychology*, 50(6), 919–932.

Chorpita, B. F., Daleiden, E. L., Park, A. L., Ward, A. M., Levy, M. C., Cromley, T., . . ., & Krull, J. L. (2017). Child STEPs in California: A cluster randomized effectiveness trial comparing modular treatment with community implemented treatment for youth with anxiety, depression, conduct problems, or traumatic stress. *Journal of Consulting and Clinical Psychology*, 85(1), 13–25.

Chorpita, B. F., & Weisz, J. R. (2009). *Modular Approach to Therapy for Children with Anxiety, Depression, Trauma, or Conduct Problems (MATCH-ADTC)*. Satellite Beach, FL: PracticeWise, LLC.

Comer, J. S., & Barlow, D. H. (2014). The occasional case against broad dissemination and implementation: Retaining a role for specialty care in the delivery of psychological treatments. *American Psychologist*, 69(1), 1–18.

Ehrenreich, J. T., Goldstein, C. M., Wright, L. R., & Barlow, D. H. (2009). Development of a unified protocol for the treatment of emotional disorders in youth. *Child & Family Behavior Therapy*, 31(1), 20–37.

Ehrenreich-May, J., Rosenfield, D., Queen, A. H., Kennedy, S. M., Remmes, C. S., & Barlow, D. H. (2017). An initial waitlist-controlled trial of the unified protocol for the treatment of emotional disorders in adolescents. *Journal of Anxiety Disorders*, 46, 46–55.

García-Escalera, J., Valiente, R. M., Sandín, B., Ehrenreich-May, J., Prieto, A., & Chorot, P. (2020). The unified protocol for transdiagnostic treatment of emotional disorders in adolescents (UP-A) adapted as a school-based anxiety and depression prevention program: An initial cluster randomized wait-list-controlled trial. *Behavior Therapy*, 51(3), 461–473.

Harpaz-Rotem, I., Leslie, D., & Rosenheck, R.A. (2004). Treatment retention among children entering a new episode of mental health care. *Psychiatric Services*, 55(9), 1022–1028.

Merikangas, K. R., He, J. P., Burstein, M., Swanson, S. A., Avenevoli, S., Cui, L., . . ., & Swendsen, J. (2010). Lifetime prevalence of mental disorders in U.S. adolescents: Results from the National Comorbidity

Survey Replication—Adolescent Supplement (NCS-A). *Journal of the American Academy of Child and Adolescent Psychiatry, 49*(10), 980–989.

Merry, S. N., Hopkins, S., Lucassen, M. F. G., Stasiak, K., Weisz, J. R., Frampton, C. M. A., . . ., & Crengle, S. (2020). Clinician training in the Modular Approach to Therapy for Children to enhance the use of empirically supported treatments and clinical outcomes: A randomized clinical trial. *JAMA Psychiatry Open, 3*(8), e2011799.

Michelson, D., Malik, K., Krishna, M., Sharma, R., Mathur, S., Bhat, B., . . ., & Patel, V. (2019). Development of a transdiagnostic, low-intensity, psychological intervention for common adolescent mental health problems in Indian secondary schools. *Behaviour Research and Therapy, 130*, 103439.

Osborn, T. L., Rodriguez, M., Wasil, A. R., Venturo-Conerly, K. E., Gau, J., Alemu, R. G., . . ., & Weisz, J.R. (2020). Single-session digital intervention for adolescent depression, anxiety and well-being: Outcomes of a randomized controlled trial with Kenyan adolescents. *Journal of Consulting and Clinical Psychology, 88*(7), 657–668.

Osborn, T., Wasil, A., Venturo-Conerly, K., Schleider, J., & Weisz, J. (2019). Group intervention for adolescent anxiety and depression: Outcomes of a randomized trial with adolescents in Kenya. *Behavior Therapy, 51*(4), 601–615.

Schleider, J., & Weisz, J. (2018). A single-session growth mindset intervention for adolescent anxiety and depression: 9-month outcomes of a randomized trial. *Journal of Child Psychology and Psychiatry, 59*(2), 160–170.

Weisz, J. R., & Bearman, S. K. (2020). *Principle-guided psychotherapy for children and adolescents: The FIRST treatment program for behavioral and emotional problems.* New York: Guilford Press.

Weisz, J. R., Bearman, S. K., Santucci, L. C., & Jensen-Doss, A. (2017). Initial test of a principle-guided approach to transdiagnostic psychotherapy with children and adolescents. *Journal of Clinical Child & Adolescent Psychology, 46*(1), 44–58.

Weisz, J. R., Bearman, S. K., Ugueto, A. M., Herren, J. A., Evans, S. C., Cheron, D. M., . . ., & Jensen-Doss, A. (2020). Testing the robustness of Child STEPs effects with children and adolescents: A randomized controlled effectiveness trial. *Journal of Clinical Child and Adolescent Psychology, 49*(6), 883–896.

Weisz, J. R., Chorpita, B. F., Frye, A., Ng, M. Y., Lau, N., Bearman, S. K., . . ., & Research Network on Youth MH. (2011). Youth top problems: Using idiographic, consumer-guided assessment to identify treatment needs and track change during psychotherapy. *Journal of Consulting and Clinical Psychology, 79*(3), 369–380.

Weisz, J. R., Chorpita, B. F., Palinkas, L. A., Schoenwald, S. K., Miranda, J., Bearman, S. K., . . ., & Research Network on Youth MH. (2012). Testing standard and modular designs for psychotherapy treating depression, anxiety, and conduct problems in youth: A randomized effectiveness trial. *Archives of General Psychiatry, 69*(3), 274–282.

Weisz, J. R., Hawley, K. M., & Jensen Doss, A. (2004). Empirically tested psychotherapies for youth internalizing and externalizing problems and disorders. *Youth and Adolescent Psychiatric Clinics of North America, 13*, 729–816.

Weisz, J. R., Kuppens, S., Ng, M. Y., Eckshtain, D., Ugueto, A. M., Vaughn-Coaxum, R., . . ., & Fordwood, S. R. (2017). What five decades of research tells us about the effects of youth psychological therapy: A multilevel meta-analysis and implications for science and practice. *American Psychologist, 72*(2), 79–117.

Weisz, J. R., Kuppens, S., Ng, M. Y., Vaughn-Coaxum, R. A., Ugueto, A. M., Eckshtain, D., & Corteselli, K. A. (2019). Are psychotherapies for young people growing stronger? Tracking trends over time for youth anxiety, depression, attention-deficit/hyperactivity disorder, and conduct problems. *Perspectives on Psychological Science, 14*(2), 216–237.

Weisz, J. R., Ng, M. Y., & Bearman, S. K. (2014). Odd couple? Reenvisioning the relation between science and practice in the dissemination-implementation era. *Clinical Psychological Science, 2*(1), 58–74.

Weisz, J. R., Vaughn-Coaxum, R. A., Evans, S. C., Thomassin, K., Hersh, J. Lee, E. H., . . ., & Mair, P. (2020). Efficient monitoring of treatment response during youth psychotherapy: The behavior and feelings survey. *Journal of Clinical Child and Adolescent Psychology, 49*(6), 737–751.

Glossary

Asynchronous Not existing or occurring at the same time. In low intensity therapy, this may refer to interventions in which elements are delivered separately; for example, the book/worksheets/online materials may be used at a different time to any guidance provided by a practitioner.

Bibliotherapy The use of books/reading materials as therapy in the treatment of mental health difficulties.

Cognitive restructuring A technique used in cognitive therapy and cognitive behaviour therapy to help the client identify their unhelpful beliefs or cognitive distortions, refute them, and then modify them so that they are adaptive and reasonable.

Condition-specific indicators A set of symptoms relating to a specific mental health diagnosis.

Cost–utility thresholds Cut-off points relating to monetary costs versus the potential benefits of the intervention, often measured in increased quality of life years.

Dissemination The process of sharing research findings with stakeholders and wider audiences.

Effect size Measures of the magnitude or meaningfulness of a relationship between two variables. For example, Cohen's d shows the number of standard deviation units between two means. Often, effect sizes are interpreted as indicating the practical significance of a research finding.

Expectancy effects The effect of one person's expectation about the behaviour of another person on the actual behaviour of that other person (interpersonal expectancy effect), or the effect of a person's expectation about his or her own behaviour on that person's actual subsequent behaviour (intrapersonal expectancy effect). Other types include experimenter expectancy effect defined as a researcher's expectations about the findings of his or her research which are inadvertently conveyed to participants and influence their responses.

Exposure response prevention A form of therapy for obsessive–compulsive disorder, involving exposure to situations or cues that trigger recurrent, intrusive, and distressing thoughts (obsessions) or provoke repetitive behaviours (compulsions), followed by abstinence from the compulsive behaviour.

Fear hierarchy Also known as an exposure hierarchy. A treatment plan that lists out specific situations or feared stimuli the patient will gradually confront during exposure therapy.

Fidelity The degree of exactness with which something is copied or reproduced, in this context the extent to which delivery of a protocol/intervention is the same across clients.

Focal treatment A form of brief psychotherapy in which a single problem is made the target of the entire course of treatment.

Gamification The application of typical elements of game playing (i.e. points scoring, competition with others) to other areas of activity, in this context psychological interventions.

Genogram A diagrammatic representation of a family that includes individual histories of illness and death. Also incorporates aspects of the interpersonal relationships between family members.

Imagery rehearsal therapy A short-term cognitive behaviour intervention for individuals experiencing chronic nightmares (used commonly in populations such as veterans with trauma-related sleep problems) in which participants write about their recurring nightmares, edit these stories (or scripts) to include more positive images, and then rehearse the images from the new, more positive scripts.

Rehearsal is both self-guided (e.g. 5–20 minutes daily) and therapist guided, and the new script eventually replaces or transforms the nightmare.

Interventionist A physician, behavioural scientist, therapist, or other professional who modifies the conditions or symptoms of a patient.

Meta-analysis A quantitative technique for synthesizing the results of multiple studies of a phenomenon into a single result by combining the effect size estimates from each study into a single estimate of the combined effect size or into a distribution of effect sizes.

Metacognition Awareness and understanding of one's own thought process awareness of one's own cognitive processes, often involving a conscious attempt to control them.

Modular approach In this context, interventions that are formed of discrete components, or 'modules' that can be combined to fit the individual needs of a client.

Neuroplasticity The ability of the nervous system to change in response to experience or environmental stimulation. For example, following an injury, remaining neurons may adopt certain functions previously performed by those that were damaged, or a change in reactivity of the nervous system and its components may result from constant, successive activations.

Phenotype The physical characteristics of something living, especially those characteristics that can be seen.

Psychoeducation An intervention involving mainly didactic knowledge transfer (i.e. teaching) to enable patients to understand more about a mental health difficulty and its treatment.

Routine outcome monitoring Repeated measurement of the progress of a client's treatment during the course of intervention, for example, through measuring symptoms or progress towards goals.

Sertraline A type of antidepressant known as a selective serotonin reuptake inhibitor. It is often used to treat depression, and also sometimes panic attacks, obsessive–compulsive disorder, and post-traumatic stress disorder.

Serious game/applied game A game primarily designed for a purpose other than entertainment.

Social learning theory The general view that learning is largely or wholly due to modelling, imitation, and other social interactions.

Socratic A process of structured inquiry and discussion between two or more people to explore the concepts and values that underlie their everyday activities and judgements. In some psychotherapies, it is a technique in which the therapist poses strategic questions designed to clarify the client's core beliefs and feelings and, in the case of cognitive therapy, to enable the client to discover the distortions in his or her habitual interpretation of a given situation.

Solution-focused brief therapy Brief psychotherapy that focuses on problems in the here and now, with specific goals that the client views as important to achieve in a limited time.

Stepped care A system of delivering and monitoring mental health treatment according to the principle that people should be offered the least intrusive intervention appropriate for their needs first. Patients are then 'stepped up' to more intensive or specialist services as required.

Task-shifted interventions In this case, transferring the task of the delivery of psychological interventions from highly qualified health workers to workers with fewer qualifications and less training.

Telehealth The use of telecommunications and information technology to provide access to health assessment, diagnosis, intervention, and information across a distance, rather than face-to-face. Also called telemedicine.

Therapeutic alliance A cooperative working relationship between client and therapist.

Transdiagnostic intervention Interventions based on therapeutic skills that can be flexibly applied across disorders.

Vignette Material (e.g. a piece of text or video) that describes a hypothetical situation, in this case usually of a patient presentation.

Waiting list control condition A group of research participants who receive the same intervention or treatment as those in the experimental group but at a later time.

Acknowledgements

We would like to thank Callum Smith, Lana Fox-Smith, and Amy Lewins for their help with compiling the glossary.

Index

For the benefit of digital users, indexed terms that span two pages (e.g., 52–53) may, on occasion, appear on only one of those pages.

Tables, figures, and boxes are indicated by *t*, *f*, and *b* following the page number